INFANTICIDE AND FILICIDE

Foundations in Maternal Mental Health Forensics

INFANTICIDE AND FILICIDE

Foundations in Maternal Mental Health Forensics

Gina Wong, Ph.D.

George Parnham, J.D.

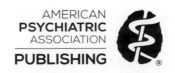

AMERICAN
PSYCHIATRIC
ASSOCIATION
PUBLISHING

Copyright © 2021 American Psychiatric Association Publishing

ALL RIGHTS RESERVED

First Edition

Manufactured in the United States of America on acid-free paper
24 23 22 21 20   5 4 3 2 1

American Psychiatric Association Publishing
800 Maine Avenue SW, Suite 900
Washington, DC 20024-2812
www.appi.org

Library of Congress Cataloging-in-Publication Data
Names: Wong, Gina, 1971- editor. | Parnham, George J., editor. | American Psychiatric Association Publishing, issuing body.
Title: Infanticide and filicide : foundations in maternal mental health forensics / [edited by] Gina Wong, George Parnham.
Description: First edition. | Washington, DC : American Psychiatric Association Publishing, [2021] | Includes bibliographical references and index.
Identifiers: LCCN 2020044380 (print) | LCCN 2020044381 (ebook) | ISBN 9781615373512 (paperback ; alk. paper) | ISBN 9781615373703 (ebook)
Subjects: MESH: Infanticide | Forensic Psychiatry—methods | Mother-Child Relations—psychology | Mental Disorders—psychology
Classification: LCC RA1148 (print) | LCC RA1148 (ebook) | NLM W 867 | DDC 614/.15—dc23
LC record available at https://lccn.loc.gov/2020044380
LC ebook record available at https://lccn.loc.gov/2020044381

British Library Cataloguing in Publication Data
A CIP record is available from the British Library.

Contents

Foundation I:
Legal Aspects Surrounding Maternal Infanticide and Filicide

Foundation II: The Impact of Perinatal Psychiatric Complications in Maternal Infanticide and Filicide

Foundation III: The Role of the Expert Witness in Maternal Infanticide and Filicide Cases

Gina Wong, Ph.D.
Kathryn Bell, M.C.

Susan Hatters Friedman, M.D., DFAPA
Daniel Riordan, MBBS, M.A., M.Sc., MRCPsych,
  FRANZCP, MInstGA
Jacqueline A. Short, M.B.Ch.B., B.A., FRCPsych,
  Affiliate RANZCP, Dip.For.Psychotherapy,
  Dip.Soc.Pol&Criminology

Foundation IV: Sociocultural
Considerations and Feminist Approaches
to Prevention and Treatment

Kimberly Rock, M.C.
Amy Corkett, M.C.
Nancy Shekarak Ghashghaei, M.C.
Gina Wong, Ph.D.

Nora L. Erickson, Ph.D.
Megan M. Julian, Ph.D.
Jonathan E. Handelzalts, Ph.D.
Gina Wong, Ph.D.
Maria Muzik, M.D., M.S.

Clinical Cases: Application of Foundations and Practical Considerations

Contributors

Franca Aceti, M.D.
Assistant Professor, Department of Human Neuroscience, Sapienza University of Rome, Rome, Italy

Diana Barnes, Psy.D., LMFT, PMH-C
The Center for Postpartum Health, Sherman Oaks, California

Kathryn Bell, M.C.
Graduate Centre for Applied Psychology, Athabasca University, Alberta, Canada

Kimberly Brandt, D.O., PMH-C
Perinatal Psychiatrist, Associate Professor of Clinical Psychiatry, Psychiatry Residency Training Director, Department of Psychiatry, University of Missouri—Columbia School of Medicine, Columbia, Missouri

Anne Buist, M.D., FRANCP
Professor of Women's Mental Health, Department of Psychiatry, Austin Health, University of Melbourne, Melbourne, Australia

Amy Corkett, M.C.
Registered Provisional Psychologist, Canadian Certified Counsellor, Alberta, Canada

Wendy Davis, Ph.D., PMH-C
Postpartum Support International, Portland, Oregon

Nora L. Erickson, Ph.D.
Psychologist, Clinician Investigator, Hennepin Healthcare Mother Baby Program, Redleaf Center for Family Healing, Minneapolis, Minnesota

Susan Benjamin Feingold, Psy.D., PMH-C
Susan Benjamin Feingold and Associates for Perinatal Mental Health, LLC, Skokie, Illinois; Advisory Council of Postpartum Support International, Illinois

Jane Fisher, AO, Ph.D., B.Sc. (Hons), MAPS, FCCLP, FCHP
Clinical Psychologist, Finkel Professor of Global Health, Head of the Division of Social Sciences, and Director of Global and Women's Health, School of Public Health and Preventive Medicine, Monash University, Melbourne, Australia; Immediate Past President, International Marcé Society for Perinatal Mental Health, Brentwood, Tennessee

Susan Hatters Friedman, M.D., DFAPA
The Phillip Resnick Professor of Forensic Psychiatry, Professor of Reproductive Biology and Pediatrics, and Adjunct Professor of Law, Case Western Reserve University, Cleveland, Ohio; Honorary Associate Professor of Psychological Medicine, University of Auckland, Auckland, New Zealand

Nancy Shekarak Ghashghaei, M.C.
Graduate Centre for Applied Psychology, Athabasca University, Alberta; Master of Arts student in clinical psychology, York University, Ontario, Canada

Nicoletta Giacchetti, M.D., Ph.D.
Psychiatrist, Department of Human Neuroscience, Sapienza University of Rome, Rome, Italy

Jonathan E. Handelzalts, Ph.D.
Clinical Psychologist, Senior Lecturer, Graduate Program in Clinical Psychology, School of Behavioral Sciences, The Academic College of Tel-Aviv Yaffo, Israel

Daniel Hoffman, B.A., B.A. (Psychology) (Hons), M.Sc. (Psychology), D.Phil.
Department of Psychiatry, School of Clinical Medicine, University of the Witwatersrand, Johannesburg, South Africa

Jane Honikman, M.S.
Postpartum Action Institute, Postpartum Support International, Portland, Oregon

Megan M. Julian, Ph.D.
Psychologist, Clinical Lecturer, Department of Psychiatry, Zero To Thrive, University of Michigan, Ann Arbor, Michigan

Amanda Kingston, M.D.
Forensic Psychiatrist, Assistant Professor of Clinical Psychiatry, Forensic Psychiatry Training Director, Department of Psychiatry, University of Missouri—Columbia School of Medicine, Columbia, Missouri

Maggie Kirkman, Ph.D., B.A. (Hons), MAPS
Academic Psychologist and Senior Research Fellow in Global and Women's Health, School of Public Health and Preventive Medicine, Monash University, Melbourne, Australia

Kirsten Kramar, Ph.D.
Instructor, Criminal Justice Program, Department of Economics, Justice and Policy Studies, Mount Royal University, Calgary, Alberta, Canada

Guido Maria Lattanzi, M.D.
Psychiatrist, Department of Human Neuroscience, Sapienza University of Rome, Rome Italy

Barry Michael Lewis, J.D.
Licensed Attorney, Law Office of Barry M. Lewis, Chicago, Illinois

Liliana Lorettu, M.D.
Assistant Professor, Department of Medical, Surgical and Experimental Sciences, University of Sassari–AOU Sassari, Sassari, Italy

Maria Muzik, M.D., M.S.
Psychiatrist, Associate Professor of Psychiatry, Obstetrics and Gynecology, and Director, Zero To Thrive and Women and Infant Mental Health Programs, Department of Psychiatry, University of Michigan, Ann Arbor, Michigan

George Parnham, J.D.
Criminal Defense Attorney, Parnham & Associates, Houston, Texas; licensed to practice in Texas and New York as well as federal courts; Board Certified in criminal law by the Texas Board of Legal Specialization, Co-Founder of the Yates Children Memorial Fund; Director Emeriti, Mental Health America of Greater Houston

Salmi Razali, M.D., M.Med. (Psychiatry), Ph.D.
Consultant Psychiatrist and Associate Professor in Psychiatry, Department of Psychological and Behavioural Medicine, Universiti Teknologi MARA, Selangor, Malaysia

Phillip Resnick, M.D.
Professor of Psychiatry, Case Western Reserve University School of Medicine, Cleveland, Ohio

Daniel Riordan, MBBS, M.A., M.Sc., MRCPsych, FRANZCP, MInstGA
Consultant Forensic Psychiatrist, Psychotherapist, Group Analyst, Austinmer Women's Unit, Forensic Hospital, Justice Health, New South Wales, Australia

Kimberly Rock, M.C.
Registered Provisional Psychologist, Saskatchewan, Canada

Tiffany Ross, M.S.S.W.
Postpartum Support International, Portland, Oregon

Jacqueline A. Short, M.B.Ch.B., B.A., FRCPsych, Affiliate RANZCP, Dip.For.Psychotherapy, Dip.Soc.Pol&Criminology
Clinical Director Forensic and Rehabilitation Service, 3DHB Mental Health, Addictions and Intellectual Disability Service; Honorary Clinical Senior Lecturer, University of Otago, Dunedin, New Zealand

Ugasvaree Subramaney, M.B.B.Ch., FCPsych(SA), M.Med. (Psychiatry), B.Sc. (Psychology) (Hons), Ph.D.
Adjunct Professor, Department of Psychiatry, School of Clinical Medicine, University of the Witwatersrand, Johannesburg, South Africa

Gina Wong, Ph.D.
Psychologist, Professor, and Program Director, Graduate Centre for Applied Psychology, Athabasca University; Director, Centre for Perinatal Psychology and Forensics International, Alberta, Canada

Introduction

> All human life on the planet is born of woman. The one uni-
> fying, incontrovertible experience shared by all women and
> men is that months-long period we spent unfolding inside a
> woman's body. Because...women not only bear and suckle
> but are assigned almost total responsibility for children, most
> of us first know both love and disappointment, power and
> tenderness, in the person of a woman.
>
> Adrienne Rich 1976, p. xi

American poet and feminist author Adrienne Rich considered all essence of human life to emerge from woman. Indeed, a mother is the root
of all life, and when she ends the life of a child she bore, it breaks a cardinal rule and violates the natural course of life. *Maternal mental health
forensics* is at the intersection of maternal mental illness and the criminal
justice system, wherein a woman comes into contact with the legal system after an alleged criminal act for which perinatal or maternal mental
illness may have been a catalyst. Before determining guilt or innocence,
courts assess for criminal responsibility in the event that an insanity plea
is warranted. A defendant is also assessed for competency to stand trial
if the defense attorney thinks the client lacks the ability to understand
the charges against her and is unable to assist in her own defense.

Maternal mental health forensics is heavily impacted by the existence or nonexistence and application of infanticide or postpartum mental health laws, as well as the legitimacy given to diagnosis of perinatal
mental disturbances. Given that representation of women in their childbearing years in our correctional system has been rising exponentially
(Hatters Friedman et al., in press), it stands to reason that maternal mental health forensics is an essential area of focus. This specialty has been
in its infancy relative to the field as a distinct discipline of study. However, reproductive and perinatal forensic psychologists and psychiatrists
have been involved for decades in the pursuit of justice for legal wrongdoings perpetrated by mothers in the perinatal and postpartum period.

The field of maternal mental health forensics comprises theories and
standards of practice that are benchmarks in the legal jurisdiction where

criminal justice is practiced. This often includes medical standards of diagnosis, such as DSM-5 (American Psychiatric Association 2013) and the *International Statistical Classification of Diseases and Related Health Problems*, 11th Revision (ICD-11; World Health Organization 2019), laws at the federal level, standards of the insanity defense, case law, existing and current knowledge bases (including research in woman's reproductive mental health and maternal mental well-being), and cultural mores as well as necessary analysis of the influence of social, gender, and race inequities and biases.

Maternal mental health forensics is advanced by professionals who work within the legal system in the area of maternal mental health or mental health in general. Experts may be psychologists, counselors, and social workers; medical professionals, such as psychiatrists, medical doctors, and obstetrician/gynecologists; or lawyers and judges (criminal experts). Professionals may be those defending, prosecuting, or assisting; assessing level of criminal responsibility or fitness to stand trial; providing expert opinions and testimony; or monitoring and treating mothers who have perpetrated filicide. It is for these professionals, and associated professions, that this book is intended.

This book provides key considerations in the successful criminal defense of mothers who commit neonaticide, infanticide, and filicide. This collection is firmly rooted in research and amplified by real case examples from more than 30 experts in the field, representing eight countries. It offers practical information and serves as an educational and training resource. *Infanticide and Filicide: Foundations in Maternal Mental Health Forensics* is an accessible read for a broad range of audiences involved in their first maternal filicide case, involved in multiple cases, or generally interested in this field. In addition, practitioners, scholars, researchers, and academics in related professions dedicated to understanding risk factors, profiles, behavioral patterns, and effective strategies to prevent maternal filicide will also appreciate this collection.

Readers already may have a wealth of education and training in perinatal mental health or may have little to no such training; they may possess specialized training in the criminal justice system or be new to understanding this area. Perinatal forensic psychiatrists and psychologists are well poised at the intersection of the two fields and optimally trained in the field of maternal mental health forensics; however, the pursuit of justice for offenses committed by mothers in the perinatal and postpartum phases involves expert witnesses with a variety of professional training backgrounds. Given the breadth of professionals who may be involved and the women's lives that hang in the balance within the criminal justice system, we in the field of maternal mental health forensics must establish chief foundations and converge upon definitions of terms and concepts; advance main clinical, legal, and cultural perspectives; and incite necessary dialogue as we move toward establishing this specialized area of forensics. Presenting the foundations of maternal mental health forensics, culminating in didactic application, is integral to this endeavor.

Filicide Terms

Historically, maternal infanticide has occurred since 4000 B.C.–2000 B.C., as documented by Babylonian and Chaldean civilizations (Meyer and Oberman 2001). It was not specific to any culture and occurred for various reasons (Putkonen et al. 2016). The killing of offspring by parents is a most intriguing and reprehensible crime; however, despite more recent focused research, its complexity continues to elude many, and it has not decreased in incidence. Adding to the challenge is that filicide terms are used interchangeably to describe the perpetration of child death by a parent, stepparent, or legal guardian. The terms *infanticide*, *neonaticide*, and *filicide* generally are distinguished by the age of the child whose life is taken by a parental figure. *Infanticide* commonly refers to the killing by a parent of an infant older than 1 day and younger than 1 year. *Neonaticide*, a concept introduced by Philip Resnick in 1969, involves the killing of a newborn within 24 hours of birth and is almost always perpetrated by a young biological mother (McKee and Bramante 2010; Meyer and Oberman 2001; Resnick 1969). *Filicide* is a complex and multifaceted term used in multiple ways in the scholarly literature. For example, some authors define filicide as taking the life of one's child who is between 1 and 18 years of age (West 2007). It is also used as an overarching term delineating the killing of a child at *any* age by a parental figure. In this book, we refer to filicide both generally, as an overarching term encompassing neonaticide and infanticide, and specifically, as the killing of one's offspring who is older than 12 months and younger than 18 years by a parental figure, namely the biological mother or father.

Prevalence of Filicide and Rate of Psychosis

The United States has the highest rate of child murder among developed nations (Resnick 2016), estimated to be 8 per 100,000 live births, which is comparatively higher than the 2.9 per 100,000 births in Canada (Hatters Friedman et al. 2005; Resnick 2016; Tang and Siu 2018). The most common perpetrators of filicide are parents; 15% of child homicides in the United States are perpetrated by parents (Mariano et al. 2014), the highest rate among industrialized nations (Hatters Friedman et al. 2005; Resnick 2016). An estimated average of 500 filicide arrests are made per year in the United States (Resnick 2016). Although the United States reportedly has the highest rate of filicide, it endorses the harshest criminal rulings. It was not until June 2018 that any of the 50 states passed infanticide legislation.

The prevalence of filicide is difficult to truly represent given the different reporting structures, inconsistent methods of data collection for child homicide among various countries, categorization of deaths (West 2007), and reality of underreporting (Koenen and Thompson 2008). Infant deaths may also go undetected or be misattributed to sudden infant death syndrome (Spinelli 2004). Child homicide is tragic at any occurrence, and the perpetration of filicide as a result of the mother's mental illness is in its own category of devastation.

Perinatal psychiatrists estimate that women are 25 times more likely to experience psychosis in the postpartum period than in any other period in their life (Marks 1996). In the first 4 weeks postpartum, women experience first-onset psychosis at a rate 23 times higher than any other period life (Bergink et al. 2016). Furthermore, in a systematic review, VanderKruik et al. (2017) confirmed the incidence rate of postpartum psychosis (PPP) to be consistent with the often-cited 1–2 in 1,000 births in the general population. Five studies reported a range from 0.89 to 2.6 in 1,000 women, and one reported a higher prevalence of 5 in 1,000 women (Vesga-López et al. 2008). The World Health Organization (2020) declared that psychosis in a mother following the birth of a child may lead to suicide or maternal filicide.

DSM-5 links postpartum psychotic episodes (with command hallucinations or severe postpartum mood episodes) with infanticide and describes postpartum psychotic episodes as occurring in relation to bipolar disorder and postpartum depression. In fact, Hatters Friedman et al. (2019), among many perinatal mental health experts, identified a previous PPP diagnosis and a history of bipolar disorder as strong indicators of future PPP diagnosis, with as much as a 50%–80% chance of a subsequent psychiatric episode. McKee and Bramante (2010) indicated that 4% of mothers with PPP may go on to commit maternal infanticide.

Although DSM-5 links psychosis in the postpartum period with infanticide, it has no formal diagnostic category for PPP. Rather, the word "postpartum" is used as a specifier that can be attached to a diagnosis if it occurs in the first 4 weeks after birth (6 weeks postpartum in ICD-11; World Health Organization 2019). However, according to researchers, the classic symptoms of puerperal psychosis are evidenced as markedly distinct from the presentation of psychosis unrelated to childbirth (Wisner et al. 1994, 2003).

Regarding the diagnostic classifications of PPP, Margaret Spinelli, a prominent forensic perinatal expert witness and a clinical professor of psychiatry at Columbia University College of Physicians and Surgeons in New York, is leading the charge to advance recognition of PPP in the formal DSM diagnostic nomenclature. What was categorized as "post-partum onset" in relation to other classifications of psychosis in DSM-5 requires upgrading to recognize PPP as a distinct classification with its own diagnostic criteria, including psychotic symptoms, mood instability, and cognitive disorganization, in the next edition of DSM.

At present, the DSM committee agreed that present specifiers were insufficient; however, they indicated they would place PPP in Section III requesting further research (personal communication, August 16, 2020). In response, Spinelli implored reconsideration. The following was her response:

Dear DSM Committee Members,

I am making this appeal for diagnostic inclusion of PPP in the DSM because this is psychiatry's opportunity to save lives and help families. In view of the facts that:

- Postpartum psychosis is the only psychiatric disorder associated with homicide (infanticide).
- The highest rate of suicide by women is in the first year postpartum using self-incineration, firearms or jumping (methods often used in psychosis).
- Many women are incarcerated for life because they were innocently afflicted with a mental illness that caused them to kill their infants.
- The diagnosis is minimized in the courtroom where it could save the lives of women and their families. (i.e. Prosecutor says, "Dr. Spinelli, isn't it correct that PPP is not a diagnosis in the DSM?")
- Because of the rarity of this illness (1–2/1000) it will take many years to collect data and provide the research that you request. We do not have mother–baby units like Europe where these women accumulate. That is why the research is limited. Should we wait another 10 or 15 years to assist these mothers?

In my 24 years evaluating women who have killed babies, not one was diagnosed or treated properly. The floridly psychotic Andrea Yates was misdiagnosed and discharged from 2 hospitalizations before she killed 5 children. A few days before she killed them she was taken off her antipsychotic because her catatonia was diagnosed as "akinesia."

This humble and good woman was a victim of this illness and must live out her life in a psychiatric facility with the fact that she killed them. She lives through every birthday reminded that they would be in college.

Postpartum psychosis was included in the DSM-2 and expunged in DSM-3 because it was incorrectly determined that it was the same as nonchildbearing psychoses. The decision to remove the diagnosis was not obtained through cognitive tests…It seems that it was a whim of a group of American psychiatrists.

I have been a researcher and clinician for more than 25 years….If a new diagnostic heading can support these criteria for acceptance, I implore those of you who undermine the importance of this diagnosis to see beyond, to accept my suggestion and protect these women and babies and save lives.

Adverse Childhood Experiences and Later-Life Psychopathology

In recent decades, research underscoring the impact of childhood adversity on adult psychological and physical health has advanced significantly (Hughes et al. 2016). In their study (N=9,508), Felliti et al. (1998) identified adverse childhood experiences (ACEs), namely abuse and household dysfunction, as having a dose-response relationship: a greater number of childhood adversities amounted to a greater risk of later-life psychopathology. Classically, the ACEs questionnaire identifies 10 childhood adverse experiences in three categories of abuse, neglect, and household dysfunction. Rates of victimization and perpetration of violence in adulthood (Centers for Disease Control and Prevention 2019) also escalate as ACEs scores increase, as does the propensity to engage in high-risk behaviors related to earlier death. Varese et al. (2012) found that childhood maltreatment such as "sexual abuse, physical abuse, emotional/psychological abuse and neglect, and experiences of parental loss and separation are risk factors for psychosis and schizophrenia" (p. 661). The possibility of being diagnosed with psychosis is decreased by 33% in persons who have not experienced any childhood traumas.

Individuals with an ACEs score ≥4, compared with those who have no ACEs, have a 4- to 12-fold risk of drug and alcohol dependency, depression, and suicidality (Felitti et al. 1998), and a score of ≥4 has been linked to a 10-fold increase in schizophrenia (Chase et al. 2019). Neurodevelopmental disruptions associated with the pathogenesis of mental disorders (Read et al. 2014) are also prevalent in those who have higher scores. Specific types of ACEs occurring at discrete neurocognitive development periods (e.g., age 3 and adolescence) inhibit brain development via the hypothalamic-pituitary-adrenal axis and the sympathetic nervous system outflow involved in the stress-brain response (Chase et al. 2019; Read et al. 2014; Ruby et al. 2014; Schalinski et al. 2018).

The traumagenic neurodevelopmental model of psychosis (see Read et al. 2014) suggests a graded relationship between the number of ACEs and later-life psychosis. In addition, higher numbers of ACEs have an enduring effect. One generation of specific childhood adversities impacts well-being in future generations because ACEs impede parental capacity to foster optimum environments for their offspring (Hughes et al. 2016; Read and Bentall 2012).

Currently, research directly linking ACEs to PPP has been amassed yet remains controversial in the psychiatric community. One study in the United Kingdom involving 208 mothers with previous PPP did not associate it with high ACEs scores (Perry et al. 2016). One of the largest population-based cohort studies to date confirmed a dose-response relationship between ACEs and development of postpartum psychiatric episodes (Meltzer-Brody et al. 2018) but did not find this to be true for the development of PPP. Researchers were limited in differentiating the specific types of postpartum psychiatric episodes, namely PPP, given the low prevalence rate. In this study (Meltzer-Brody et al. 2018), childhood physical and sexual abuse—identified as strong risk factors for psychosis and schizophrenia in adulthood (Varese et al. 2012)—were not among the eight ACEs assessed. Such research variables may have skewed the findings of association between ACEs and PPP.

In addition, the study by Meltzer-Brody et al. (2018) did not account for attachment-related childhood traumas, identified by Barone et al. (2014) as pervasive among filicidal women. In their European study of 121 women (normative group $n=61$; maternal mental illness group $n=37$; and filicide group $n=23$), they found that early traumatic experiences, low socioeconomic status, and mental illness did not increase relative risk to filicide, but that attachment styles were significant. That is, although ACEs absent of attachment traumas did not yield significant difference between the filicide and maternal mental illness groups, a hostile-hopeless attachment pattern involving unresolved traumatic attachment experiences differentiated the filicide group from the others. As such, attachment variables must be further investigated and considered for their role in the collection of risk factors linking ACEs to PPP and maternal filicide.

Impetus for This Book

This book pays homage to George Parnham, J.D., and honors the legacy of his work—fighting for, giving voice to, and supporting mothers who take the lives of their children whilst in the throes of maternal mental illness. Outstanding in his profession, with 50 years of legal practice, George is honored in this book for his contribution, service, and social justice advocacy on behalf of mothers who are thrust into the criminal justice system as a result of taking the lives of their children, when these mothers are as much a victim to their mental disturbance as their children. George is heralded and revered for his courage and the impact he has made on the lives of so many. The role of mental illness in maternal filicide was less understood before the Andrea Yates case in 2001, which George successfully defended. From public disdain for Andrea after she drowned her five children to mobilized understanding of the impact of maternal mental illness, namely PPP, the world caught a glimpse of the life of a mentally ill mother, and many cultivated compassion for her, the likes of which had not been experienced before. Given this, our book is also a tribute to Andrea Yates.

George Parnham: A Man of Scruples

I feel you whispering
across my heart today
reminding me that
you're still there
holding my fractured pieces
lovingly in your little hands.

Andren 2018

My (G.P.) life as a criminal lawyer, a defender of the underdog, had its genesis and evolution in my seminary experiences. My folks were strongly bonded by a deep love for each other and for their children. They enrolled me in parochial school when I was young, which was where I quickly gravitated to Catholicism and the priesthood. On Sundays, I would pretend to be a priest, setting up an altar in my room and, with prayer book in hand, saying Mass.

At the ripe age of 13, I said goodbye to my parents and joined the seminary. There, we had no contact from regular civilization and were self-sufficient. Located far in the Alabama Piney Woods, we grew our own crops and built much of the infrastructure with our bare hands. We enjoyed a beautiful baseball field and basketball gym, but, above all, I rejoiced in the chapel, where a large percentage of each day was spent in prayer. One day, after 7 years, I was stunned and bewildered when Father Doyle told me I was to leave the seminary because of my extreme scrupulosity. My mentors saw my rigidity to the church and believed that my fear of doing wrong in the eyes of God would thwart me from becoming the man I could be. The next day, the priests, chaplain, and my fellow seminarians lined up in a tearful goodbye, and I was set out into the real world. It was only in later years that I could understand and appreciate why I was asked to leave.

Over time, my scrupulosity to religious scriptures subsided. Nevertheless, as a criminal defense lawyer, I became scrupulous in my dedication to and pursuit of defending those accused of some of the most heinous crimes. Although the road from extreme religious scrupulosity to defending murderers is seemingly unbidden and inconceivable, it was most fortuitous and natural for me. I had been denied the priesthood due to my overzealous adherence to rules, but my calling to attend to those who might feel lost and in pain remained strong. Certainly, they could be viewed as allegedly doing wrong in the eyes of God, and defending them was—and is—my priesthood. My involvement in the legal defense of mothers who take the lives of their children has been the most challenging among all the cases in my many years of practice. However, bringing about education and awareness, and a changing attitude for the better, in the area of maternal mental health has been one of the most rewarding aspects of my career.

Gina Wong: Forging Ahead

> Memories saturate my heart and the story of you spills from my eyes.
>
>   Andren 2018, p. 11

In 2003, as a young psychologist and early academic, I (G. W.) continued seeing perinatal and postpartum women in clinical practice. I trained with Postpartum Support International (PSI) to diagnose and treat women experiencing perinatal mood and anxiety disorders. My publications in motherhood scholarship focused on deconstructing the damaging cultural ideologies and institutions that regulate mothers' lives. Many women struggle with mental illness and personalize issues to themselves, remaining silent and internalizing societal madness rather than locating it in the systems, cultural beliefs and practices, institutions, and ideologies of mothers within our society.

My foray into the role of perinatal expert witness in maternal filicide cases in Canada began in 2017 when I was called to a case in which a young mother had stabbed her three children and herself. As a psychologist who specialized in maternal mental health, assessing and working with mothers was in concert with my training; however, I languished in my knowledge of the legal ramifications of maternal filicide and my understanding of criminal processes involved in court cases. As a fledgling expert witness in Canada, I recognized a dearth of understanding surrounding maternal filicide and of dialogue, training, and community resources. I sought to highlight wisdom gleaned from the veteran experts in the field with whom I met in my quest to successfully fulfill the role. I felt profound meaning in this work, and the impetus to bring together a collection that would serve as a training resource was born.

Wendy Davis, executive director of PSI, connected me with veterans in the field, specifically Diana Barnes, who became my greatest mentor and has met with me over the years and provided insight and guidance as well as friendship. I also spoke often with Margaret Spinelli, who graciously gave her time. I consulted with George Parnham regarding legal understanding of maternal filicide cases. He mentored me and unequivocally offered his expertise. George and I delivered key conference presentations together that inspired our recognition that a book in the field of maternal mental health forensics was urgently needed.

Available Resources

Several publications about mental health and the criminal justice system are available. Notably, *Experts in Court: Reconciling Law, Science, and Professional Knowledge* by Sales and Shuman (2005) examines the use of expert testimony across the legal system, including the pitfalls and the possible perception of mental health expert testimony as nonobjective. *The Psychiatrist as Expert Witness*, edited by Gutheil (2009), is another well-used resource in psychiatry training programs. Likewise, *Psychological Evaluation for the Courts: A Handbook for Mental Health Professionals and Lawyers* by Melton et al. (2018) is a compendium that guides readers through many contradictory perspectives in translating clinical expertise for applicability within criminal justice. Although these books inform expert witnesses, they do not focus explicitly on maternal mental health experts in maternal filicide court cases. Books such as *Models of Madness: Psychological, Social and Biological Approaches to Psychosis*, edited by Read and Dillon (2013), and *Psychosis, Trauma and Dissociation: Emerging Perspectives on Severe Psychopathology*, edited by Moskowitz et al. (2008), address childhood adversity and trauma. However, few books specifically address trauma and attachment as they relate to perinatal mood and anxiety disorders—and more specifically PPP—in infanticide and filicide cases. This is a gap that our book begins to fill, with several chapters elucidating these perspectives.

The most resounding publication our book aims to complement is *Infanticide: Psychosocial and Legal Perspectives on Mothers Who Kill*, edited by Spinelli (2003). It is the most authoritative resource examining the legal, medical, and psychosocial aspects of mothers who take the lives of their infants. A chapter by Macfarlane describes criminal defense theories of diminished capacity, involuntary acts, and insanity pleas in relation to infanticide, filicide, and neonaticide (Spinelli 2003). The book addresses criminal defense in infanticide and neonaticide and the medical, biological, and legal determinants of postpartum psychiatric disorders and offers discussion of treatment, prevention, and rehabilitation. Our book underscores and extends Spinelli's ideas by including deeper discussion surrounding ACEs and trauma related to perinatal mental health outcomes. Spinelli's book informs our understanding of filicide and the pivotal dimensions of a woman's psychological state of mind that contribute to enacting filicide.

Dawn of New Hope

The timeliness of this book comes from a recognition that we are entering a new dawn in time, an era of hope in the United States and internationally for mothers and for postpartum mental illness–related filicide. Twenty years after the Andrea Yates tragedy, we continue addressing maternal mental illness and its intersection with criminal justice in ways far greater than before. We stand at the precipice of change that will have lasting impact, in which maternal mental health forensics is underscored as an essential subspecialty area.

The first revelation toward a new dawn of hope is the understanding that childhood adversity relates to adult psychopathology and greater risk for psychosis-related mental illness. Although some controversy exists regarding the association of ACEs with PPP, a convincing body of research is developing. Continued research examining attachment-related childhood trauma, specifically the hostile-hopeless attachment pattern characterized by unresolved attachment injuries, will further understanding of the types of childhood adversities that increase the risk of PPP and elevate the risk of filicide. Furthermore, research including childhood physical or sexual abuse as variables of ACEs, as well as research noting the impact of ACEs on developing parts of the brain at discrete developmental stages in childhood, is needed.

Such awareness will galvanize intervention efforts aimed to support families at risk by reducing specific types of child adversities at critical neurological brain development periods. Furthermore, a life course perspective (Hughes et al. 2016) applied to understanding maternal filicide is needed to advance our ability to see the evolution of postpartum mental illness relative to childhood (and intergenerational) experiences. A life course framework can elicit in-depth understanding of the intergenerational effects of childhood adversity and improve outcomes for future generations. The World Health Organization's (2013) *Comprehensive Mental Health Action Plan 2013–2020* underscores the need to focus on mental well-being as part of its overarching goal and advocates a life course approach empowering early intervention in adverse childhood circumstances.

The second major shift comes with the possible inclusion of PPP in the next edition of DSM, with Spinelli's involvement advocating PPP as a distinct classification. Such a shift would provide legitimacy to a PPP diagnosis in the courtroom and could save the lives of countless women. The third indicator of change was the passage of a postpartum law in Illinois in 2018, which is a seismic shift in the United States regarding harsh laws for maternal filicide acts. In Chapter 3, the authors detail their successful advocacy work lobbying for the Illinois postpartum law to pass in the state senate. Feingold and Lewis (2020) wrote about how this postpartum law amends the Criminal Code of Corrections to consider postpartum depression and PPP as "mitigating factors" in sentencing when women commit offenses whilst gripped with postpartum mental illness. They also advanced HD 1736 in Massachusetts in 2019; however, it has not yet passed legislation.

Chapters in This Book

This collection brings together a cadre of esteemed professionals to advance the field of maternal mental health forensics in light of a new dawn of hope and to provide an educational and training resource with scholarly underpinnings. We approach maternal mental health forensics based on the four foundations upon which the book is structured. Case illustrations are offered throughout the book. Each chapter culminates with a didactic section wherein main clinical/legal and cultural points and practice and discussion questions for professionals are offered. In Chapters 16 and 17, two additional clinical presentations of maternal infanticide are provided that illustrate application of foundations and practical considerations. A glossary at the end of the book contains key terms and concepts discussed throughout the chapters.

The first part of the book, "Foundation I: Legal Aspects Surrounding Maternal Infanticide and Filicide," begins with an anchoring chapter. I (G.P.) reflect upon the Andrea Yates case and my involvement as a criminal defense attorney in Chapter 1, "Honoring the Legacy of the Andrea

Yates Case." Chapter 2, "Becoming a Legal Expert in Infanticide and Filicide Cases in the United States," delineates my work defending mothers whose mental illness has resulted in the commission of the filicidal act. Having been involved in nearly a dozen maternal filicide cases in my 50 years as a defense attorney, I draw on the need to legitimize maternal mental disorders in these cases and give shape to the necessary understanding for successful criminal defense of these mothers. Furthermore, the chapter explicitly speaks to the dire need for more compassionate laws in the United States.

In Chapter 3, "A Groundbreaking Illinois Postpartum Law Brings Hope for Change in the United States," Susan Feingold, a licensed psychologist, and Barry Lewis, an attorney at law, who together published *Advocating for Women With Postpartum Mental Illness: A Guide to Changing the Law and the National Climate* (Feingold and Lewis 2020), discuss their involvement in passing the postpartum law PA100-0574 in Illinois in 2018. PA100-0574 is groundbreaking because it is the first postpartum criminal legislation in the United States, and Illinois is the first state to recognize the role of perinatal mental illness in maternal filicide. Overall, this chapter addresses legal considerations in maternal filicide in the United States and the need to continue this advocacy in all states.

In Chapter 4, "Delineating the Meaning of *Disturbance of Mind* in Canadian Infanticide Law," Kirsten Kramar, a criminologist and sociolegal studies scholar in Canada and author of *Unwilling Mothers, Unwanted Babies: Infanticide in Canada* (Kramar 2005), describes the evolution of the Canadian Infanticide Law and offers an authoritative perspective on related and relevant legal issues. Kramar cites Canadian case law and summarizes what lawyers and perinatal expert witnesses need to know about its current application in the criminal justice system in Canada.

Chapter 5, "Fathers and Filicide: Mental Illness and Outcomes," is authored by Susan Hatters Friedman, a renowned perinatal forensic psychiatrist in the United States who edited *Family Murder: Pathologies of Love and Hate* (2018). Her chapter here elucidates paternal filicide and highlights the gender disparities in legal outcomes for male perpetrators with mental illness. She also integrates research results identifying the profiles of men who commit filicide. Hatters Friedman invites discernment as well as recognition of the similarities between the genders when it comes to evaluation and criminal justice.

These chapters are followed by "Foundation II: The Impact of Perinatal Psychiatric Complications in Maternal Infanticide and Filicide." In Chapter 6, "Role of Perinatal Psychiatric Complications in Infanticide and Filicide," Kimberly Brandt, a perinatal psychiatrist, and Amanda Kingston, a forensic psychiatrist, both in the United States, relay the peri-

natal mental illnesses commonly identified in maternal infanticide and
filicide and present three cases to illustrate best practices in forensic assessment and differentiate between potentially confusing mental illness
presentation in mothers.

Chapter 7, "Altruistic Filicide: A Trauma Informed Perspective" is
authored by Diana Barnes, an award-winning perinatal psychologist in
the United States and the editor of *Women's Reproductive Mental Health
Across the Lifespan* (2014). Barnes examines the impact of childhood
trauma on a mother's sense of safety and protection for her own children, which may lead to altruistic filicide and a subsequent charge of
murder. She advances a biopsychosocial perspective that is exemplified
in clinical cases from her work as a perinatal expert witness. Barnes also
co-authors Chapter 8, "Understanding the Mysteries of Pregnancy Denial," with Anne Buist, a psychiatrist and professor of women's health
in Australia. They explore clinical presentations of neonaticide and the
psychological underpinnings of pregnancy denial. Barnes' examples
from her case files, coupled with Buist's 30-year understanding of neonaticide in Australia, amplify similarities and differences between the
United States and Australia in cultural perspectives as well as legal outcomes of maternal filicide cases. Together, they examine sociocultural,
medical, psychological, and psychiatric considerations to inform lawyers and expert witnesses relative to pregnancy denial and neonaticide.

"Foundation III: The Role of the Expert Witness in Maternal Infanticide and Filicide Cases," begins with a chapter by Phillip Resnick, who
is a renowned forensic psychiatrist and forefather in the field, with more
than 50 years of expertise progressing the field of filicide. Resnick poignantly articulates his foray into the role of an expert witness in the Andrea Yates case in Chapter 9, "Reflections of an Expert Witness in the
Andrea Yates Case." He reveals his strategy, thoughts, and opinions for
both trials, which occurred in 2002 and 2006. He presents and expounds
upon his early writings on the topic of filicide, particularly outlining the
five typologies of apparent motives behind why mothers kill their children (Resnick 1969, 1970, 2016).

This is followed by Chapter 10, "Becoming an Expert Witness in Maternal Filicide Cases," wherein Canadian researcher Kathryn Bell and I
(G.W.) present a research study funded through the Social Sciences and
Humanities Council of Canada. We elucidate our research involving six
novice and four veteran expert witnesses, each of whom were involved
in at least 1 or as many as 60 maternal filicide cases in the United States
or Canada. Three domains of competencies are identified as essential to
the role of the expert witness. We reveal how experts gained these competencies, their initiation to their first case, necessary supports to this

role, and the meaning derived from working as expert witnesses. This research will inform the development of competency-based curriculum for becoming a maternal mental health expert witness and may support guidelines developed to establish the high level of professional competence this role necessitates.

Chapter 11, "Writing the Maternal Filicide Report: Pearls of Wisdom for Expert Witnesses" offers practical considerations grounded in scholarship. Susan Hatters Friedman, along with Daniel Riordan, a forensic psychiatrist in New South Wales, Australia, and Jacqueline Short, a forensic psychiatrist in New Zealand, share their wisdom about the essentials for a forensic mental health professional who is inexperienced in filicide cases or a maternal mental health professional who is first venturing into the forensic arena. They present guidelines for conducting expert witness assessments and clinical interviews and provide excerpts redacted from real reports to illustrate key points.

The fourth part of the book, "Foundation IV: Sociocultural Considerations and Feminist Approaches to Prevention and Treatment," begins with Chapter 12, "Maternal Filicide in Canadian News: A Decade in Review." Canadian researchers Kimberly Rock, Amy Corkett, Nancy Shekarak Ghashghaei, and I (G.W.) delineate an ethnographic content analysis of 95 electronic news articles from the *Toronto Star*, *Globe and Mail*, and *National Post* encompassing a 10-year period between January 1, 2008 and April 26, 2018. We consider how Canadian media representations of mothers who kill their children impact, and are informed by, social and legal perspectives of the crime. We reveal what journalists most often report and focus on when writing about maternal filicide in Canadian news.

Chapter 13, "Trauma and Attachment: Preventing Maternal Filicide Through the Generations," explores childhood trauma and attachment and how such foci contribute to maternal filicide prevention through understanding intergenerational patterns. Authors Nora Erickson and Megan Julian, clinical psychologists in the United States; Jonathan Handelzalts, a clinical psychologist in Israel; myself (G.W.), a psychologist and professor in Canada; and Maria Muzik, a psychiatrist and associate professor in the United States, write about the significance of secure-base attachment relationships in early life and childhood traumas that, when supported and processed effectively, safeguard against mental illness in adulthood. Fundamentally, we show the necessity of fortifying supportive caregiver relationships in childhood as fundamental to prevention of maternal filicide.

In Chapter 14, "Maternal Filicide in Malaysia: Structural Inequality and Cultural Disparity," Salmi Razali, a psychiatrist and academic in Malaysia, and Jane Fisher and Maggie Kirkman, who are both psychologists and academics in Australia, share their pioneering research. They present secondary analysis of national data and qualitative interviews with women incarcerated for infanticide or filicide in Malaysia, as well as interviews with associated professionals in that country. They identify that Malay women are often punished for filicidal crimes for which they were not solely or, in some cases, at all responsible. In describing their results, they examine maternal filicide through the lenses of social contexts, structural and gender inequities, and human rights and present narratives of three mothers convicted of filicide in Malaysia.

Foundation IV concludes with Chapter 15, "Postpartum Support International: A Leading Resource Center for Maternal Filicide in the United States," in which Jane Honikman, founder of Postpartum Support International (PSI); Tiffany Ross, social worker; and Wendy Davis, PSI executive director and psychologist, bring to light the evolution of one of the world's largest nonprofit organization, which since 1987 has been dedicated to helping women and families experiencing perinatal mental health disorders. PSI has been advocating for greater understanding and compassion for maternal filicide across the globe. The PSI Justice and Advocacy Program offers recorded training materials and a Checklist for Attorneys and is developing further resources for maternal mental health specialists and legal experts involved in these cases.

> my voice was silent
> but my tears spoke eloquently
> each quiet drop a story of you.
>
> Andren 2018, p. 23

The final part of the book, "Clinical Cases: Application of Foundations and Practical Considerations," narrates the maternal filicide case of Greta in Chapter 16, "The Dark Side of Mother: A Clinical Case in Italy," authored by Nicoletta Giacchetti, psychiatrist; Liliana Lorettu, assistant professor; Guido Maria Lattanzi, psychiatrist; and Franca Aceti, assistant professor, all from Rome, Italy. They share the results of their clinical interview and assessments, including evaluations of Greta's early attachment and childhood traumas. Chapter 17, "Falling Between the Cracks of Medical Care: A Case of Maternal Infanticide in South Africa," by Ugasvaree Subramaney, psychiatrist, and Daniel Hoffman, clinical psychologist, both from Johannesburg, South Africa, describes the case of MM, a young woman who presented to a psychiatric facility following a charge of first-degree murder. MM had committed infanticide and was assessed to be under the influence of a mood disorder and PPP at the time. The insanity defense was applied, and MM received psychiatric care, treatment, and rehabilitation under a section of the Mental Health Care Act. Both of these cases demonstrate compassion in countries where psychiatric treatment for mentally ill mothers is prioritized over punitive action and imprisonment.

Future Directions

Although this book covers key foundations in *maternal mental health forensics* specifically addressing maternal infanticide and filicide, a call for further exploration of the topic is warranted. For instance, we advance discussions about ACEs, the neurobiology of trauma, and the importance of childhood attachments; however, the neurohormonal and biological bases of PPP, for example, are essential topics that should not be overlooked. Amplifying discussions of feminist and race deconstruction is the significant work of Razali, Fisher, and Kirkman (Chapter 14), who call attention to the structural inequities and cultural disparities in Malaysia. They delineate how gender inequality and rigid cultural and religious mores confine girls and women. Such oppression is essential to recognize in all parts of the world because it relates to the ways in which women's lives are regulated. It is also critical not only to highlight how such oppression contributes to the psychological sequelae of a mother who enacts filicide but also to analyze how it contributes to inequities within criminal justice processes and decisions. Hatters Friedman lays groundwork in Chapter 5 for continued dialogue in this area. She underscores that the gender, race, and socioeconomic status of parents may unduly influence societal perspectives and court rulings of filicide. The need to focus on gender, cultural, and racial disparities in the area of maternal mental health forensics is imperative. In addition, it is crucial to examine the role of visible and invisible disabilities and limitations a mother may face concomitant to a perinatal psychiatric disturbance, when considering equity issues.

Finally, further expanding on this collection, the need for a trauma-informed framework and attachment-minded perspective in examining maternal mental illness within the criminal justice system is fundamental. As previously stated, research examining ACEs from a life-course perspective (Hughes et al. 2016) in maternal mental health and criminality is crucial to advance the field.

No Longer It "Depends"

Determining the criminal responsibility and the guilt or innocence of a woman who commits maternal infanticide or filicide *depends*. It *depends* because of the wide range of opinions, levels of understanding, and inconsistent practices. It behooves us to highlight and converge on foundations in maternal mental health forensics in filicide cases. Women's and their families' lives hang in the balance of, or are altered as a result of, conditions for which little variability should exist. Too often the outcome of a mother's life

- *Depends* on the country, region, or state relative to whether infanticide or postpartum laws exist and how they are applied;
- *Depends* on the definition and cultural understanding of maternal filicide;
- *Depends* on systemic, gender, ethnicity, and race issues;
- *Depends* on the lawyers, defense teams, prosecutors, juries, expert witnesses, and judges involved, who are variable in their knowledge and insight into maternal filicide;
- *Depends* on how many other cases have been tried around the same time, their outcome, and public perception of those cases;
- *Depends* on societal compassion and a woman's understanding of the crime and her culpability related to maternal mental health; and
- *Depends* on her access to resources (e.g., criminal lawyer).

Keeping in mind that there will always be inconsistencies, it is prudent to mitigate what is within our control. Understanding, educating, recognizing commonalities; continuing to develop foundations of maternal mental health forensics along with standards, benchmarks, protocols, and assessments; and continually updating information based on evidence-based research are essential. Our book is a step in this direction.

An Invitation to Forge Ahead Together

We invite our readers into a mindset to "forge ahead together." Such a framework underscores the need, despite inconsistencies, to move forward together in unity. Spinelli (2004) initiated this intent, stating the need for enhanced knowledge exchange between maternal mental health specialists and legal experts regarding mental illness in mothers that may lead to noxious acts such as filicide. Whether prosecution or defense, understanding maternal or paternal filicide and the multiple motivations, potential psychiatric underpinnings, and legal outcomes is essential to *forge ahead together* despite differences in opinions, theories, and conceptualizations. Maternal filicide may be an outcome not only of untreated perinatal mental illness but also of treated (albeit poorly) mental illness, as evidenced by many of the clinical cases presented in this volume. Maternal filicide is also a tragic symptom of systemic issues. Forging ahead together involves examining the ways that culture may impinge upon women and maternal well-being. In doing so, this book serves as a necessary step toward canonizing the field of maternal mental health forensics and toward continued understanding. As we reduce the circumstances for *it depends,* we do so entering this new dawn in time in which the field of maternal mental health forensics brings together essential knowledge and understanding to address, advance, and advocate on behalf of mothers, their children, their families, and the generations to come.

> Oh, to be free
> like the wildflower
> to bask in surrender
> under the wide open
> forgiving sky

Andren 2018, p. 170

References

American Psychiatric Association: Diagnostic and Statistical Manual of Mental Disorders, 5th Edition. Arlington, VA, American Psychiatric Association, 2013

Andren G: Speaking in Tears: The Poetry in Grief. Kansas City, MO, AnCor Press, 2018

Barnes D (ed): Women's Reproductive Mental Health Across the Lifespan. Basel, Switzerland, Springer International Publishing, 2014

Barone L, Bramante A, Lionetti F, Pastore M: Mothers who murdered their child: an attachment-based study on filicide. Child Abuse Negl 38(9):1468–1477, 2014

Bergink V, Rasgon N, Wisner KL: Postpartum psychosis: madness, mania, and melancholia in motherhood. Am J Psychiatry 173(12):1179–1188, 2016

Centers for Disease Control and Prevention: Adverse Childhood Experiences (ACEs). Atlanta, GA, Centers for Disease Control and Prevention, 2019. Available at: https://www.cdc.gov/violenceprevention/childabuseandneglect/acestudy/index.html. Accessed January 15, 2020.

Chase KA, Melbourne JK, Rosen C, et al: Traumagenics: at the intersect of childhood trauma, immunity and psychosis. Psychiatry Res 273:369–377, 2019

Feingold SB, Lewis BM: Advocating for Women With Postpartum Mental Illness: A Guide to Changing the Law and the National Climate. Lanham, MD, Rowman and Littlefield, 2020

Felitti VJ, Anda RF, Nordenberg D, et al: Relationship of childhood abuse and household dysfunction to many of the leading causes of death in adults: The Adverse Childhood Experiences (ACE) Study. Am J Prev Med 14(4):245–258, 1998

Gutheil TG: The Psychiatrist as Expert Witness, 2nd Edition. Washington, DC, American Psychiatric Publishing, 2009

Hatters Friedman S (ed): Family Murder: Pathologies of Love and Hate. Washington, DC, American Psychiatric Association Publishing, 2018

Hatters Friedman S, Horwitz SM, Resnick PJ: Child murder by mothers: a critical analysis of the current state of knowledge and a research agenda. Am J Psychiatry 162:1578–1587, 2005

Hatters Friedman S, Prakash C, Nagle-Yang S: Postpartum psychosis: protecting mother and infant. Curr Psychiatry 18(4):12–31, 2019

Hatters Friedman S, Kaempf A, Landess J, Kauffman S: Forensic issues in reproductive psychiatry, in The American Psychiatric Association Publishing Publishing Textbook of Women's Reproductive Mental Health. Edited by Hutner L, Catapano L, Nagle-Yang S, et al. Washington, DC, American Psychiatric Association Publishing, in press

Hughes K, Lowey H, Quigg Z, Bellis MA: Relationships between adverse childhood experiences and adult mental well-being: results from an English national household survey. BMC Public Health 16(1):222, 2016

Kendell R, Chalmers J, Platz C: Epidemiology of puerperal psychoses. Br J Psychiatry 150(5):662–673, 1987

Koenen MA, Thompson JW Jr: Filicide: historical review and prevention of child death by parent. Infant Ment Health J 29:61–75, 2008

Kramar KJ: Unwilling Mothers, Unwanted Babies: Infanticide in Canada (Law and Society Series). Vancouver, Canada, UBC Press, 2005

Macfarlane J: Criminal defense in cases of infanticide and neonaticide, in Infanticide: Psychosocial and Legal Perspectives on Mothers Who Kill. Edited by Spinelli M. Washington, DC, American Psychiatric Publishing, 2003, pp 167–184

Mariano TY, Chan HC, Myers WC: Toward a more holistic understanding of filicide: a multidisciplinary analysis of 32 years of U.S. arrest data. Forens Sci Int 236:46–53, 2014

Marks MN: Characteristics and causes of infanticide in Britain. Int Rev Psychiatry 8(1):99–106, 1996

McKee GR, Bramante A: Maternal filicide and mental illness in Italy: a comparative study. J Psychiatry Law 38(3):271–282, 2010

Melton GB, Petrila J, Poythress NG, et al: Psychological Evaluation for the Courts: A Handbook for Mental Health Professionals and Lawyers, Professionals and Lawyers, 4th Edition. New York, Guilford, 2018

Meltzer-Brody S, Larsen JT, Petersen L, et al: Adverse life events increase risk for postpartum psychiatric episodes: a population-based epidemiologic study. Depress Anxiety 35(2):160–167, 2018

Meyer CL, Oberman M: Mothers Who Kill Their Children: Understanding the Acts of Moms From Susan Smith to the "Prom Mom." New York, NYU Press, 2001

Moskowitz A, Schäfer I, Dorahy MJ (eds): Psychosis, Trauma and Dissociation: Emerging Perspectives on Severe Psychopathology. Hoboken, NJ, John Wiley and Sons, 2008

Munk-Olsen T, Laursen TM, Pedersen CB, et al: New parents and mental disorders: a population-based register study. JAMA 296(21):2582–2589, 2006

Perry A, Gordon-Smith K, Di Florio A, et al: Adverse childhood life events and postpartum psychosis in bipolar disorder. J Affect Disord 205:69–72, 2016

Putkonen H, Amon S, Weizmann-Henelius G, et al: Classifying filicide. Int J Forensic Ment Health 15:198–210, 2016

Read J, Bentall RP: Childhood experiences and mental health: theoretical, clinical and primary prevention implications. Br J Psychiatry 200:89–91, 2012

Read J, Dillon J (eds): Models of Madness: Psychological, Social and Biological Approaches to Psychosis, 2nd Edition. Abingdon, UK, Routledge, 2013

Read J, Fosse R, Moskowitz A, Perry B: The traumagenic neurodevelopmental model of psychosis revisited. Neuropsychiatry 4:65–79, 2014

Resnick PJ: Child murder by parents: a psychiatric review of filicide. Am J Psychiatry 126(3):325–334, 1969

Resnick PJ: Murder of the newborn: a psychiatric review of neonaticide. Am J Psychiatry 126(10):1414–1420, 1970

Resnick PJ: Filicide in the United States. Indian J Psychiatry 58(6):203–209, 2016

Rich A: Of Woman Born: Motherhood as Experience and Institution. New York, W.W. Norton and Company, 1976

Ruby E, Polito S, McMahon K, et al: Pathways associating childhood trauma to the neurobiology of schizophrenia. Front Psychol Behav Sci 3(1):1–17, 2014

Sales BD, Shuman DW: Experts in Court: Reconciling Law, Science, and Professional Knowledge. Washington, DC, American Psychological Association, 2005

Schalinski I, Teicher MH, Carolus AM, Rockstroh B: Defining the impact of childhood adversities on cognitive deficits in psychosis: an exploratory analysis. Schizophr Res 192:351–356, 2018

Spinelli MG (ed): Infanticide: Psychosocial and Legal Perspectives on Mothers Who Kill. Washington, DC, American Psychiatric Publishing, 2003

Spinelli MG: Maternal infanticide associated with mental illness: prevention and the promise of saved lives. Am J Psychiatry 161(9):1548–1557, 2004

Tang D, Siu B: Maternal infanticide and filicide in a psychiatric custodial institution in Hong Kong [online]. East Asian Archives of Psychiatry 28(4):139–143, 2018

VanderKruik R, Barreix M, Chou D, Allen T: The global prevalence of postpartum psychosis: a systematic review. BMC Psychiatry 17(1):272, 2017

Varese F, Smeets F, Drukker M, et al: Childhood adversities increase the risk of psychosis: a meta-analysis of patient-control, prospective- and cross-sectional cohort studies. Schizophr Bull 38(4):661–671, 2012

Vesga-López O, Blanco C, Keyes K, et al: Psychiatric disorders in pregnant and postpartum women in the United States. Arch Gen Psychiatry 65(7):805–815, 2008

West SG: Review: an overview of filicide. Psychiatry 4(2):48–57, 2007

Wisner KL, Peindl KS, Hanusa BH: Symptomatology of affective and psychotic illnesses related to childbearing. J Affect Disord 30(2):77–87, 1994

Wisner KL, Gracious BL, Piontek CM, et al: Postpartum disorders: phenomenology, treatment approaches, and relationship to infanticide, in Infanticide: Psychosocial and Legal Perspectives on Mothers Who Kill. Edited by Spinelli MG. Washington, DC, American Psychiatric Publishing, 2003

World Health Organization: Comprehensive Mental Health Action Plan 2013–2020. Geneva, World Health Organization, 2013

World Health Organization: International Statistical Classification of Diseases and Related Health Problems, 11th Edition. Geneva, World Health Organization, 2019

World Health Organization: Maternal mental health, 2020. Available at: https://www.who.int/mental_health/maternal-child/maternal_mental_health/en. Accessed January 30, 2020.

FOUNDATION I

Legal Aspects Surrounding Maternal Infanticide and Filicide

CHAPTER 1

Honoring the Legacy of the Andrea Yates Case

George Parnham, J.D.

The Fateful Day

June 20, 2001, was just another typical Wednesday in Houston for me: sweltering hot and fast paced. With temperatures expected to reach the high 80s, the blistering heat and humidity are what Texans live and breathe in the "city on the bayou." On this particular morning, driving to the Harris County Criminal Courthouse to file a motion, I was early for my day. I took my time, planning the strategy for the felony charge, and savored the rush of air conditioning before the anticipated yet unwelcome day-long perspiration ahead.

As usual on my drive to the courthouse, I tuned my radio to the easy listening station. A little after 9:30 A.M., breaking news interrupted, announcing that a mother in Clear Lake City had killed her children by drowning each of them in the family bathtub. My stomach instantly tightened, and I changed the station. At that time, I had been practicing for approximately 30 years and been exposed to every reprehensible, unimaginable act known to humankind, but the thought of a mother harming a child brings its own kind of bewilderment. Really, how could a mother harm the very people to whom she gave life?

However, changing the station made no difference. The airwaves were filled with venom and vitriol about this mother. Callers volunteered to drown the murderous mom, sparing the taxpayers of Harris County the expense of a trial and endless appeals—and her ultimate and inevitable execution by the State of Texas. News reporters conjured up images that were too distressing for me to stomach. I turned off the radio and popped in a CD. After all, I had a client in court to worry about who deserved my undivided attention. As I reached the courts and crowded elevators and hallways, calls of "Did you hear about the mother?" were a relentless buzz and constant distraction.

At the back of my mind murmured a "What if…?" that I shook away. As a veteran Texas defense attorney, I knew I could well be on the short list of possible defenders for this mother. While I had shuddered initially at the crime, my firm belief is that everyone has the right to the presumption of innocence and effective counsel. I have a deep commitment and sense of duty to defend against governmental authority, whose burden it is to prove its allegations of wrongdoing beyond a reasonable doubt. Yet now I wondered: in this situation, with this mother, what would I do if I got the call? The day unfolded as a typical defense attorney day, except for the lingering possibility that quietly gnawed at me in unexpected moments.

That night, when I arrived home, a message was waiting for me on the answering machine. It was John O'Sullivan. In 1998, John, then a young lawyer, had asked me to help him defend a man accused of murder. I agreed, and we had proceeded to a jury trial that ended in conviction. I had not heard from John since then except in passing in the courthouse. His message to return his call now sounded urgent, and the "What if…?" murmurs in my mind became deafening. First, I spoke with my wife to consider her thoughts, and then I made my decision. When I returned the call, John explained that he was involved in another matter that drew him close to the mother who had drowned her children, and she was in need of a defense attorney as soon as possible. My hunch was right: he asked if I would consider meeting with the family. True to the values fashioned from my days in the seminary, I agreed without a moment's hesitation and was retained on the case.

I can calculate the influence of the seminary on my life as a criminal defense attorney, fighting for the underdog—for no one in a courtroom setting fits that role more than the person accused. To search for and find an element of value in an individual accused of the most factually horrible crime is personally rewarding; to then paint the picture for the jury of this newfound virtue is a goal worth pursuing. In the seminary and in my legal practice, I was helping my fellow man. I saw spirituality, intangible at best, as a common denominator in both religious life and lawyer life. The holdover area (where lawyers meet with the accused in jail) was in many ways my "confessional."

The summer of 2001 in Houston was the summer of the great flood. Rising water had invaded the new criminal courthouse, displacing prisoners and judges from their natural habitats. It was memorable for me because Andrea Yates was confined in the Harris County Jail and attended by a makeshift staff of mental health professionals. The next morning, as I rounded the bend across the bridge over the bayou to meet Ms. Yates, I knew that this experience would forever change me. Little did I know just how much.

A mass of reporters surrounded the jail facility, and satellite dish trucks from both local and national networks swarmed the area. I had never seen the likes of it. Everyone wanted to know any and all details about the case and about this mother. As I walked across the bridge, I saw a dead snake that had washed up on the bridge as the floodwaters receded. An NBC affiliate seized the moment: Phil, a hardworking reporter with impeccable integrity, noticed the proximity of the snake to the courthouse and quipped, "How appropriate," referring to defense attorneys who stand behind their clients. As I made my way through the sea of cameras and reporters to the steps of the jail, a cameraman I knew silently mouthed, "Is it you?" I shook my head and proceeded through the front doors, aware that if they knew I had been retained, I would have had to fight my way to my first visit with my new client. Once inside, I saw the lobby was crowded with attorneys and family members of inmates and sheriff's personnel, not unlike any other day.

FACE TO FACE WITH ANDREA YATES

Yet this day was quite different. There was discernible chatter about the mother on the third floor who had killed her children. Ms. Yates's family was in the crowded lobby. I thought how important it would be for the family to show a united front in supporting her. Securing that unity would likely prove to be tough. However, meeting with the defendant was the priority. The family also was there to visit with Ms. Yates, except for her husband, Rusty Yates (a telltale sign of possible disruption in the family). They were ushered upstairs by the deputies to a deserted third floor of the jail, with me in tow. The other inmates from that floor were shuttered in their cells, their visitors long ago dismissed. Mr. Yates appeared at last, and when all was secure, the steel jail door opened, breaking the silence.

I caught a glimpse of a frail figure in an orange jumpsuit. Andrea Yates appeared on the opposite side of the plexiglass window. The space behind her was darkened, giving her a shadowy appearance that added to the macabre scene and heightened my nerves. I focused first on meeting the family. As I talked with Andrea's oldest brother, I watched out of the corner of my eye as Rusty talked to his wife. His words were muffled and indiscernible but were obviously words of comfort. His wife, my new client, pressed her head against the plexiglass and stared silently ahead. At the end of our conversation, her brother whispered, "Andrea told me she was Satan."

When the family visit ended, I spoke briefly with Dr. Melissa Ferguson, the psychiatrist who had been on duty when Andrea was arrested. Dr. Ferguson informed me of her initial assessment. I did not comprehend much of what she said, but I knew enough to know that Andrea Yates was severely mentally ill. After my discussion with the psychiatrist, it was my turn to meet with Andrea. I sat in the attorney/client booth, no longer surrounded by her family or the deputies. Andrea appeared as the door to the prisoner's side opened. I saw her unkempt hair, clenched cheeks, and dark and sunken eyes—darkened, with no discernible pupils. My initial thought was that she had eyes like a shark. Soon after, I recognized that those vacant eyes were symptomatic of psychosis.

Two days later, on June 22, at 7:30 A.M., I again met with Andrea, who remained the buzz of rumor and speculation. I had with me a medical history request form that required her signature. Completing it meant I could query her past mental and physical health records, which is always procured in these cases. I gave the consent form to the jail worker to pass on to her, and as Andrea's eyes scanned the paper, I realized she had no idea what she was looking at or being asked to do. It would be futile to explain the importance of signing the form; it was clearly beyond her capability to sign, at least on that day.

A SOLEMN PROMISE

I told Andrea I would return the next day, thinking she might sign after a night's reflection. As I turned to leave, I realized that the pen in her hand could be used to hurt herself. I wondered why the jail attendant would leave a pen with her when she was on suicide watch. I brought this to the guard's attention, and he soon retrieved the pen, much to my relief. I reflected that many people would not want this mother to end her life and thus be absolved of her wrongdoings, but I, on the other hand, was genuinely concerned for her welfare.

As I stood to leave, Andrea hunched forward, laying her forehead against the plexiglass and mumbling inaudibly. I leaned forward, my right ear pressed firmly against the plexiglass, and heard her barely audible whisper, "Please don't leave me alone." In that moment, I realized how alone she felt and that the isolation in her world, both physically and within her psychotic mind, must have been excruciating. My seminarian past and lawyer present dovetailed. Without a moment's hesitation, and although intensely perspiring from the heat and my serious focus on her, I dropped all plans to leave. I spoke to Andrea, expecting nothing in return. Nothing else mattered. She was my client, and she needed me to stay with her. From that moment on, I knew I would not leave her; I would always be there for her in her defense and in the defense of other mothers with maternal mental illness. I ended my visit with a promise to return the next day. I headed back to the lobby of the jail, and while I was talking with family members, the strangest thing happened. Rusty came up from behind and tapped me on the shoulder. He shook my hand with a smile and said, "Well, I guess it's welcome to the team." I had been retained and accepted to defend Andrea Yates. I was a legal team of one and sorely in need of teammates.

I immediately contacted my office mate, Wendell Odom. Wendell's easygoing nature and calm demeanor disguised an extremely brilliant mind able to cut through complex legal layers. He agreed to join me, knowing as I did that it was going to be the most publicized case of our lives. We also welcomed his sister, Molly, to our team. With no road map to guide us except common-sense experience, our knowledge of the law, and our bootstrap determination, we took on the case. We had no idea how much more was to come in learning about maternal infanticide and filicide offenses.

A Media Maelstrom

After my baptism of journalistic fire at the steps of the jail house, I began a long, fruitful, and mostly enjoyable relationship with the media. Despite this rapport, many leaked terrible rumors about Andrea and the deaths of her children. Often, by the time the false stories surfaced, they would indelibly be set in stone in the public's mind—even to this day. I set out to try to level the playing field of public perception. There was no question to me that Andrea Yates was a severely mentally ill mother and not the cold-blooded, monstrous killer the media depicted. I pored over DSM and read up on postpartum depression and the most extreme biological and gender-based illness: postpartum psychosis. Then I hit the airwaves. I took every opportunity afforded to educate the community—the potential jury pool—about the difficulty of understanding my client's mental state. I suspected that after the weekend of media blitz, a court-imposed "gag order" would soon be ordered, which would mean no more vilifying of Andrea in the media but also no more advocacy for her. My time was running out to correct public perception.

The morning talk shows on NBC, ABC, CBS, CNN, and Fox all contacted me, and I was eager to speak. I set up shop at Total Video, a Houston media center used by all national and some local television affiliates for Houston-based stories. The owners ran a tight ship, and through this process, we became dear friends. By Sunday evening I was utterly exhausted. Monday provided more platforms to discuss mental health issues, Andrea, and her beloved children, but my instinct about the gag order was correct: I received a call from the court to be in the chambers of Judge Belinda Hill of the 230th District Court first thing Tuesday morning. I, as Andrea's mouthpiece, was to be legally shut—but I had made my points.

A quickly circulating rumor in the media was that Andrea was pregnant, which made it imperative that she sign the medical history consent form. Each media source wanted an exclusive interview to confirm this news. Someone within the jail personnel evidently had suggested to a media representative that the mandatory pregnancy test given to female inmates had come up positive for Andrea. I had to learn the truth immediately, but without a signed consent form, the doctors would neither confirm nor deny anything. Urgency demanded action. If the story aired, more degradation of this already demonized mother would make a guilty verdict all the more satisfying to the general public. I was able to convince a source knowledgeable about the pregnancy test that I had a "need to know" basis for information, with or without a signed consent form. After all, it was painfully apparent that Andrea—despite her keen intelligence and educational background—had no idea what she was being asked to sign and therefore in all probability would never sign.

As it turned out, the pregnancy rumor was false, but how could I alert the media that the story they were about to air was simply not true? After all, the ink on the gag order had barely dried. I decided that arranging a shorthand, confidential communication with Phil of Channel 2 would be appropriate given the circumstances. After my third jail visit with my client, as I passed his parked television van, Phil simply shouted a rhetorical question to "no one" in particular: "Is the rabbit alive or dead?" A thumbs-up meant alive and a thumbs-down was my signal for dead. Thumbs up it was; the rabbit was alive, and Andrea was not pregnant. The "story" of Andrea's pregnancy, with one exception, never aired. I later discovered that Channel 13, the ABC affiliate, had aired the scintillating matter without determining its credibility. Phil, in a later story, was able to dispel the rumor without revealing his source. In hindsight, I am certain that the letter of the gag order was not obeyed, but although the judge was well aware of this, I was never chastised by the court for such a violation. Priorities sometimes demand creative ingenuity.

Learning From the Andrea Yates Case

The horrific circumstances surrounding the Andrea Yates case and the deaths of her five children present a multitude of complex issues that are legal as well as emotional, both professional and personal in nature. The foremost task as Andrea's defense lawyer was managing my own shock and bewilderment about the offense, but once I understood the nature of mental illness and its potential to significantly warp the reality of the mind, I knew that Andrea, too, was a victim. Because she had physically caused the children's deaths, the entire family was in duress, with the potential for divisive and catastrophic results that would erode the very foundation of a support system that I, her lawyer, sought to create and solidify. In a case with such overwhelming notoriety, public perception of family unity was crucial to compel the compassion I hoped to garner from the public. Adding to the state's leverage was the fact that the insanity defense was the least understood and probably the most difficult to present and persuade a jury to accept.

The Yates case exemplified both personal and professional failures within the systems, as well as legal and medical missteps in managing severe mental health issues. The tragic deaths of Noah, John, Paul, Luke, and Mary Yates were the inevitable and unfortunate result of those failures. To know and understand what happened and why, as dark and uncomfortable as this situation was, enables us not only to properly deal with mental illness in the criminal justice system but also, we hope, to prevent reoccurrences of June 20, 2001.

It is not easy to review from afar the reasons behind the tragedies of that fateful day and the manner in which the justice system reacted to the mental illness of Andrea Yates. However, we must review them here, if for no other purpose than to answer the question, "Why?" Before the drowning of the children, all the signs were there, to be recognized by the professionals and the nonprofessionals alike. There was no question that Andrea Yates had the most severe form of postpartum illness: postpartum psychosis. Her medical records were replete with references to, and diagnoses of, postpartum mental illness. From the severity of her depression after Luke's birth in 1999, doctors documented Andrea's fears that she might hurt the children or that they would all go to hell and recorded the physical effects of her mental illness—catatonia, mutism, severe psychomotor retardation—that were all present. Andrea's first hospitalization at Methodist Hospital on July 21, 1999, had been under the care of Dr. Starbranch, her psychiatrist. Dr. Starbranch had noted observations that Andrea "hadn't eaten in days. [Has a] bald spot on her scalp where she had been scratching," and, finally, made a diagnosis of postpartum depression with psychosis (probable delusions). Dr. Starbranch had also noted that "any additional pregnancy will surely guarantee future psychotic depression" and prescribed the harsh antipsychotic Haldol. This medication worked, and her symptoms abated.

Andrea was admitted into Devereux Hospital for her second hospitalization on March 31, 2001. She had stopped taking Haldol and had given birth to her fifth child, Mary, the preceding December. Andrea physically presented the same symptoms as with her hospitalization after Luke was born. The admitting psychiatrist, Dr. Albritton, indicated that she was catatonic and had flat affect, severe psychomotor retardation, and so on. Dr. Albritton tried to get a medical history from Andrea and her husband, but Andrea could not speak due to her condition, and Rusty was unable to recall the positive effects of Haldol in the previous hospitalization. Andrea was subsequently admitted with a diagnosis of major depressive disorder, postpartum onset (rule out psychotic features). The insurance company relied on a precoded determination and allotted 11–13 days for the hospital stay before withdrawing financial assistance.

Dr. Saeed was Andrea's treating physician during this second as well as a third hospital stay at Devereux Hospital. She had been released on April 13, 2001, and been readmitted the third time a little more than 2 weeks later on May 4. There had been no communication between Dr. Saeed and Dr. Starbranch the entire time that Dr. Saeed was her psychiatrist. During Andrea's second stay at Devereux Hospital, after Rusty informed Dr. Saeed that Andrea had previously been placed on Haldol and it was successful, a fax was sent to Dr. Starbranch's office for medical records, but it was unclear whether those records were received, for they were never mentioned in her treatment plan at Devereux. Nonetheless, at Rusty's suggestion, Dr. Saeed placed Andrea temporarily on Haldol.

On June 4, after Andrea was discharged from Devereux Hospital, Dr. Saeed decided to take her off of Haldol. On June 18, Rusty brought his nearly catatonic wife to Dr. Saeed's office for an outpatient visit. Instead of administering an antipsychotic, Dr. Saeed gave Andrea a "pep" talk—"You must begin to think 'happy thoughts'"—and sent her home with a slight modification in her antidepressant medication. Two days later, her five children were dead.

On June 20, 2001, sometime after 9:00 A.M. (about the same time I was stepping into my car to drive to Harris County Criminal Courthouse), Andrea, alone with her children ages 6 months to 7 years, drowned each child in the bathtub, one by one. After their deaths, she dialed 911 and requested police assistance. When officers arrived and discovered the children's bodies, she was immediately arrested. Andrea confessed her actions in an unemotional statement to City of Houston homicide detective Eric Mehl. Afterward, she was placed on suicide watch in the psychiatric ward of the Harris County Jail, where I first met her.

The Trial

The State of Texas charged Andrea Yates with capital murder and gave notice that it would seek the death penalty. Our legal team immediately filed its notice to utilize the insanity defense. Andrea Yates was determined by a jury to be competent to stand trial, and in February 2002, she was tried on three of the five deaths of the children and was convicted of capital murder. When the guilty verdict was announced (after only 1 hour of deliberation), it was devastating to everyone involved with Andrea's defense, including the attorneys, clerks, expert witnesses, and, of course, her family. Andrea herself remained reserved. With the sentencing phase still facing us, however, we had no time to grieve. We now were literally fighting for her life.

At sentencing, the jury rejected the State's plea for the death penalty, thereby automatically sentencing Andrea to life in the penitentiary. Although life in prison is by all accounts a harsh sentence, in retrospect it is a more favorable verdict than the ultimate penalty, execution. Andrea again showed little emotion compared with me and my staff when the sentencing phase of the trial concluded. "Euphoric" best describes our reaction; for the effort we had put forth in this case, of all cases, success at saving her life was by far the best resolution.

THE APPEAL

Pending her appeal to the First Court of Appeals of Texas, Andrea was placed at the Skyview Unit in the Texas Department of Criminal Justice, a facility for mentally ill individuals within the penitentiary system. Andrea was incarcerated at Skyview for more than 3 years while her appeal was pending. The court of appeals granted oral arguments in the case as requested in our brief. Regarding a particular "point of error" in the defense's appellate brief and taking almost 1 year after arguments to make their decision, the court agreed with the defense that the State's expert witness, Dr. Park Dietz, had been untruthful during his testimony. He had testified under oath that an episode of *Law and Order*, for which he was a consultant, had involved a woman who killed her children, pled not guilty, and was acquitted. He testified further that the show had aired in the Houston area shortly before Andrea killed her children. The jury already was aware that Rusty and Andrea regularly watched *Law and Order*. Yet Dr. Dietz's testimony was false, and the defense argued that the perjured testimony had been used in the cross-examination of a defense witness and again during the State's closing arguments. Defense also argued that this testimony had been weighed heavily during jury deliberations and had helped the jury reach its verdict of guilty. Ultimately, the First Court of Appeals agreed and reversed the guilty verdict, sending the case back to the trial court for a retrial—basically starting from "square one."

Andrea was returned to the Harris County Jail to await retrial. The State was precluded from again seeking the death penalty in the second trial because the issue of future dangerousness (needed to sentence someone to death) had already been decided by the first jury and was not in dispute on appeal. Pending retrial, a bond was placed, and the defense arranged as a condition of bond that Andrea be sent to a state mental health facility at Rusk State Hospital in Rusk, Texas, where she was voluntarily committed as a mental health patient awaiting retrial.

The challenge as a defense attorney was to educate the jury about the unreal world of the person on trial, who had been experiencing a psychotic delusion on the day of the offense. A person who is delusional has a different mindset and decision-making process than one who is not delusional. However, the delusional individual may be able to perform certain tasks and make certain decisions that indicate an awareness of the nonpsychotic reality. For instance, Andrea had planned to drown her children well in advance, had waited until her husband and mother-in-law were absent from the home, had called 911 and asked for the police to come, had confessed to the homicide sergeant, and had admitted that she knew her actions were wrong. At the same time, Andrea had believed unequivocally that ending her children's lives was the right thing for them. By taking their lives at a tender age, she was saving their souls from eternal damnation. Andrea had known that the criminal justice system would punish her, and therefore had known that it was legally wrong (a wrongful act) to do what she did. She had wished to be executed so the Governor of the State of Texas would be the one to "slay Satan," who singularly lived within her. Through her own execution, she had believed that she would save the world from Satan.

Another challenge as a defense attorney is in raising awareness in the minds of jurors, who decide the fate of mothers such as Andrea, about the general, as well as specific, experiences of the mother–child relationship in order to counterbalance the bizarre nature of a mother taking the lives of her children. Normally—although there are exceptions—the nature of the mother–child bond embodies protection and love, which, in fact, is often quite evident in the relationship of the mother to her children prior to the filicide event. If anything, that knowledge embodies the distinction between the unreal reality of what occurred and the true nature of the mother and child relationship, which can be helpful for jurors to have as a barometer for just how much Andrea was not in her right state of mind.

THE SECOND TRIAL

On July 26, 2006, a non-death qualified jury, after 2.5 days of deliberation, adjudged Andrea Yates as not guilty by reason of insanity (NGRI). She was sent to a state mental health hospital in Vernon, Texas, which is the initial facility for assessment once a defendant is found NGRI in Texas. She was assessed semiannually to determine whether she constituted a danger to herself or others. This assessment includes evaluation regarding self-harming, homicidal, or suicidal ideations. After her first assessment, Andrea was able to be moved to a less secure facility and remains there today. She also remains under the jurisdiction of the court and comes up for annual reviews.

Present-Day Reflections

Looking back, the Andrea Yates case was a landmark for maternal mental health awareness not only in the State of Texas but also nationally and internationally. Prosecutors are now more acutely aware of mental illness and the impact it has on criminal behavior. In October 2002, the Mental Health Association of Houston agreed to sponsor an effort to establish a memorial for the Yates children: Noah, John, Paul, Luke, and Mary. The Yates Children Memorial Fund was founded for the purpose of raising education and awareness in the community about the reality and ravages of postpartum mental illness and has conducted seminars on women's mental health, as well as the law relating to insanity and its inadequacy in addressing postpartum issues, for groups across the country. If future lives are spared, the Yates children will not have died in vain.

I take every opportunity possible to speak to groups because of my devotion to this issue, yet so much more awareness is still needed today. Nineteen years later, I remain steadfast in lobbying for awareness of maternal filicide and legal expertise for mothers who take the lives of their children while in the grips of psychiatric illness. I held true to my promise to Andrea that second day of our meeting: I have not left her. I continue my relationship with her and hold her dear to my heart. This book is emblematic of my desire to honor Andrea and my continued drive to educate and guide others in this field.

MAIN CLINICAL/LEGAL POINTS AND CULTURAL PERSPECTIVES

- A lawyer's perception of the client's offense must be through the eyes of the mentally ill defendant and the reality she held at the time of the crime.
- Public perception that those closest to the mother are fully supportive of her is vital to compel compassion and understanding.
- Legally, the ability to distinguish the different meaning of *to know* and *wrongful act* as it pertains to the case is foundational.
- Core competencies of legal experts involved in maternal filicide cases include
  - Greater awareness and appreciation of mental illness as a legitimate reality that potentially can trigger maternal filicide
  - Enhancement of law enforcement's as well as mental health professionals' ability to understand mental illness and its role in criminality
  - Development of an appreciation of the indicators of mental illness that separate the mentally ill from those who are criminally responsible for their actions

Practice and Discussion Questions

1. Reflect on your own experiences and belief systems that might impact whether you would take a maternal filicide case. What support and resources would help you in this endeavor?
2. What is your knowledge of the *Diagnostic and Statistical Manual of Mental Disorders* (DSM), and how can you ensure you are aware of the classification of mental disorders relevant to maternal filicide?

3. Should the actions of Andrea Yates and her ultimate prosecution for the drowning deaths of her children be governed by the *Webster's Dictionary* definition of the word *know* or by the reality of her psychotic world, in which she protected the children she loved from a danger that was real to her but was nonexistent to minds absent from mental illness?

Media Coverage

Bernstein M, Bridgers R, Chaisson S, et al (executive producers): The State of Texas vs. Andrea Yates [television series episode]. Crimes of the Century. CNN, July 21, 2013

Burka P: It's crazy. Texas Monthly, July 2002. Available at: https://www.texasmonthly.com/articles/its-crazy. Accessed September 2020.

Dunham N: He defended the woman who drowned her five children—then dedicated his life to making sure it never happens again. Narratively, August 1, 2017. Available at: https://narratively.com/he-defended-the-woman-who-drowned-her-five-children-then-dedicated-his-life-to-making-sure-it-never-happens-again/?utm_source=Week. Accessed September 2020.

Hollandsworth S: Her dark places. Texas Monthly, August 2001. Available at: https://www.texasmonthly.com/articles/her-dark-places. Accessed September 2020.

Hollandsworth S: The satanic versus. Texas Monthly, September 2006. Available at: https://www.texasmonthly.com/articles/the-satanic-versus. Accessed September 2020.

Morgan M: Insanity plea successful in Andrea Yates retrial. Psychiatric News, August 18, 2006. Available at: https://psychnews.psychiatryonline.org/doi/full/10.1176/pn.41.16.0002. Accessed September 2020.

Newman M: Yates found not guilty by reason of insanity. The New York Times, July 26, 2006. Available at: https://www.nytimes.com/2006/07/26/us/26cnd-yates.html. Accessed September 2020.

O'Malley S: Are You There Alone? The Unspeakable Crimes of Andrea Yates. New York, Simon and Schuster, 2004

CHAPTER 2

Becoming a Legal Expert in Infanticide and Filicide Cases in the United States

George Parnham, J.D.

In this chapter, I hope to shed light on defending mothers whose mental illnesses have resulted in the commission of a criminal filicidal act that places them in the criminal justice system. Greater awareness and appreciation of mental disorder as a legitimate illness and the need for law enforcement and forensic expert witnesses to better understand mental illness and its effects, particularly in the criminal defense of mothers, are crucial. The information presented here is essential to assist those in the judicial system, such as judges, prosecutors, defense attorneys, and forensic experts, in understanding the reality of mental illness behind maternal filicide.

When a mother takes the life of a child, regardless of the reason, the very definition of the symbol we hold most dear is distorted. The archetype of the Madonna is embedded in the fabric of our culture. In 50 years of criminal defense practice, I have defended nearly a dozen mothers who committed infanticide or filicide in the throes of mental illness. In every one of these cases, I have found that their maternal instincts remain intact—that is, they nurture, love, and protect their young from danger. In altruistic filicide, in fact, mothers kill in order to save and protect their children.

In the Andrea Yates case, all of the natural elements of motherhood existed. She loved her five children and nurtured and protected them from danger. Yet in the psychotic world in which she lived, the danger

17

she perceived (unreal to the nonpsychotic mind) was real. The Andrea Yates case was a landmark in demonstrating how a mother's unconditional love for her children can be distorted by psychosis. Andrea Yates believed that her children's souls were doomed to hell unless she took their lives at a young age to prevent them from sinning. Indeed, the cruelest of all mental illnesses causes a mother to see danger where, in reality, there is none.

Although many strides have been made by medical science to sufficiently document the reality of postpartum mental illness, more understanding is needed by the legal and forensic communities of the United States and other countries. It has been nearly two decades since the Andrea Yates case, yet mothers continue to be disadvantaged in the courts. What was a hot topic at the time remains a hot topic today. We should have advanced much further in the criminal justice system by now.

Harsh Sentencing

Sentences of death or life imprisonment for mothers who ended the lives of their children while in a mentally ill state continue to be a reality. We do not have to look far to see cases, such as Carol Coronado in California, who is currently serving a life sentence for the deaths of her children despite raising a defense of insanity due to postpartum mental illness. I am currently involved in a case in Missouri in which a mother is accused of killing one of her children and attempting to kill another. She then attempted suicide, did not succeed, and was arrested. She has been incarcerated for more than 2 years now, and the state has recently announced that it will seek the death penalty if the defendant proceeds to trial in lieu of pleading to life in the penitentiary. This case is currently set for trial in March 2021.

My previous caseload includes a mother with a well-documented history of mental illness and postpartum psychosis (PPP) who was hospitalized after the birth of her first child and then reunited with her family. She had a second child and unfortunately took his life when he was 2 months old. Tried and convicted of capital murder in a Houston courtroom, she is serving a life sentence. Several years ago I assisted in the case of a Louisiana mother who was charged with capital murder in the deaths of her two children. She also had attempted suicide. There was overwhelming evidence, as testified to by expert witnesses for the defense, that mental illness issues had prompted these tragedies, but the jury rejected her defense of insanity, and this mother is also serving a life sentence.

Herein, I clarify the meaning and present realities of the law pertaining to the mental illness defense in the United States. For the insanity defense to apply, a mother must have committed the act. Furthermore, the insanity defense is perceived by the public at large and by most prosecutors in general as a last resort to absolve criminal culpability of a defendant who has no other defense to rely upon. In reality, approximately less than 3% of all criminal cases tried involve an insanity defense, and less than 1% of those are successful. This documented lack of success itself deters criminal lawyers from using the insanity defense, sometimes even when it is warranted. Although I refer to "mothers" exclusively, this chapter could also apply to fathers who commit filicide precipitated by mental illness (see Chapter 5).

The Insanity Defense

One challenge for an insanity defense is that the act of filicide may be particularly gruesome, which invariably brings a crush of public opinion against a mother who has taken the life of her child. Adding to the state's leverage is the fact that the insanity defense is the least understood and probably the most difficult to present and persuade a jury to accept. Finally, in most instances, jurors are not informed before rendering a verdict about the effect of a not guilty by reason of insanity (NGRI) result. This permits a lay person to believe that if the jury finds in favor of an NGRI verdict, that unstable mother who is capable of killing may ride down the courthouse elevator with them (see Chapter 9). This, of course, is not the case. Mothers determined by the courts to be NGRI are normally transferred to a mental health facility where they receive treatment and are not released until they have been assessed as not being a risk and now safe to integrate back into society.

Generally, mothers who take the life of a child are treated by the U.S. judicial system without any mental health consideration due to the nature of their unfathomable act. In some cases, objective circumstances of the event may support prosecution, such as insurance motives, fetal maltreatment, or spousal revenge. However, the criminalization of maternal mental illness is particularly disheartening and disturbing when a mother, due to her own suffering, takes the life of her child and thus becomes involved in a judicial process that may lead to a life sentence or execution.

Postpartum mental illness is real, as is the importance of the innocent lives of the children taken. Yet the added political pressure of an outraged community focused only on the lives taken and the magnitude of what has happened can influence a state's attorney's office to seek the harshest penalty. It is as though the nature of the event closes the mind to the severity and reality of postpartum mental illnesses. In the United States, there are far too many cases in which the mother's grotesque and bizarre perpetration of filicide renders invisible the clear evidence of PPP, and innocent mothers are thus imprisoned for life or sentenced to death. In preparation for the defense, any demonstrable history that can be used as a juxtaposition to show how bizarre the mother's actions were on the day in question in comparison with her interactions with the child in years prior is essential to develop. It is key for drawing the jury to appreciate the distinction between *abhorrent* behavior (repugnant, detestable) and *aberrant* behavior (departing from the norm).

The following information is derived in large part from my personal experiences defending Andrea Yates and in my years since, advocating and mentoring others about this essential topic.

LESSONS LEARNED FROM THE ANDREA YATES CASE

After the drownings of the five Yates children, the investigator at the scene and later at the homicide division of the Houston Police Department reported that Andrea's affect was flat, her voice was monotone, and she was devoid of any emotion. She answered their questions correctly, displaying unimpaired memory of important dates and events in her life and that of her family. When she was called to provide statistical responses, her statements were correct and unequivocal. Yet when a detective asked the only question that demanded abstract thinking—"Andrea, why did you drown your children?"—she became completely silent and was incapable of answering or connecting the dots. The detective had to break the silence. He later testified in trial that at the end of the interview he realized he only had "half the picture." Following Andrea's statement (or lack thereof), she was placed in the psychiatric ward of the Harris County Jail on suicide watch. It is an understatement to say that it is *vital* for a jury determining the ultimate guilt or innocence of a filicidal mother to be presented with the whole picture.

Within the psychotic world of Andrea Yates on June 20, 2001—her "real" world—her children were doomed to the eternal fires of hell unless she stepped in to stop their downward spiral into Satan's clutches. In her mind, she had to take their lives to save their souls. She even went a step further: she wanted to be sentenced to death and executed so that Satan, who singularly resided within the tabernacle of her body, could be slain by the ruler, the chief executive of the State of Texas. With her execution, the world would be saved from "the evil one."

NATURE OF THE ACT OR CASE

As in many cases like Andrea's, the State attempts to bifurcate the definition of *insanity* with respect to whether mental illness caused the defendants not to know that what they were doing was wrong. The State will likely stipulate that a mother was severely mentally ill but that she still "knew what she was doing was wrong." Such was the case in the Yates appeal, *Andrea Yates vs. State of Texas* (2005). The State's appellate brief to the First Court of Appeals on page 4 indicates

> There is no question that the appellant's evidence of her delusions was extensive. However, this does not resolve the question of the appellant's legal sanity. See *Bigby v. State* (1994). Although there may be some dispute as to the type and severity of the appellant's mental disease before and during the time that she committed the charged offenses, there is no real dispute that the appellant was suffering from a severe mental disease or defect at the time of the charged offenses. Consequently, the only real dispute in this case centers around whether the appellant knew that her conduct was wrong when she killed her children.

This position can be misleading and undermine the reality of mental illness in which a mother *knows* the act is wrong but is compelled to perform it because of the warped reality of her mental illness. When a psychotic individual commits an act that results in that person becoming a defendant in the criminal justice system, discounting the reality of that person's world and judging her actions based on interpretation of the word *know* as seen through the objective eyes of the state's expert forensic psychiatrist is duplicitous at best. The legal expert must condition the jury to view the act and evidence through the *mother's* eyes.

Should the actions of a mother such as Andrea Yates, and her ultimate prosecution for the drowning deaths of her children, be governed by an objective, standard definition of *know* or by the reality of her own psychotic world, in which she was protecting her beloved children from a danger that was real to her but was nonexistent to minds absent from mental illness? Unfortunately, the law has not kept pace with matters involving the actions of mothers with postpartum mental health issues. Many civilized societies have incorporated into their legal structure the defense of *infanticide*, which is available to a mother with postpartum illness who takes the life of her child within 12 months of the child's birth. Yet no U.S. state recognized an infanticide defense until 2018, when Illinois passed PA 100-0574, a groundbreaking postpartum law that recognizes the mental illness of the mother in the culpability of filicide. Since passage of PA 100-0574, Feingold and Lewis (see Chapter 3) have joined with advocates in other states, such as Massachusetts, to create broad postpartum legislation. Public attitudes in the United States are gradually changing, and there is hope for judicial compassion and for changing the public perception of defendant mothers in the criminal justice system.

Mental Illness and Insanity Standards in the United States

An understanding of the insanity standards within the individual state jurisdictions is vital. To attempt to analyze the reasons for the inequities existing within the criminal justice system in conjunction with women's mental health, one must begin at the roots of the judicial process and its handling of mental illness in general. In the United States, there are approximately 44 different state standards, but all have common denominators: the nature of the act or case, to know or appreciate the nature of the case, and the wrongfulness of the action.

NATURE OF THE ACT OR CASE

On June 20, 2001, Andrea Yates called 911 and stated, "please send an officer." An officer responded to the residence. Andrea opened the door, and the officer saw that she was dripping wet. After the officer's introduction, Andrea stated, "I've just drowned my children."

In a typical homicide case, there are, of course, unchanging factors—the death of an individual (victim) and the presentation of possible defenses. A distinct difference between filicide and other homicides can best be illustrated thus: a jury can envision a bar fight that results in the death of a participant, as well as other homicides, such as an intoxicated driver who has an accident and causes the death of another. In the case of a mother who takes the life of her child, however, jurors may intuitively relate to a parent becoming angry with a child but can never envision taking the life of that child. The nature of the case itself renders it difficult for jurors to comprehend how this could occur. Again, the defense expert must emphasize the most important factor—the reality as it was lived and experienced through the eyes of the mentally ill mother.

TO KNOW OR APPRECIATE THE NATURE OF THE CASE AND CONSEQUENCES OF ACTIONS

As described earlier, the state has to prove *knowing* and compel the jury to see that the defendant *knew* she was taking the life of her child and that it was wrong. To *appreciate* is a broader standard because it allows the defense to speak in terms of all the circumstances that surrounded and impacted the mind of the mother beyond the objective determination of *know*. Andrea Yates *knew* she was taking the lives of her children, but she failed to appreciate the *consequences* of the action. She thought she was sending them to heaven before they reached an age at which they could not be saved. She believed she would then be charged in the legal system with capital murder and executed, thus ridding the world of Satan (who lived within her). She believed as a result of her biblical readings that only the ruler—in this case the governor of Texas—could kill the evil one, "Satan."

Juries, in many instances, are not informed what "to know" means in a legal context (as in "to know" the difference between right and wrong). As a consequence, the State's forensic expert is able to opine about the wrongfulness of the mother's actions using the *Webster's Dictionary* definition of the word *know*. To counteract this inequity, the defense must be prepared to demonstrate what the psychotic mother "knew" within her world of mental illness and present this view of wrongfulness through that mother's eyes. Only with the assistance of the clinician, an expert in postpartum illnesses, can this be achieved.

As an example, were one to have tapped Andrea Yates on the shoulder during the drowning and asked, "Andrea, don't you know it is illegal to take the life of your child?" she would have probably responded, "Yes, I'm aware of that, but don't you see I know what's best for my children? I am doing the right thing, because I'm saving their souls by sending them to heaven in their innocent years before Satan corrupts them and takes them to hell for all eternity." She was prepared to suffer the legal consequences of doing what she knew to be right—thus the horrific nature of PPP.

THE WRONGFULNESS OF THE ACTION

Simply put, unless the act committed by an accused person is "illegal," that person will not be prosecuted. Thus, a defense that the accused lacked knowledge that the act was wrong is unnecessary. The wrongfulness of the act is a foregone conclusion—to become a defendant in the criminal justice system, one's actions must be legally wrong. Therefore, the issue of what factually happened is undeniable. However, the defendant's mindset is vital.

Without considering the mental state of the defendant, there would be sufficient evidence for a jury to convict for capital murder. The mindset of the person charged with capital murder is thus paramount to a legal and successful defense. For example: Mr. Anju lives next door to Mr. Lau. Mr. Anju believed Mr. Lau's house was filled with aliens who intended to attack Mr. Anju. Mr. Anju then proceeds to set fire to Mr. Lau's house, which is an illegal act. However, Mr. Anju's mental state remains a key element of the defense that he lacked the *intent* to harm Mr. Lau. Mr. Anju also used his credit card to buy cement and build a runway for his own friendly aliens, which is not illegal, but for all the wrong reasons. Therefore, all these rational legal acts have an absurd conclusion. In his mind, if he *knows* his actions are illegal, the counterbalancing of his mindset—his belief that what he was doing was right—overcomes the illegality of what has occurred (in his mind). Objectively viewed, however, his actions will always appear to be illegal.

In Andrea's case, as described earlier, what mother would not want to save her children from burning in hell? In her maternal love, she was saving their souls from eternal damnation. The prosecution will use any motive it can to establish a rationale unrelated to the mental illness of the person charged, such as spousal revenge, life insurance of the children, neglect, abuse, lack of medical care for the children (also negligence, but this goes more directly to the mother's intent to take the child's life), and any previous actions such as neglect or positive attempts to take the child's life.

The M'Naghten Rule

Unfortunately, the United States has a litany of insanity standards. Each state is free to decide what language governs the criminal consequences of the matter on trial. However, as stated earlier, most definitions of insanity have some common denominators. Those principles are derived from the source of almost all insanity standards applied in each state's criminal jurisprudence: the M'Naghten rule. *M'Naghten's Case* (1843) is the bedrock of all current insanity standards in the United States. Jurors must be told that in order to establish a defense on the grounds of insanity, the defense must clearly prove that at the time of committing the act, the accused was laboring under such a defect of reason or disease of the mind as to not know the nature and quality of his or her actions or did not know that the actions were wrong.

Seventeen states and the federal government have incorporated the M'Naghten rule to some degree. The portion of the rule that addresses a person's inability to understand the nature and quality of his or her actions due to mental illness is referred to as the "cognitive" prong. The second portion, the "moral" prong, interprets that even though a person is able to understand the nature of his or her actions as a result of a severe mental disease or defect, that person did not "know" that those actions were "wrong." (Some state standards incorporate the language "distinguish between right and wrong.") Only Alaska has the cognitive prong as its standard, and 10 states have only the moral prong, or the moral incapacity test.

To illustrate, Eric Michael Clark shot and killed a police officer in Flagstaff, Arizona. It was uncontested that Clark had paranoid schizophrenia and was acutely psychotic around the time of the shooting. His defense was insanity. The Arizona definition of insanity is mirrored after the "moral" prong of M'Naghten, and the burden is on the defendant to offer clear and convincing evidence. The defense had to prove that his mental illness resulted in Clark not knowing his actions were wrong. As the Supreme Court stated in *Clark v. Arizona* (2006), four basic "principles" are incorporated in the various states' standards (and federal standard) that deal with mental illness within the criminal justice systems:

1. *Cognitive incapacity*: Did the severity of the mental illness cause the person to fail to appreciate the nature and quality of his or her actions? (M'Naghten's first prong)
2. *Moral incapacity*: Did the severity of mental illness result in the person not knowing the actions were wrong? (M'Naghten's second prong)
3. *Volitional incapacity*: Did the severe mental illness cause the person to be unable to control his or her actions (also known as *irresistible impulse*)? (M'Naghten's third prong)
4. *Product of mental illness*: Simply put, were the person's actions a product of mental illness?

M'Naghten in its various forms had not been revised until after the shooting of President Reagan and the ultimate acquittal of John Hinckley Jr. based on his mental illness. A collective legislative backlash occurred to change the federal insanity standard, resulting in the Insanity Defense Reform Act of 1984. Several states also rewrote their statutes regarding the insanity defense and in some cases eliminated it altogether. Basically, these federal and state reforms eliminated defendants' ability to conform their conduct to the law. Legislators wanted to do away with "irresistible impulse"—that, in essence, defendants may know their actions are wrong, may know they are not supposed to do what they are doing because it is wrong, but may have an impulse that is absolutely irresistible. This is an element of nature that falls within M'Naghten.

Sanity is invariably presumed, and the burden of proof is on the defense to prove otherwise. This burden can differ from jurisdiction to jurisdiction. Most states have a "preponderance of evidence" standard—that is, the greater weight of credible evidence should "rule the day." Some employ a "clear and convincing" standard, a burden greater than the preponderance burden. The distinction is to a large degree meaningless if the defense of insanity for a mother with postpartum illness has been properly prepared and presented. That brings about the necessity of incorporating into the defense a clinician trained in postpartum issues who can clearly and comprehensibly articulate to a jury—through an equally educated defense counsel—the reality of the illness and the thought processes of the mentally ill mother.

In *Clark*, the defense attacked the *mens rea* element of the offense, arguing that the defendant did not intend to kill a human being (it was uncontested that Clark believed aliens who were out to kill him were frequently using the identity of government agents). Hypothetically, if Clark did not *intend* to kill a police officer, his defense—absent the insanity defense—should have been successful. The problem was in the trial court's prohibition of expert psychiatric testimony about Clark's mental illness on the issue of *mens rea*. On appeal, Clark argued that the trial court's exclusion of evidence of mental illness in attacking the *mens rea* element was a denial of due process. The Supreme Court rejected this argument and stressed the right of the states to establish individual standards of insanity and admissibility of psychiatric evidence on the *mens rea* element of an offense. In effect, it sustained the lower court's prohibition of psychiatric testimony on the *mens rea* intent issue.

Unfortunately, the court in its opinion went out of its way to denigrate psychiatry and its ability to link uncontested mental illness with the defendant's thought process at the time of the act. By prohibiting mental illness testimony, the court emphasized that dueling psychiatric experts can easily mislead the jury to the wrong verdict:

> [Alt]hough mental disease evidence is certainly not condemned wholesale, the consequence of this professional ferment (the mental illness diagnoses and the debate over the "very contours of the mental disease itself") is a general caution in treating psychological classifications as predicates for excusing otherwise criminal conduct. (*Clark v. Arizona* 2006, p. 10)

By its own language, the court—perhaps unwittingly and by infer-ence—opened the door for trial courts and psychiatry to raise the bar when making a legal determination of who is and is not qualified to tes-tify as an expert in matters dealing with mental health. The argument can be made that only experts who have a foundation in postpartum ill-nesses should be permitted to render an opinion as to whether a mother on trial appreciated the nature and quality of the act she was commit-ting or "knew" that her conduct was "wrong." In Andrea Yates's second trial, an amicus brief supporting this proposition was filed with the trial court; however, the state's expert witness, Dr. Dietz, did not have this qualification. Dr. Dietz admitted he was not an expert in women's men-tal health and judged both sexes' mental illness by the same standards.

Jurors are legally entitled to informed testimony from qualified ex-perts. Mentally ill defendants must be judged not on the basis of specu-lation and conjecture but on scientific fact and informed expert analysis. Therefore, *amici curiae* respectfully suggest specific criteria pursuant to *Kelly v. Texas* (1992) as utilized in both *Sexton v. State* (2002) and *E.I. Du-Pont de Nemours and Co. v. Robinson* (1996) that apply to expert witnesses testifying to the mental state of mothers with PPP. Under the particular facts of the Yates case, this proposed standard required that only mental health experts with significant experience in PPP be permitted to testify as to whether Andrea knew that her conduct was wrong.

As indicated, states' standards are diverse and depend on a variety of factors and legal concepts, ignoring for the most part the reality of mental illness and its effect on the thought processes of the particular de-fendant. The American Law Institute Model Penal Code Section 4.01 (1) (1962) incorporates the following definition: "A person is not responsible for criminal conduct if at the time of such conduct as a result of mental illness or defect he lacks substantial capacity either to appreciate the criminality (wrongfulness) of his conduct or to conform his conduct to the requirements of the law."

An individual state's right to determine its way of dealing with the acts of mentally ill mothers is given priority over the illness itself, even when those mothers share the same mental illness. Fourteen states have adopted a form of this standard. Three states use a combination of voli-tional incapacity and the M'Naghten standard. Only one state uses the "product of mental illness test," and four states have no insanity standard at all.

A standard has been incorporated for a lesser included pragmatic alternative to an insanity defense: *guilty but mentally ill* (GBMI; wording may vary slightly from state to state, e.g., "guilty except for mental ill-ness"). Generally, if the defense fails to meet its burden on insanity (either by a preponderance of evidence [meaning more likely than not] or clear and convincing evidence) on any of the issues presented in the insanity definition, then the judge or jury can return a verdict of GBMI. The defendant is transported to a mental health facility until he or she is no longer deemed a danger to self or others and then taken to general prison population to serve the sentence imposed. (A person found NGRI would be transferred to a mental health facility and then integrated back into the community when well, not transferred to a jail or prison facility.) Interestingly, evidence of mental illness is admissible on the issue of *mens rea* in the four states that do not have an insanity defense. The distinction between NGRI and GBMI is that although both result in mental health treatment, GBMI includes a conviction and often penitentiary time and NGRI does not.

Defending the Mentally Ill

A large percentage of situations that demand the involvement of law enforcement have, at their core, an ingredient of mental illness. Domestic disputes, fathers who physically abuse their children, and mothers who take the lives of their children are all examples—although certainly not exhaustive—of conflicts in which mental illness frequently plays a part. Obviously, not all situations of this nature are caused by mental illness, and it behooves the law enforcement officer or team who initially confronts a potentially violent offender to be aware of the indicators of mental illness and know how to respond accordingly.

Legal experts are wise to visit with the client as soon as possible after being retained. If it appears through observation, conversation, or both or a review of the offense report and any available mental health records that the client has signs of maternal mental health issues, consider taking at least these four actions:

1. Ensure the mother is receiving mental health treatment while incarcerated.
2. Ensure the medical professionals involved in the mother's care document and write copious notes, including the types and dosages of prescribed medications.
3. Find the most qualified psychiatrist/psychologist available to evaluate the mother. This professional should have competence in maternal mental health. Too often, U.S. courts permit forensic experts who are untrained in women's mental health issues to testify about their opinions as to whether the defendant mother qualifies for an insanity

defense. Such was the case in both murder trials of Andrea Yates. In part, this resulted from a lack of understanding and appreciation of the reality of postpartum illness. In general, the judicial system simply does not acknowledge mental health differences between men and women, depriving jurors of the ability to judge the actions of defendants with PPP.

4. Video record the mother as soon as possible in the assessment. If she is psychotic, it will be evident in her presentation. In all likelihood, after she takes prescribed medication, her mental illness will be less apparent. In some cases, she may appear to be well and "sane." The more time that elapses between the index event and the video recording, the more "normal" she will likely present. Along with this point, video recording is only meaningful if the jury is made aware of the signs of psychosis in an individual. The decision to record a client is obviously based on a determination by defense counsel that she is mentally ill. As such, the legal expert must educate the courts to observe for flat affect, dull speech, dilated pupils, and so forth. Video recordings of Andrea Yates immediately after the crime, which were shown in court, captured her floridly psychotic and provided visual evidence of her mental illness.

DEFENSE COUNSEL

Research the track record of the prosecution's forensic experts to review their testimony in other cases. This enables you to avoid the land mines that sometimes exist when a defense lawyer confronts the state's expert head to head. One example is the expert's motive for testifying. In the Yates trial, I learned that Dr. Dietz was a businessman who had blanketed the Houston area weeks before the trial with brochures about his services. When I cross-examined him, I inquired whether any of his activities as a forensic witness for the state included expertise in or mention of women's mental health. He had to admit in the negative. This lack of expertise in maternal mental health is a profound gap in understanding, and the prosecution was disadvantaged as a result. As I posed these questions to Dr. Dietz, although I was not confronting him with his evaluation of my client and the accuracy of his opinion, he became hostile, as though I were attempting to belittle him in the eyes of the jury by questioning his credentials. Dr. Dietz has since stated that he was upset I did not ask him "important, relevant questions" pertaining to resolving the most difficult issues.

When I questioned him about his role as a consultant for the NBC television series *Law and Order*, Dr. Dietz saw his chance to regain his power and put me in my place. When asked if the show had an episode about a mother killing her children, he responded that such an episode existed and described his consultation on an episode in which a mother was found NGRI that (he claimed) had aired a few days prior to the deaths of the Yates children. (Rusty Yates, Andrea's husband, had testified earlier that he and Andrea frequently watched *Law and Order*.) He sealed Andrea's fate on this falsehood (*Yates* 2005, p. 92). Later, Dr. Dietz stated he had confused the Yates case, in that moment, with another. His response to my question was not only untrue, it was damning and damaging because it was used by the State in cross-examining one of our experts and also in summation, suggesting to the jury that Andrea had watched the show and come up with a plan to get out of a trapped marriage. The result of this false testimony was initially a conviction and then a rejection by the jury of the death sentence. It later meant reversal on appeal by the First Court of Appeals, allowing a new trial.

In her second trial, on July 26, 2006, a non-death qualified jury adjudged Andrea Yates to be NGRI. This was a victory not only for Andrea and the defense team but also for the citizens of the United States because it elevated maternal mental health to a legally acceptance level and gave credibility to mothers with postpartum depression or PPP. Ironically, the severity of Andrea's mental illness was never contested because the State of Texas had stipulated to it. Yet the State's ignorance of the implication of her mental illness on her actions was emphasized when they voiced, "Let the State be clear. The Appellant (Yates) is and was severely mentally ill. There is absolutely no legitimate question about that. The only question lies in whether the appellant should be held criminally responsible for killing her children" (*Andrea Yates vs. State of Texas* 2005, p. 63). This is not part of the statutory insanity standard but is a crucial part of a defense of mental illness. In overturning the guilty verdict in the second trial, the jury applied the Texas Insanity Standard (Penal Code Section 8.01): "It is an affirmative defense to prosecution that, at the time of the conduct charged, the actor, as a result of a severe mental disease or defect, did not know that his conduct was wrong."

THE DEFENSE EXPERT WITNESS

It is essential to consider the impact on the jury of a forensic expert's witness testimony for either side and to prepare for the direct or cross examination of that expert. Keep one step ahead of the prosecution's expert witnesses. This can be accomplished by obtaining from the State, pretrial, the background of the experts, including the cases in which they have testified. Frequently, a pretrial hearing will be necessary to determine the qualifications, or lack thereof, of the experts and their ability to testify in the matter at hand. Be aware of motive (have the experts ever testified for the defense?). Be fully aware of depositions or recorded interviews in previous cases. Obtain the experts' prior testimonies before judges or juries; transcripts can be obtained, for a fee, by contacting the court reporter for those cases. Also, determine any allegations against the experts (i.e., lying under oath, not being prepared). Be cautious of introducing specific case analogies unless the legal defense has previous testimony in direct conflict on specific case-related issues.

Beware of the state's forensic experts having an agenda to convict the mother simply because they have been hired by the state to do so. Evidence "shaping" is more prevalent in an insanity defense case than in any other, from my perspective. There is so much subjectivity in dealing with the actions of an ill mind. Expert witnesses for the state will invariably tell the jury that their report (if one exists) has been "peer reviewed," thereby suggesting that not only the expert but also their peers have reviewed the report and determined its accuracy in support of the expert's opinion. With this in mind, the defense attorney needs to find out, pretrial, who those peers were, and if possible, check their backgrounds. It is likely that the peers are in some way financially connected to the expert. Furthermore, the peer likely has only reviewed the written report in conjunction with a conversation with the expert and has never reached his or her own conclusion by interviewing the defendant mother or other witnesses. Rarely, if ever, will the peer have read any medical evidence related to the case. The peer examines only the expert's completed report and concludes that the expert's rationale is accurate, which of course can be called into question.

An expert witness must review all of the factors of the client's life and the relationship that existed between mother and child and extended family as well. For instance, forensic experts should review medical records that exist and visit the treating medical personnel. In most cases, the state's expert witness will not have talked with the nurses, attendants, and so on. I also firmly believe an expert witness benefits from going to the scene of the offense. It is not a common practice, but much can be gleaned from the defense lawyer and possibly the expert witness going out to the location. Questions raised during the trial about the scene will reflect to the jury that not only does the defense lawyer have factual knowledge about the issue but that the defense lawyer and expert witness thought enough about the defense of the case to make the extra effort. Having the opportunity to talk with the family's neighbors is also key; in the Yates case, Andrea's neighbors talked about how quiet she was (not in the least the type to take the lives of her children).

The expert witness becomes an extension of the crime scene investigator and relies upon the investigator's report, which should include all of the investigation (i.e., background of the defendant; state of mind before, during, and after the "event"). Forensic expert opinions are frequently rendered before judges and juries based on the situational circumstances accumulated during law enforcement investigations.

BECOME FAMILIAR WITH PSYCHIATRIC TERMINOLOGY

Defense attorneys should be conversant in the various types of mental illnesses in order to stay one step ahead during cross-examination. For instance, what defines schizophrenia? How does clinical depression impact the thought process of the actor? What constitutes a delusion or a hallucination, both verbal and auditory? What is the difference between an *obsession* and a *thought insertion*? Can an act be both intentional and premeditated and the accused still be legally insane? How do any of the mental illnesses or symptoms thereof affect an otherwise logical thought process?

The forensic expert witness will be able to guide the lawyer in this regard. Consult the most recent edition of the *Diagnostic and Statistical Manual of Mental Disorders* (DSM), which every criminal defense lawyer should have on hand. In DSM, schizophrenia, schizoaffective disorder, delusional disorder, brief psychotic disorder, shared psychotic disorder, psychotic disorder due to a general medical condition, substance abuse-induced psychotic disorder, and psychotic disorder not otherwise specified are all mental illnesses that could well apply to the mother. PPP is under consideration as a distinct classification for the sixth edition of DSM, which will then substantiate the reality of this mental illness in the court system.

Pay close attention to researching and understanding delusions and psychosis. Although different meanings have been applied to a psychotic condition, one layman's definition might be "out of touch with reality." The name of the illness is somewhat important, but the symptoms are what count; if more than one expert is being used, ensure they are all on the same page with their diagnoses. The commonly used term *psychotic* refers to delusions, any prominent hallucinations, disorganized speech, or disorganized or catatonic behavior when the illness is schizophrenia, schizoaffective disorder, or a brief psychotic disorder. In a psychotic disorder due to a general medication condition, *psychotic* refers to delusions or only those hallucinations that are not accompanied by insight. In a delusional disorder, or shared psychotic disorder, *psychotic* is equivalent to delusional.

THE STATE'S FORENSIC EXPERT

An undeniable trend exists within the U.S. court systems that lessens the importance of mental health medicine in the judicial trial process and replaces it with sanitized but artificial "logical" explanations of the actions of the mentally ill. Too often, the treating physician, the person with the most intimate knowledge of the mental health of the patient on trial, is discarded by the forensic expert as a witness who is more interested in the patient's well-being than in being a "truth seeker." As an unfair consequence, a direct conflict arises between the "objective" opinion of the forensic expert and the "subjectively tainted" opinion of the treating psychiatric expert.

"PIERCING THE VEIL OF PSYCHOBABBLE"

In almost every instance, to arrive at an opinion adverse to the insanity defense, the expert witness will have evaluated the wrongfulness of the defendant's actions and her knowledge of such by combining the content of her interviews with the uncontradicted factual circumstances of the offense. The state's expert witness will have determined that the defendant was sane at the time of the act and then interpret the facts to support that opinion. For instance, a mother can know it is legally wrong to commit an act, but again, the definition of *knowing* in the mind of a psychotic mother is disputable. In Andrea Yates's case, after she drowned her children, she called 911. The State used that as a foundation to argue that, by calling 911, she must have *known* what she was doing was wrong because she knew to reach out and report the crime. On the other hand, calling 911 to report the deaths can also be evidence of her mental illness and her immediate mindset, which in this case indicated that she was still protecting her children by calling law enforcement, by calling for help. She called for help instead of fleeing the scene or fabricating a story to hide the truth.

In my opinion, calling 911 was evidence of at least two issues: What does one do when there are dead bodies at the house? The 911 call is an initial step toward her prosecution and ultimate execution, and as such, a reflection into her psychotic state.

Also demonstrating differences in perceptions or conclusions, Dr. Dietz argued that Andrea's action of covering her children's bodies with a sheet indicated her sanity because she felt shame and remorse and did not want the children to see what was happening and what their fate was to be. However, my conclusion of the same action was that covering a dead body with a sheet is a cultural practice. I also asked about what the placing of Mary's body on John's shoulder and the protective intertwining of John's arm around Mary indicated. Dr. Dietz never gave me an opinion for that one.

The state's expert witnesses will do their best to convince the jury that they have objectively reviewed all the facts and rendered an opinion that the mother is sane. They will attempt to skew the evidence to support their conclusion of sanity. For example, Dr. Dietz claimed that Andrea had obsessive-compulsive disorder (OCD) and not PPP. OCD would not qualify for an insanity defense. Dr. Dietz argued that the idea to take the lives of her children was the result of OCD in which the compulsive or intrusive thoughts were the product of Andrea's own mind (ego-dystonic). That is, her compulsive/intrusive thoughts were nonpsychotic, whereas *thought insertions* equaled psychosis. This distinction can be difficult, given that an obsession or intrusive thought from OCD can turn into a thought insertion (evidence of psychosis) and be objectively classified depending on the severity of the person's mental illness. What might be an *intrusive* thought in a mood disorder can become a thought inserted into that person's psychotic world. Dr. Dietz wanted the jury to believe that the thought of drowning her children came into Andrea's mind from within. He knew that if the jury believed that the thoughts came from an outside source, they would believe she was afflicted with psychosis.

To demonstrate the difference, Dr. Dietz used the solitary example of Andrea's urge to take the lives of her children as an example of an obsession, which evidenced OCD. However, he did not give the jury the full DSM diagnostic criteria for OCD, that individuals are able to recognize that their compulsive thoughts are imposed from within (ego-dystonic). When I challenged him on cross-examination, he begrudgingly admitted that Andrea had told him a number of times that Satan had put the thoughts in her head to kill her children (ego-syntonic). When psychosis is involved, consider the following:

- The psychotic mother's experience of reality is fundamentally different from normal human experience.
- The intent to commit the act of filicide does not automatically render one legally sane.
- Psychotic delusions may ebb and flow as a result of life stressors or psychiatric medications but cannot be willed away.

- Awareness of the illegality of the act does not necessarily mean that the actor *knew* it was wrong.
- When a person is experiencing a full (psychotic) delusion, that person holds it with absolute conviction, and no evidence or argument will change his or her mind. In New Zealand, for example, "moral wrongfulness" is spelled out in the statute: someone may know that the act of killing one's children is illegal (and wrong) yet may believe it is the morally right thing to do because they are enacting God's command.

THROUGH THE EYES OF THE MOTHER

I believe defendants should not testify when an insanity defense is being used. Testifying in hindsight about what occurred during a psychotic event opens the door to an extensive cross-examination from a logical perspective about what happened. However, the case must be founded on the mother's perspective at the time of the event. The foundation of good cross-examination of a forensic expert in an insanity defense is to always be mindful that the wrongfulness of the actions must be viewed through the mother's eyes. Her perceived reality must be the thread that connects every issue on cross-examination. The logic of the expert who objectively views the circumstances of the offense is not what counts; it is only the mindset of the mentally ill defendant mother and what she "knew" in her unreal world of postpartum mental illness that matters. The jury must be reminded of this issue in *voir dire* as well as in the opening argument and throughout the lawyer's questioning of witnesses. Again, the concept of "obsessions" versus "thought insertions" is a perfect example.

LASTLY, EMBRACE THE VICTIM(S)

Competent presentation of women's mental health issues to judges and juries engaged in the criminal justice system is never more critical than in the tragic case of a mother who takes the life of her child as a direct result of a postpartum disorder. To make the various standards applicable to the acts of the mentally ill mother and persuade a jury of this reality is a daunting task. My aim in this chapter has been to summarize the major barriers limiting the fair trial and sentencing of these mothers as a result of the legal realities of the United States.

The true victims in maternal infanticide and filicide cases, when maternal mental illness is at play, are the mothers and their children (both living and deceased). Yet we must also not forget the pain in the family and the loss that we as a society experience not only when the mother is not supported in the criminal justice system but also because prevention efforts are in continued need. The true defendant is the mental illness that drove the mother to commit acts she would never have perpetrated if she were free of mental illness. A mother can know it is legally wrong to commit an act, but again, the definition of *knowing* in the mind of a psychotic mother is disputable. Andrea Yates has been a beacon of light shining on the sidelines of this endeavor in the United States since her acquittal. Andrea is one of the most congenial individuals I am honored to know; she presently is no risk to society whatsoever. She was never a true risk to anyone except on that fateful day when the psychosis that descended was not treated with proper medication and her grip on reality was lost.

MAIN CLINICAL/LEGAL POINTS AND CULTURAL PERSPECTIVES

- Public perception of family support of the defendant is important to compel more compassionate understanding of the offense.
- The ability to distinguish the different meanings of *to know* and *wrongful* act as they pertain to the case is crucial.
- A lawyer's perception of the offense must be through the eyes of the mentally ill mother and the reality she held at the time of the crime.
- The enhancement of law enforcement's and mental health care professionals' ability to understand mental illness and its role in criminality cannot be overlooked.
- It is prudent to develop an appreciation of the indicators of mental illness and the postpartum mental health realities that separate the mentally ill from those who are criminally responsible for their actions.

Practice and Discussion Questions

1. Reflect on your own experiences and belief systems that could impact whether you would involve yourself in a case like that of Andrea Yates and what supportive people and resources may help you in this endeavor. Although this statement has previously been addressed, it is important to re-emphasize the attorney's perspective.

2. Lawyers and forensic expert witnesses having greater awareness and appreciation of mental illness, particularly maternal mental illness, is essential. What are your thoughts about the necessity to require that only professionals with knowledge of maternal mental illness be involved in these court cases?

3. What is your knowledge of the most recent edition of the *Diagnostic and Statistical Manual of Mental Disorders* (DSM), and how can you ensure you are aware of the classification of mental disorders that pertain to postpartum psychiatric disorders? How might the addition of postpartum psychosis to the next edition of DSM advantage or disadvantage mothers who enact infanticide or filicide?

4. Discuss the insanity defense as it pertains to your country and region. Are change and advocacy needed? What are the laws? See Chapter 3 for ways to enact change for a postpartum mental illness law.

5. What strategies would allow you to see *abhorrent* behavior as *aberrant* in the tragedy of maternal filicide?

References

Andrea Yates v. State of Texas, 171 S.W.3d 215 (Tex.App.-Houston [1st Dist.] 2005)

Bigby v. State, 892 S.W.2d 864, 878 (Tex. Crim. App. 1994)

Clark v. Arizona, 548 U.S.735 (2006)

E.I. DuPont de Nemours and Co. v. Robinson, 923 S.W.2d 549 (Tex. 1996)

Kelly v. Texas, 824 S.W.2d 568 (Tex. Crim. App. 1992)

M'Naghten's Case (10 C1. & Fin., at 210, 8 Eng. Rep., at 722 [1843])

Sexton v. State, 93 S.W.3d 96 (Tex. Crim. App. 2002)

Model Penal Code, Section 4.01 (P.O.D. 1962)

CHAPTER 3

A Groundbreaking Illinois Postpartum Law Brings Hope for Change in the United States

Susan Benjamin Feingold, Psy.D., PMH-C

Barry Michael Lewis, J.D.

The objective of this chapter is to explain the need for and promote the development of compassionate and rational laws pertaining to special issues regarding the interface of perinatal mental illness and criminal law in the United States. Recognizing the unique nature of the illness, more than 30 countries have written specific laws for mothers who have been victims of an outdated criminal justice system, including Australia, Austria, Brazil, Canada, Colombia, England, Finland, Germany, Greece, Hong Kong, India, Italy, Japan, Korea, New Zealand, Norway, Philippines, Sweden, Switzerland, Turkey, Wales, and many others. It is long past time for the United States to join them.

Maternal Mental Illness Is a Crisis Affecting Millions Worldwide

Maternal mental illness is not what new mothers and fathers anticipate when they dream of becoming a family. Pregnant women and their

---

Feingold and Lewis share the goal of advocating for perinatal criminal laws state by state and are coauthors of *Advocating for Women with Postpartum Mental Illness: A Guide to Changing the Law and the National Climate* (2020) published by Rowman and Littlefield. It is second book for each and their first together.

partners are often not informed of the risks of perinatal mood and anxiety disorders and can be completely unaware of them, although these disorders are the most common complication of pregnancy and childbirth. Indeed, mothers and families rarely contemplate mental illness when dreaming of and preparing for a baby.

The reality is that approximately 800,000 women a year in the United States experience maternal mental illness. In both the United States and worldwide, it has been estimated that 10%–15% of women experience significant symptoms of depression, anxiety, or both during their pregnancy or the postpartum period (O'Hara and Swain 1996). Postpartum Support International (2019) estimates that 1–2 women in 1,000 experience the most severe form: postpartum psychosis (PPP). In a study of the global prevalence of PPP, it was concluded that the range was 0.89–2.6 in 1,000 childbearing women and perhaps as high as 5% (VanderKruik et al. 2017). Various genetic, endocrine, biochemical, hormonal, and psychosocial risk factors have been identified that increase the probability of maternal mental illness. Prevention and being proactive with a perinatal treatment plan may help lower the risk.

Women with a personal or family history of bipolar disorder, depression, OCD, or anxiety disorders must be monitored closely. Their likelihood of illness is greater than for those without a history of a mood disorder; however, this does not guarantee that a woman with no mental health problems will not experience a first episode of a mood disorder surrounding childbirth. Many perinatal women do (Feingold and Lewis 2020). Thus, every woman and partner, every doctor—in fact, everyone— must be aware of the potential for this illness. Although the overall numbers indicate that most women with PPP *do not* commit suicide or harm their infants or their children, the risk is still there. Meyer and Oberman (2008) estimated conservatively that there were 120 cases of infanticide or neonaticide yearly in the United States alone.

At-Risk Mothers Need a Prevention and Treatment Plan

In those with a greater risk profile due to premorbid symptomatology, a risk-benefit analysis is essential to consider various pharmacological as well as psychotherapeutic approaches for prevention and treatment of maternal mental illness. A preemptive plan is beneficial. An individualized treatment plan is critical in circumstances when symptoms manifest. All treatment should involve collaboration between the woman and her health care providers. It is advisable to include others in related disciplines (i.e., doulas, lactation consultants, childbirth educators, nutritionists) who could support the pregnant woman or new mother, as well as her partners and family members. Education of the mother, her spouse or partner, and involved family members is vital. All medical providers working with perinatal women must be knowledgeable about and inform their patients of this common complication of pregnancy and childbirth.

More laws are being enacted throughout the United States that require providers to screen and refer high-risk or symptomatic pregnant and postpartum patients for treatment. A necessary step toward prevention and early detection is screening and monitoring all childbearing women, not only during the 40 weeks of pregnancy but also throughout the "fourth trimester" following childbirth, at a minimum. Best practices would include periodic screenings throughout the first year after delivery and beyond. DSM-5 (American Psychiatric Association 2013) defines postpartum mental illness as occurring within 4–6 weeks of childbirth; however, perinatal mental health specialists agree this is inaccurate. Psychiatric symptoms can present during pregnancy or anytime in the first year after delivery (Mayo Clinic 2019). As mentioned, complex multidimensional factors, including biological and genetic underpinnings, massive endocrine changes, and psychosocial and societal expectations during pregnancy, lactation, and delivery, all contribute to a mother's risk profile.

Postpartum Psychiatric Disorders and Mothers Who Commit Filicide

What happens when detection and treatment fail? In some tragic circumstances, women with maternal mental illness—particularly those with severe depression or PPP—commit crimes. Of those women, many who find themselves involved with the criminal justice system have not experienced mental illness prior to pregnancy or childbirth. For example, Cynthia Wachenheim (Belluck 2014) had no prior mental illness or criminal record (see "Suicide Versus Life in Prison" later).

It is particularly difficult for a defense attorney to establish an insanity defense for a mother who has no prior history of mental illness or whose illness waxes and wanes. As a result, women with PPP who commit filicide can be at a disadvantage over defendants who have a history of mental illness and records of psychiatric treatment. A change in criminal law is therefore essential. In the United States, women with maternal mental illness who commit crimes such as filicide commonly receive harsh and often irrevocable sentences. It does not seem rational for mothers with PPP, a temporary mental illness, to be sentenced to life imprisonment or the death penalty. It is unjustifiable to have laws that punish mentally ill mothers with penalties that are similar to or harsher than those given to psychopathic criminals who kill for personal gain or pleasure. We share a belief with many in the perinatal and forensic communities that the only sensible solution to the unique issues of individuals with perinatal mental illness is a change in the law. In a survey of 34 countries, almost all indicated that infanticide is a mitigated form of homicide, punishable by an average maximum of 6 years imprisonment (Smit et al. 2012). Contrast these survey results with cases in the United States, in which a life term without parole is often mandatory.

New efforts to understand filicide were the focus of the Marcé Society's special edition in 2019. In the article "Filicide Research in the Twenty First Century" (Klier et al. 2018), co-author Margaret Spinelli described her commitment as an expert witness, recognizing that the insanity defense in the United States is antiquated and was established in 1843. She also "makes the case that this reliance on outdated notions about mental health, added to the lack of clarity of the DSM, are systematically disadvantaging women who are severely mentally ill and facing a murder charge" (Klier et al. 2018, p. 136). Women with maternal mental illness are subjected to the most severe penalty allowed in each and every one of the 50 states, even the death penalty or life imprisonment without the possibility of parole. No direct consequence of carrying a child to term in the womb should result in an extended penitentiary sentence (Lewis 2018), yet it does, as we have seen too many times. In Illinois alone, more than 20 women are serving life sentences or decades behind bars as a result of their perinatal mental illness.

Criminal Laws Throughout History

> Anyone who strikes a man and kills him shall surely be put to death. However, if he does not do it intentionally,… he is to flee to a place I will designate. But if a man schemes and kills another man deliberately, take him away from my altar and put him to death.
>
> Exodus 21:12–15

Since biblical times, a generalized distinction has been made between grades of homicide. Historically, various codes in differing nations and states developed degrees of homicide. For as long as written language has existed, written laws have distinguished "lesser" homicides from murder. We insist that a crime caused by the biological, biochemical, and social stresses of motherhood itself against the child of her creation calls for this distinction.

U.S. LAWS TRACE THEIR ORIGIN TO THE COMMON LAW

In early England, laws developed in a piecemeal fashion. There was a Northumbrian law, a Devonshire law, and laws particular to any king or baron who was capable of imposing them. Then in 1066 came the Norman Conquest. William the Conqueror chose to impose his rule over the entire land by decreeing a particular set of laws throughout the kingdom, written laws common to the entire realm. This became known as the *common law*.

Each state's law had its starting point with the common law as it existed in a particular year in England (typically the date of statehood or the date of the Declaration of Independence). William the Conqueror's laws were based upon Greek and Roman antecedents. The Roman laws at the end of its empire were written down by Justinian in the sixth century. As interpreted by William the Conqueror, murder required an act causing death and a certain intent, called *malice aforethought* or *premeditation*. That terminology had a certain amount of flexibility; juries could determine within certain limitations just what constituted premeditation. However, over the centuries, this pliability was removed. Premeditation and malice aforethought were eliminated from the definition of murder and were replaced by more specific definitions and limitations. The definition of murder became solidified and specific. The various forms of homicides that were considered to involve lesser culpability were written into U.S. laws with titles such as second-degree, third-degree, voluntary manslaughter, involuntary manslaughter, and reckless homicide.

We have come a long way from the Bible's version of murder that included one form of murder and only two possible punishments, death or banishment. The path we have taken has not universally led us to fair laws, however. *Murder* is now defined as the intentional killing of a person without legal justification. Generally, this is inarguable, yet there are some problems within certain classes of homicide.

FORMS OF MURDER AND HOMICIDE

Unfortunately, lesser forms of homicide do not apply in cases associated with postpartum illness. Murder in the first degree includes all situations wherein the person acts with the intent to kill or to cause great bodily harm, and death results. Most filicides would fit into that category. Considering murder, we draw from Shakespeare: "The quality of mercy is not strained. It droppeth as the gentle rain from heaven. Upon the place beneath…. It is an attribute to God himself" (*Merchant of Venice*, Act IV, Scene 1). There is no room for "the quality of mercy" in the written law relative to postpartum illness and any resulting crimes. Manslaughter does not fit. *Manslaughter* applies to a self-defense claim with certain defects or to provocation by the victim sufficient to overwhelm reason in the average person. A claim of self-defense is an absurdity in any situation between a mother and her infant. Jurors would not agree the acts of an infant would be sufficient provocation to justify homicide.

THE DEFENSE OF MENTAL ILLNESS

Mental illness is a defense in limited circumstances in almost every state. Its acceptance has the uniformity of a pendulum, swinging back and forth following one notorious murder after another. Vastly inconsistent verdicts result from current insanity laws. The mental illness defense, or insanity defense, is usually traced back in time to the 1843 *M'Naghten* case. Before *M'Naghten*, the rule was that individuals who had no understanding or memory of what they had done, any more than a wild beast or an infant, were insane and not criminally responsible (Asokain 2016). Daniel M'Naghten was acquitted of the murder of a man whom he had mistaken for his intended target, England's Prime Minister Peel. Because this result was unpopular, the British Parliament took up the issue of defining *insanity*. As a result, the insanity defense became restricted in such a fashion that M'Naghten himself would have been found guilty.

Following *M'Naghten*, individuals were deemed insane or not criminally responsible if, due to mental illness, they either did not know what they were doing or did not know their actions were wrong. Later, the pendulum swung again as the public perceived that the M'Naghten rule was too restrictive. The American Law Institute created a Model Penal Code (MPC) that broadened the M'Naghten rule to include mental illness that resulted in a "lack of substantial capacity" to understand or control one's conduct. The MPC gained acceptance.

In 1981, John Hinckley Jr. shot President Ronald Reagan and others, including press secretary John Brady. Hinckley was bizarre and delusional, and the jury's insanity verdict was completely justifiable. However, that verdict was unpopular. Thus, the pendulum swung back from the MPC to the more restrictive M'Naghten standard. This was devastating to the application of insanity laws to postpartum mental illness, because there was no longer room for leniency. Under the MPC standard, if the illness caused the mother to lack substantial capacity to conform her conduct to the requirements of the law, the defense could be applied. The return to the M'Naghten standard of knowing right from wrong virtually eliminated the insanity defense in the postpartum context. Even in the extreme case of a command hallucination to kill, showing that a mother knew it was wrong or illegal to kill could defeat an insanity defense. In another example, obtaining a knife or potent drugs to cause death would plainly demonstrate planning to kill; this planning would diminish the chance for a successful insanity defense. In the Andrea Yates case (see Chapters 1 and 9), the successful insanity defense in her second trial required the combination of a diligent and highly talented attorney who himself garnered the necessary funding, the timely enough discovery of perjury by the prosecution's expert witness, and an experienced and talented expert witness.

The result of these more restrictive laws (M'Naghten) was evident in the 1999 case of Calandra Hulitt in Illinois. Ms. Hulitt was 6 days postpartum when she caused the death of her 2.5-year-old child. The trial attorneys could afford only one expert witness for their proposed insanity defense. That witness stated that due to the defendant's peripartum illness, she lacked substantial capacity to conform her conduct to the requirements of the law. The judge correctly noted that that standard had been eradicated after Hinckley, and therefore decided that no evidence of insanity or even of her mental state could be presented by the defendant's expert witness. Furthermore, the prosecution successfully argued that the expert could not testify because everyone knows what depression is (*People v. Hulitt* 2005, 2012).

The Harshness of Present Law

At present, according to U.S. laws, the outcome of a trial by a judge or jury who find the defendant guilty is a conviction of murder and decades in the penitentiary or a mental institution, even in the case of the most severe postpartum depression (PPD) or PPP. This is far from the likely result under either a malice aforethought standard or the MPC. It is harsh and wrong, as illustrated by the following cases.

WRONGFULNESS OF ACT

Andrea Yates faced the death penalty despite her mental illness. The State argued that she "was not insane when she killed her children… [she] knew it was a sin, knew it was legally wrong and knew society would disapprove of her actions" (Newman 2006). Yet she was obviously mentally ill. In a 2-year period, Ms. Yates had been hospitalized four times for treatment of her mental illness and for her repeated suicide attempts. Diagnosed with PPP following the birth of her fourth child, her doctor told her not to have any more children because if she birthed another child, she would likely have a psychotic break again. Nevertheless, she had another child because her religious beliefs urged having "as many children as nature would provide" (Denno 2017). Following her fifth delivery, Yates was stable until her father died 4 months after that birth. That loss precipitated her downward spiral.

Inexplicably, on June 4, 2001, her psychiatrist discontinued Yates's prescription of the antipsychotic medication Haldol. Two weeks later, she drowned her five children so they would not spend eternity in hell. Her interpretation of the Bible convinced her that hell could only be avoided by killing the children before they reached the age of responsibility. In her psychotic viewpoint, this was to protect them and save them from eternal damnation. Yet on some level, she knew it was wrong and would be disapproved of by society. The first jury concluded that because Yates knew her actions were wrong, she was guilty under the M'Naghten standard (but not the MPC).

SUICIDE VERSUS LIFE IN PRISON

In another case, Cynthia Wachenheim was an outstanding lawyer who wrote opinions for judges in New York. In 2013, she had her first child, over whom she doted and worried. Her principal worry was that her child was damaged. She believed he had seizures and other health issues and that it was her fault because she had failed to protect him from the minor falls that are commonplace for children. Wachenheim brought her child to pediatric neurologists and to his pediatrician countless times. They told her that the child was healthy and that she was just a worried first-time mother. They did not detect that she was having delusions or psychotic thinking. They reassured her that the child was not defective (Belluck 2014).

One morning, she called her husband, saying she needed his help right away. He was at his office and could not rush home. Wachenheim tried to focus on her usual task of writing; she had written many opinions and briefs with remarkable clarity and precision. Yet this day was different. Her delusional beliefs overwhelmed her. She needed to protect her son from having a miserable life due to his defects. She wrote a rambling suicide note explaining her conduct and her failure to protect her son. Believing she was saving her 10-month-old child, she strapped him to her chest and jumped from her eighth-floor window. Wachenheim landed on her back and died, but the child, who was protected by his mother's body, suffered only bruises. If the reverse had happened and the child had taken the weight of the fall, he would have died and Wachenheim would have been sentenced to decades in prison. An insanity defense would likely have failed because no signs of psychosis had been detected by Wachenheim's gynecologist or her husband or by the baby's pediatrician.

PREPARATION, NOT PERPETRATION

Heather[1] had decided to end her life. She had bipolar illness, a noted risk factor in PPP. She believed her older children could make it without her, but her younger ones would have to come with her to their deaths. No one was aware or suspicious of how deeply depressed and disturbed she was. Heather's plan was a murder-suicide, which she planned to implement by ingesting pills and having her younger children drink a fatal dose mixed with a flavored beverage. Lacking rational thought, she enlisted her friend's help to carry out the plan. Instead, her friend confiscated the pills and took Heather to a hospital. Had Heather carried out her plan, given that no evidence of insanity had been observed and prior psychotic behavior was lacking, an insanity defense would have been far more difficult than in the Yates case. Heather's decision to spare her older children would, in prosecutors' minds, have shown logical thought, premeditation, and that Heather knew murder was wrong. In short, her thinking, although not rational, would have been used to show sanity and plainly demonstrate her intent was murderous and not insane.

Heather was fortunate that she had not yet committed a crime; a charge of attempted murder requires a substantial step of perpetration, not merely preparation. She had done all of her planning, but she had not mixed the pills, thus she made no act of perpetration.

The U.S. System of Laws

The law is supposed to be reasoned and its application reasonable. Yet postpartum mental illness cases routinely result in unprincipled and unjust applications. It often comes down to fortune and timing. PPP cases that are resolved under the common law, absent modifications for filicide, are arbitrary and inconsistent. This is the opposite of the intended

---

[1]"Heather" is a pseudonym and certain details have been omitted to protect her privacy.

result of the common law, which was meant to result in consistent and equal treatment of all who are in equivalent situations. The limitations of the insanity defense are especially unsuitable for mothers with postpartum illnesses. Sentences are harsh.

Heather avoided jail because her friend's intervention was fortunate, lifesaving, timely, and well handled. She had not yet committed a *substantial step of perpetration*. Cynthia Wachenheim's fate was to die from her injuries, which ultimately protected her child from death. Had she survived instead of her son, she would likely have been convicted of murder. Timing was also a factor in Andrea Yates's fate; her conviction after her first trial was reversed by the timely discovery of the perjury.

A TRAVESTY OF JUSTICE

Another notorious case from 2014 is that of Carol Coronado of California. Coronado stabbed her three daughters, who were ages 2.5 years, 16 months, and 2 months old, respectively. As may have been expected with her history of trauma and mental illness, Coronado was at high risk for maternal mental illness and had a classic case of PPP. When police arrived, they saw a devastating scene; Coronado was naked and trying to pry open her self-inflicted stab wound with her hands. She was lying next to the bodies of her dead children, with a vacant stare. She appeared to be protecting them, huddled, with her arms around them. She was not capable of responding to police commands (Artemis Rising Foundation 2019).

The conclusion of the first psychiatrist the state hired was that Coronado was psychotic and insane at the time of the homicides. However, the prosecutor dismissed that expert and hired another. That second evaluation was more compatible with the prosecutor's desired outcome, which was that Coronado was indeed sane at the time of the stabbings. The prosecution's new expert witness held the opinion that Coronado was not psychotic at all but may have been mildly depressed at the time of the homicides. This opinion is nonsensical. She was suicidal, unresponsive, and could not recall recent events, such as phoning urgently for her mother. That is far more than mildly depressed. It is not uncommon for state expert witnesses to be selected because of their willingness to color their opinion in favor of the prosecution. Meanwhile, the prosecution treats defense experts as hired guns.

The presiding judge at trial, Ocampo, recognized the inconsistency between the testimony of the state's expert and the facts of the case. He concluded that Coronado needed mental health treatment and decreed she could receive that psychiatric treatment in prison. He assured sufficient time for that treatment by sentencing her to three consecutive life terms in the penitentiary. A law allowing three consecutive life sentences without the possibility of parole makes no sense whatsoever, but the appellate court upheld the conviction and the sentence (*People v. Coronado* 2018). The California Supreme Court refused to hear the case, allowing this injustice to stand.

I (B.M.L.) wrote to many of the people who were involved in Coronado's trial. Attached to the letter were my credentials for the inquiry: more than 40 years as a litigator, author of the cover page article "Postpartum Disorders: A New Law Offers Hope" in *The Champion* (see Lewis 2018), and a speaker on the subject of legal advocacy in perinatal mood disorders at the annual meeting of the American Psychological Association. It was not merely a general inquiry of the curious. The judge's response was kind but firm: judicial ethics meant he should not comment. We may never learn why he ruled the way he did. What we do know is that a conviction of murder and a penitentiary sentence are the norm in these cases. A few in authority act with mercy, but they are not many. This is not enough. It is the obligation of the law as a whole, throughout the nation, to show mercy and compassion.

THE NECESSITY OF CHANGING THE CRIMINAL LAW IN THE UNITED STATES

A defendant with the classic symptoms of PPP is often found guilty of first-degree murder. These cases are not the exception; they are the result of a systemic error, a fundamental failure of the U.S. judicial system to accept medical science and the plight of victims of postpartum illnesses. This failure leaves even sympathetic jurors with few options. At the conclusion of the evidence, the judge provides the jurors with written instructions that they must follow. In most states, these instructions are based on M'Naghten standards, which require jurors to find the defendant not guilty by reason of insanity (NGRI) *only if* the proof shows that the defendant, because of a severe mental illness, did not know what he or she was doing or did not know it was wrong. At trial, proof of psychosis alone does not reduce culpability. Furthermore, in most states the defense has the burden of proving insanity. Four states—Idaho, Kansas, Montana, and Utah—do not offer the insanity defense at all.

The lack of consistency across the United States is apparent in the range of results in the courthouse, from not guilty, to NGRI, to life imprisonment or even death. It is a discredit to any criminal justice system that, in identical conditions, with equivalent defendants and victims, there is such a wide disparity of outcomes. Such unpredictable variability is entirely contrary to the fundamental requirement of jurisprudence: that all who are similarly situated should receive equal treatment and similar outcomes. It is for this reason that we have judges, juries, courtrooms, and attorneys who are charged to maintain consistency and fairness. It is the mechanism whereby the law is to be equally applied to all. Yet it breaks down when dealing with certain circumstances, such as postpartum illness. As some have said, the judicial system is broken. This statement could not be more true than with respect to its dealings with maternal mental illness.

LEGISLATIVE CHANGES BEGAN IN BRITAIN IN 1922

It is imperative that the United States take a lesson from the more understanding populace in England that brought about the Infanticide Act of 1922. That Act eliminated the death penalty for mothers who committed infanticide. Even a century ago, judges and jurors in England were not interested in convicting mothers, recognizing that causes of infanticide were medical and societal. Sixteen years later, the revised and updated British Infanticide Act of 1938 further reduced the penalty for mothers who committed crimes such as filicide. It changed the offense from murder to manslaughter, which vastly reduced the defendant's sentence and even allowed the option of probation. Treatment, not punishment, was emphasized.

The expanded British Infanticide Act of 1938 was so reasoned and successful that it has spread around the globe. The number of countries with similar laws continues to grow. At last count, this included more than 30 countries. The law states (after minor revisions over the years) in its opening paragraph:

> Where a woman by any willful act or omission causes the death of her child being a child under the age of twelve months, but at the time of the act or omission the balance of her mind was disturbed by reason of her not having fully recovered from the effect of giving birth to the child or by reason of the effect of lactation consequent upon the birth of the child, then, if the circumstances were such that but for this Act the offence would have amounted to murder or manslaughter, she shall be guilty of felony, to wit of infanticide, and may for such offence be dealt with and punished as if she had been guilty of the offence of manslaughter of the child. (Infanticide Act 1938)

This infanticide law mitigates the problems of the grossly disparate treatment of persons in identical circumstances and the mistreatment of persons with a curable mental illness. Instead of having to prove insanity, the focus became whether "the balance of her mind was disturbed" by the consequences of motherhood. This emphasis can result in a favorable outcome in expert witness testimony, as discussed in other chapters. A manslaughter conviction also opens the door to treatment rather than punishment. Once the mother has recovered from the effects of her "disturbed mind," she is no longer mentally ill or a danger to her family. After recovery and under controlled and safe circumstances, the mother can integrate back into society and be reunited with her loved ones.

Treatment is also far less expensive than incarceration. Federal statistics confirm that a lifetime of incarceration for a woman of childbearing age costs in excess of $1 million (Bureau of Prisons 2018). Raising children in foster care or orphanages costs additional dollars and imposes further punitive effects on any surviving children. Exposing these children to their mother in prison facilities has another cost more difficult to ascertain; they are often already traumatized, and not letting them see their mother can lead to other serious problems that are equally difficult to determine.

It is not merely a matter of dollars and cents, although we are speaking not of dollars but of millions of dollars. This is a fundamental issue of justice and the aberration of treating identical crimes differently. It is objectionable to take two equivalent postpartum cases and have one woman institutionalized in the penitentiary for life and the other receive some form of probation or conditional release allowing for mental health treatment until cured. There is inconsistency from case to case throughout the United States.

A Groundbreaking Law in Illinois Is a Model for Change

In 2018, Public Act (PA) 100-0574 was passed in Illinois, the first postpartum criminal law in the nation. It is a reasonable and modest beginning. Although not as comprehensive as the British Infanticide Act, its modest provisions allowed for its passage. PA100-0574 has become the catalyst for more comprehensive legislation being introduced in other states. Before PA100-0574, no state had passed laws concerning crimes committed by mothers who have mental illness related to childbirth. Transformation of antiquated laws is a process; judicial change is evolving nationwide.

PA100-0574 amended the Code of Corrections to consider PPD and PPP as "mitigating factors" in sentencing when women commit crimes while experiencing these illnesses. In Illinois, as of June 1, 2018, the law allowed incarcerated women who had PPD or PPP at the time of their crime to file for resentencing under the stipulation that their postpartum illness was not previously identified, treated, or presented at the time of their trial or initial sentencing.

The postpartum infanticide law, as it is sometimes known, is a start and the first time an exception has been considered in Illinois allowing a new sentencing hearing when a valid sentence had been previously imposed. Following the passage of PA100-0574, more than 20 incarcerated women in Illinois serving long or lifetime sentences have hope for reduced sentences and possible freedom. It has been estimated that about 1,000 women are incarcerated in the United States for crimes associated with pregnancy, lactation, or delivery, most often filicide.

AN AMAZING GRASSROOTS FEAT

Particularly inspiring about the passage of the Illinois law was that only a handful of people with no advocacy training or legislative experience effected this change. Novice advocates ushered the first postpartum criminal law through the Illinois legislature, which began a movement to change perinatal criminal laws across the United States. This began with a retired assistant deputy director of the Illinois Department of Children and Family Services, Bill Ryan. Ryan spent his retirement visiting inmates throughout the state, seeking prison reform and advocating for justice. In 2017, he encouraged two incarcerated women to draft legislation for the new postpartum law. These women were best friends at Logan Correctional Facility in Lincoln, Illinois. Both had received prison sentences of natural life without parole and had been in prison for more than 30 years. One had PPP and could possibly benefit from the new law, getting a reduced sentence. The other could not benefit; she had been incarcerated due to a domestic abuse–related homicide. Ryan took the legislation's draft to the state capitol in Springfield.

THE PROCESS OF THE BILL [ILLINOIS HB 1764] BECOMING LAW

Ryan found a sponsor in Representative Linda Chapa LaVia, who formally introduced the bill in 2017. PA 100-0574, then known as HB 1764, was referred to the Rules Committee and thereafter assigned to the Judiciary-Criminal Committee in the Illinois House of Representatives. It was amended and debated until the end of March 2017 and was then set for a formal hearing and final vote in the committee. This was the first critical phase for the bill. At this point, a request was made for expert testimony in support of it. With minimal notice, I (S.B.F.) and Lita Simanis, coordinator of the Pregnancy and Postpartum Mood and Anxiety Disorder Program at Amita Health, headed to the state capitol to testify to the committee as perinatal mental health experts. After our testimony, the bill passed unanimously on March 28, 2017.

In accordance with parliamentary procedure, the bill moved to the full house for a short debate, vote, and unanimous passage on April 5, 2017. At this juncture, it gained a senate sponsor, Senator Toi Hutchinson. The next critical step was when the bill was brought up for a vote in the Senate Criminal Law Committee. At that point, the lobbyist for the State's Attorney's offices claimed the bill was unconstitutional. Barry (Lewis) became involved, and his legal background and expertise became essential. We joined forces, and with Barry's written brief and my oral testimony, the bill sailed through the senate committee and continued to gain traction. At each step we learned more about the process of advocating for the new law. Eventually HB 1764 moved through the legislative process, overcoming numerous threats and challenges. Repeatedly, impediments arose that might have put an end to the legislation had it not been for our scrutiny and resolve. Along the way, we learned the lessons of advocacy, including determination and persistence. The bill was finally signed into law by the Illinois governor in January 2018.

Since its passage, we have continued working together with the goal of helping to introduce comprehensive postpartum criminal laws in all other jurisdictions throughout the United States. Illinois was the beginning. We joined together to author *Advocating for Women with Postpartum Mental Illness: A Guide to Changing the Law and the National Climate* (Feingold and Lewis 2020), a how-to-guide for advocates and a source of useful information for legal defense teams, attorneys, judges, legislators, and anyone seeking to advocate for responsible laws. Detailed information is included about the process of changing the criminal law to assist advocates and others interested in the topic of maternal mental illness, forensics, and criminal law. PA100-0574 is a great start. More comprehensive legislation is contemplated for Illinois as well as other states. The law in Illinois has its benefits and shortcomings, some of which are described later in this chapter.

Our aim in the book was, and is, to provide essential guidance to advocates. Other state sponsors and stakeholders can use Illinois's PA100-0574 as a model. Alternatively, they can incorporate the broader, more comprehensive legislation that we, with a small group of other advocates, created in 2018 for the Commonwealth of Massachusetts. That legislation, known as HD 1736, An Act Relative to the Well-Being of New Mothers and Infants (2019), was sponsored by Representative James O'Day. We anticipate the Commonwealth of Massachusetts may be the second state to enact a postpartum criminal law. However, to date, that legislation has not become law.

THE PURPOSE AND LIMITATIONS OF PA100-0574

The law's purpose is to provide a new sentencing hearing and allow testimony of PPD or PPP to be introduced at that hearing if, for various reasons, it was not previously diagnosed, treated, or presented to the court. It recognizes postpartum mental illness (PPD or PPP) as a specific mitigating factor in all sentencing hearings and is the first criminal law in the nation to recognize the unique nature of PPD and PPP. Of great importance, it is the first criminal law in the United States to identify postpartum mental illnesses, thereby making it a model for the rest of the nation.

However, this groundbreaking law has some important limitations. First, the law does not reduce any of the state's mandatory minimum sentences, regardless of the severity of the mental illness. The minimum sentence for murder in Illinois is 20 years; for the murder of more than one person, the minimum is a life sentence without the possibility of parole. Second, it does not make it any easier to reduce a homicide from murder to something less, such as manslaughter. Third, the law does not attempt to change any of the rules regarding the defense of insanity. It neither shifts the burden of proof to the prosecution nor incorporates the more lenient insanity rules under the MPC, which were previously part of the Illinois law. It does not incorporate the British Infanticide Act's lenient requirement only that "the balance of her mind was disturbed by reason of" childbirth or lactation. Finally, and most essential, it does not incorporate conditional release or treatment programs.

Conclusion and the Future of Postpartum Criminal Laws

Our hope is that the future will bring compassion and justice to an often harsh judicial system. The overhaul of mental health laws in general is beyond the scope of this chapter. With respect to maternal mental illness, PPD, and PPP, the need for enhanced opportunities for screening, treatment, and reduced sentences is abundantly clear. Maternal mental illness is unique and temporary, and those who have it rarely, if ever, present a threat to the general public. A fundament of criminal jurisprudence is that serious long-term threats to the general public call for extended penitentiary sentences. Others do not. A temporary risk does not justify an extended sentence, especially when the option of a short-term hospitalization alleviates the problem. Maternal mental illness is beyond the woman's control, responds well to treatment, and is the actual by-product of motherhood itself.

We envision a future in which every state and every country recognizes the uniqueness of maternal mental illness and calls for specific ameliorative laws. Advocates for these laws must gain public and legislative support. The right name will help, one that engenders support from the public and legislators as well as professionals and professional organizations. Giving the law a name such as "The New Moms and Infants Well-Being Act" is far superior to calling it "The Infanticide Act" simply because the phrase "infanticide act" is provocative and carries an unfavorable suggestion, bringing attention to the crime rather than health and protection. The proposed law ideally will be comprehensive, incorporating treatment and a conditional release program and allowing for punishment less severe than that for murder. Passing postpartum legislation acknowledges the complexities of maternal mental illness, due to the neurohormonal and biological underpinnings and huge endocrine changes that take place for women surrounding childbirth. A crucial step necessitates designating different laws and less punitive sentences when crimes result from perinatal illness.

Mothers with PPP who commit crimes such as filicide within 1 year of delivery due to lack of identification and mental health treatment should not be subject to state homicide laws and severe sentences. New laws in the United States will bring hope for generations of childbearing women and families to come.

MAIN CLINICAL/LEGAL POINTS AND CULTURAL PERSPECTIVES

- Laws in the United States regarding maternal mental illness (depression and psychosis) do not acknowledge their complexities.
- Postpartum depression (PPD) and postpartum psychosis (PPP) are unique psychiatric illnesses due to the neurohormonal and biological underpinnings and huge endocrine changes that take place for women surrounding childbirth.
- Throughout history, the insane are not held responsible for their crimes.

- The defense of insanity is particularly difficult to establish in postpartum filicide cases.
- More than 30 nations have adopted some form of the British Infanticide Act of 1938, which emphasized treatment over punishment in filicide cases.
- Illinois is the only state that has a criminal law recognizing PPD and PPP and allowing mitigation in cases of filicide. Although limited in scope, it is a model for the rest of the United States.
- We envision a future in which every state and every country recognizes the uniqueness of maternal mental illness and enacts specific ameliorative laws.

Practice and Discussion Questions

1. Why should insanity be a defense to a crime?
2. If insanity should be a defense, under what circumstances?
3. Why is it difficult for women with postpartum mental illness to be treated fairly within the current criminal justice system in the United States?
4. Do you think postpartum mental illness deserves unique treatment under the law?
5. How can we encourage mental health providers, perinatal experts, and laypersons to become advocates for perinatal screening, treatment, and criminal laws in their own state legislatures?
6. What is the process of drafting legislation and getting a law passed in your home state?
7. There is a definite shortage of perinatal forensic experts able to testify in cases of filicide. How can we encourage mental health and early career professionals to become interested in the perinatal specialty area, including the application of forensics and criminal law?

References

American Psychiatric Association: Diagnostic and Statistical Manual of Mental Disorders, 5th Edition. Arlington, VA, American Psychiatric Association, 2013
An Act Relative to the Well-Being of New Mothers and Infants (Mass. HD 1736), petition, 2019
Artemis Rising Foundation: Not Carol. Directed by Harrington E, Watkin J. Malibu, CA, Planet Grande Pictures, 2019

Asokain TV: The insanity defense: related issues. Indian J Psychiatry 58(suppl):S191–S198, 2016

Belluck P: A case study in maternal mental illness.The New York Times, June 16, 2014, sec D, p 1

Bureau of Prisons: Annual determination of average cost of incarceration. Fed Regist 83(83):18863, 2018

Denno D: Andrea Yates: a continuing story about insanity, in The Insanity Defense: Multidisciplinary Views on Its History, Trends, and Controversies. Edited by White M. Santa Barbara, CA, Prager, 2017, pp 367–416

Feingold S, Lewis B: Advocating for Women With Postpartum Mental Illness: A Guide to Changing the Law and the National Climate. Lanham, MD, Rowman and Littlefield, 2020

Infanticide Act, 1938, Second Reading, House of Lords Hansard, 22 March 1938

Klier CM, Fisher J, Chandra PS, Spinelli M: Filicide research in the twenty-first century. Arch Womens Ment Health 22(1):135–137, 2018

Lewis B: Postpartum disorders: a new law offers hope. The Champion, March 2018

Mayo Clinic: Postpartum depression. MayoClinic.org, 2019. Available at: https://www.mayoclinic.org/diseases-conditions/postpartum-depression/symptoms-causes/syc-20376617. Accessed December 14, 2019.

Meyer C, Oberman M: When Mothers Kill: Interviews From Prison. New York, NYU Press, 2008

Newman M: Yates found not guilty by reason of insanity. The New York Times, July 26, 2006. Available at: https://www.nytimes.com/2006/07/26/us/26cnd-yates.html. Accessed December 17, 2019.

O'Hara MW, Swain AM: Rates and risk of postpartum depression: a meta-analysis. Int Rev Psychiatry 8:37–54, 1996

People v. Coronado, No. B269983 California Court of Appeal, 2018

People v. Hulitt, 361 Ill. App. 3d 634. (2005)

People v. Hulitt IL App (1st) 092595-U (2012)

Postpartum Support International: Postpartum psychosis. Postpartum.net, 2019. Available at: https://www.postpartum.net/learn-more/postpartum-psychosis. Accessed December 17, 2019.

Public Act 100-0574 HB 1764 Enrolled LRB100 04687 RLC 14693 b (Ill. 2018)

Smit P, de Jong R, Bijleveld C: Homicide data in Europe: definitions, sources, and statistics, in Handbook of European Homicide Research: Patterns, Explanations, and Country Studies. Edited by Liem MCA, Pridemore WA. Berlin, Germany, Springer Science+Business Media, 2012, pp 5–24

VanderKruik R, Barreix M, Chou D, et al: The global prevalence of postpartum psychosis: a systemic review. BMC Psychiatry 17(1):272, 2017

CHAPTER 4

Delineating the Meaning of *Disturbance of Mind* in Canadian Infanticide Law

Kirsten Kramar, Ph.D.

This chapter describes the history of the prosecution of women who commit maternal neonaticide and the use of the Canadian infanticide law to mitigate a conviction for murder. The interpretation and use of the infanticide offense/defense have had an uneven development in Canadian common law. Key cases illustrate the initial problems with the infanticide law that led to legislative reforms, giving rise to additional legal hurdles for addressing this issue in criminal cases. In 2016, the Supreme Court of Canada clarified the specific burden of proof required for the *mens rea* and *actus reus* elements of the infanticide law, thereby settling longstanding debates about the medicolegal aspect of the infanticide mitigation framework. Over the past 20 years, as a criminologist and academic, I have conducted research on the legislative and common-law history of the Canadian infanticide provision to inform its application by the courts in these cases. Herein, I provide an authoritative perspective on the current application of the infanticide law in the Canadian justice system, along with case exemplars, and what those involved in maternal filicide cases that meet infanticide law criteria need to know about its use and applicability in the court system. Notably, re-

Kirsten Kramar is the author of *Unwilling Mothers, Unwanted Babies: Infanticide in Canada* (2005) published by UBC Press. Her research on Canadian infanticide law has informed courts across Canada.

search underscores the underutilization of the infanticide charge in Canada, which I explore in this chapter.

History

Since its passage into law in 1948, the Canadian infanticide law has been poorly understood and unevenly applied in cases identified as maternal neonaticide. *Maternal neonaticide* is the term used in Canada when a biological mother ends the life of an infant less than 1 year of age (defined in Canada as *newly born*). The law was added to the homicide framework to assist prosecution in securing a lesser included offense that recognized the special socioeconomic circumstances of young, unmarried mothers who kill their babies at birth. Reluctant to impose the death penalty in these cases, judges and juries had been unwilling to convict these women of murder. The range of ancillary charges available to prosecutors failed to recognize that the life of an infant had been lost due to the mother's actions or omissions. The infanticide law was intended to address these issues by providing a lesser punishment framework that recognized these women's circumstances and offered a more humanitarian prosecutorial approach.

In 2016, the Supreme Court of Canada heard arguments on the elements of the infanticide offense in *R. v. Borowiec* (2016) (Table 4–1). Here the court heard an appeal from the Crown of a judgment by the Alberta Court of Appeal in which Meredith Borowiec was convicted for the lesser crime of infanticide after the discovery of a baby crying in a dumpster in 2010. Borowiec admitted giving birth to the rescued child, who survived, and later admitted to delivering two other babies in 2008 and 2009 and leaving both babies in dumpsters to die. She was charged with two counts of second-degree murder for the deaths of the deceased newborns (*R. v. Borowiec* 2016). The Crown sought to have the court articulate a new legal standard for *disturbance of the mind*, set out as one of the specific criteria for an infanticide charge, and a more restrictive medicolegal category that required proof of mental disorder or disease of the mind and that the disturbed mental state be declared as part of the *mens rea* of the offense in order to sustain a conviction on the lesser charge of infanticide (Factum of the Appellant, Attorney General of Alberta 2016).

The appellant sought to have the court introduce restrictions that would limit the use of the infanticide law by defense, arguing that "society's views have changed" and that society would be better served by a criminal law policy that allowed the courts to more harshly punish any woman who kills her children (Factum of the Appellant, Attorney

TABLE 4-1.   Summary of relevant cases

R. v. L.B. (2008, 2011)

This case involved the homicide of two babies born 4 years apart. Both deaths were ruled sudden infant death syndrome/sudden unexplained death syndrome by the coroner. The first child had been killed at 4.5 months of age when the mother was 17 years old. The second child had been killed at 10 months of age when the mother was 21 years old. The accused was charged with two counts of first-degree murder after she confessed to the killings while undergoing psychiatric treatment in a secure mental health facility. At the time, she had two living children. At trial, L.B. was acquitted of the murder charges but convicted for the lesser included offense of infanticide. The Ontario Court of Appeal dismissed the Crown's appeal. Because L.B. was a young offender at the time of the first offense, a publication ban required under the *Youth Criminal Justice Act* (2003) prevents the use of her full name. The case involved the interpretation of the *mens rea* required for infanticide. The court concluded that the onus is on the Crown to prove a "willful act or omission" and that if the *actus reus* elements of the defense are present, then an infanticide verdict is proper.

R. v. Boroweic (2015, 2016)

This case dealt with the meaning of the phrase "her mind is then disturbed" in the context of a mother who was convicted of infanticide of her newborns delivered in 2008 and 2009. Both babies were never discovered after the accused disposed of each in a dumpster after delivery. Following the discovery of a third baby found crying in a dumpster in 2010, Borowiec confessed to the earlier crimes and was charged with two counts of second-degree murder. At trial, she was acquitted of the murder charges and convicted for the lesser included offense of infanticide. The Alberta Court of Appeal dismissed the appeal, finding that the trial judge had properly applied the infanticide law in rendering the verdict. The Crown then appealed the case to the Supreme Court of Canada. In 2016, in a 7–0 decision, the Supreme Court set out a definitive statement on the necessary elements for an infanticide verdict and dismissed the Crown's appeal.

R. v. Marchello (1951)

Marchello was the first reported case after the passage of the Canadian infanticide law in 1948. The trial judge refused to allow the jury to consider a substituted verdict of infanticide because he would not allow a 4.5-month-old child to be defined as newly born. The jury acquitted the woman on account of insanity (today not criminally responsible on account of mental disorder) as a result, likely because they were unwilling to convict a woman for murder, which carried the death penalty at the time. Canadian law prohibits canvassing juries for their reasoning. Parliament would later pass an amendment to define a *newly born* child as one who had not yet had their first birthday.

TABLE 4-1. *(continued)*   Summary of relevant cases

R. v. Jacobs (1952)

Jacobs was the first reported case in which the initial charge laid was infanticide. The trial court refused to convict for infanticide because the Crown had established that the accused was acting rationally at the time of the offense (the act or omission was willful). The Crown lost its case because they had proven that the act was willful in an attempt to secure a conviction. In doing so, they failed to prove what was mistakenly understood to be the mental element of the crime: that the balance of her mind was disturbed. The trial judge misunderstood the infanticide framework, which allowed for a conviction once the Crown proved willfulness (the *mens rea* requirement for a conviction). The case led to the amendment of the *Criminal Code* infanticide framework in 1954 to add the provision entitled "no acquittal unless act or omission not willful."

R. v. Swain (1991)

A leading constitutional decision of the Supreme Court of Canada, *R. v. Swain* involved the due process rights of the mentally ill. The case dealt with a challenge to the common-law rule permitting the indeterminate detention of an accused who is found not guilty by reason of insanity. It led to the overhaul of the entire legislative scheme dealing with the mental disorder defense in Canada adopted in 1992. These amendments led to further misconceptions about the "disturbance of mind" requirement for infanticide, leading trial courts, Crown prosecutors, and defenses to believe that expert mental health testimony was required to establish a threshold *mens rea* for an infanticide verdict.

General of Alberta 2016). The Women's Legal Education Action Fund (LEAF), one of three intervenors in this case, sought to ensure that the Canadian Parliament's intention was preserved by continuing to read the infanticide law through the lens of the unique sex-based disadvantages associated with reproduction and motherhood, because these issues remain relevant today. LEAF sought to ensure that the availability of the statutory criminal law offense/defense continued to operate to promote the substantive equality of women (Factum of the Intervenor, Women's Legal and Education Action Fund Inc. 2016). In this case, the Attorney General for Ontario sought clarification from the highest court on the proper interpretation and essential elements of the *disturbed mind* element, recognizing it as "a legal concept with a medical dimension" to avoid further confusion at trial (Factum of the Intervenor, Attorney General for Ontario 2016). The Criminal Lawyers' Association of Ontario (CLA) objected to the appellant's use of the appeals process to "read new restrictions into a statutory defense in order to limit its availability" and suggested a change in societal views, arguing instead that the abolition of the infanticide law requires an act of Parliament (Factum of the Inter-venor, Criminal Trial Lawyers' Association 2016).

Section 233 of the *Criminal Code of Canada* (1985) provides a mitiga-tion framework for infanticide that has been part of the criminal law since 1948:

> A female person commits infanticide when by a willful act or omission she causes the death of her newly born child, if at the time of the act or omission she is not fully recovered from the effects of giving birth to the child and by reason thereof or of the effect of lactation consequent on the birth of the child her mind is then disturbed. (c. C-46)

In the *Criminal Code of Canada* (1985), infanticide is a form of culpable homicide, one of only two offenses that applies exclusively to women. The other offense, neglecting to obtain assistance in childbirth, is often used in conjunction with murder, concealment of birth, or infanticide charges.[1] The infanticide offense operates both alone and as a partial de-fense to murder. It requires a mother–child relationship between perpe-trator and victim, and the mental state of the mother must be disturbed as a consequence of the effects of childbirth and/or lactation. The infant must *not* be older than 12 months of age to meet the definition of a newly born child. Since its adoption into the criminal law in Canada, the mental disturbance element has formed part of the *actus reus* of the offense, *not* the *mens rea* (*R. v. Borowiec* 2016).

LEGISLATIVE HISTORY

At the time the infanticide law was added to the *Criminal Code* (1985), the penalty on a murder conviction was death.[2] The new provision was

---

[1]Section 242 of the *Criminal Code of Canada* (1985) reads:

> A female person who, being pregnant and about to be delivered, with the intent that the child shall not live or with intent to conceal the birth of the child, fails to make provision for reasonable assistance in respect of her delivery is, if the child is permanently injured as a result of the failure or dies immediately before, during or in a short time after birth, as a result of the failure, guilty of an indict-able offence and liable to imprisonment for a term of not more than five years; or an offence punishable by summary conviction (c. C-46).

[2]Capital punishment was abolished in Canada in 1976, except for certain mili-tary offenses under the *National Defence Act* (1985, c. N-5). Canada eliminated capital punishment for these military offenses in 1998 and is now a fully aboli-tionist country.

added to the homicide framework to allow for a humanitarian approach to addressing maternal neonaticide while achieving a conviction for homicide with a lesser punishment framework in cases in which women, typically young and unmarried, take the life of their unwanted babies, usually at birth. According to the Canadian minister of justice at the time, the Hon. J. L. Ilsley (1948), the law was intended to apply to

> cases where the mother kills her newborn child, and that in the normal case of that kind it is useless to lay a charge of murder against the women, because invariably juries will not bring in a verdict of guilty. They have sympathy with the mother because of the situation in which she has found herself. Therefore, crown prosecutors, and those who lay charges, if they are to obtain convictions lay charges of concealment of birth; or a charge that is equal to concealment of birth. (p. 5185)

The infanticide law provided for circumstances in which a "slightly deranged, distressed mother" (Ilsley 1948, p. 5187) could be convicted for the lesser crime of infanticide. This new law created a lesser homicide offense that recognized the socioeconomic conditions of unwanted motherhood in order to harmonize its prosecution across the Canadian provinces.

Throughout the late nineteenth and early twentieth centuries, Crown prosecutors in various provinces across Canada relied on a variety of criminal charges to address maternal neonaticide, resulting in uneven punishments and *ad hoc* outcomes. Prior to 1948, the available criminal charges were murder, concealment of birth, failure to obtain assistance at birth, and failure to provide the necessaries of life. A Canadian woman in one provincial county could be charged and convicted for murder and face a mandatory penalty of death, whereas a woman in another provincial county could be charged and convicted for concealment of birth and face no jail time whatsoever. The infanticide law was therefore viewed as a solution that would rationalize the prosecution of similar cases and provide for fairer outcomes through the even application of punishment.

EARLY MEDICOLEGAL HURDLES

The charges of concealment of birth, failure to obtain assistance in childbirth, and failure to provide the necessaries of life were often relied upon when forensic medical testimony failed to establish a live birth, as required for a homicide charge, which was exceedingly difficult to prove under the circumstances. Women who gave birth unattended often asserted that the baby had been stillborn. In my experience, proof of live birth in cases of maternal neonaticide continues to be a significant hurdle for prosecutors looking to charge murder.

Establishing a live birth at autopsy can rarely, if ever, meet the burden of proof required for a criminal conviction. Because a live birth is the threshold test for criminal legal action, autopsy results must show that the newly born child had been born alive to be considered a human being. It must be established that the infant was breathing through its own lungs alone and was not deriving any of its power of living from connection with the mother. In the absence of a witness, the test for establishing live birth was the floating lung, or hydrostatic test. However, this test was discredited as far back as the eighteenth century because of the many ways in which air can enter the lungs both during and after birth. Noted medical expert William Hunter warned against relying on this test for conviction in a 1784 article entitled "On the Uncertainty of the Signs of Death" published in *Medical Observations and Inquiries*. Hunter described the ways air could enter a stillborn baby's lungs that could raise reasonable doubt as to live birth (Lacqueur 1989). For instance, a child may breathe in utero after the amniotic membrane has been ruptured during a difficult birth; the mother may breathe air into the child's lungs in an attempt to resuscitate a stillborn infant; the "lungs may float" as a consequence of "putrefaction" (Kramar 2005; Lacqueur 1989); or a child may fail to breathe once fully born alive but only remain alive because it is attached to the mother by way of the umbilical cord. In the absence of any witnesses or visible signs of trauma on the child's body, the forensic presumption remains one of stillbirth (Kramar 2005).

Once the infanticide provision was added to the homicide framework, problems with prosecution arose almost immediately. In addition to the difficulty of determining live birth, understanding and proving beyond a reasonable doubt the connection between childbirth and/or lactation and the disturbance of the mother's mind, all of which form the *actus reus* elements of the infanticide offense, were also problematic. Unlike the English Infanticide Act of 1922 (revised in 1938), which mitigated punishment on a murder conviction, the Canadian law imported that provision as a stand-alone charge. This created the odd situation in which a mother could be *acquitted* on an originating charge of infanticide when the Crown failed to prove beyond a reasonable doubt that her mind was disturbed. Women found to be of sound mind at the time of the act or omission could be acquitted on a stand-alone charge of infanticide, although potentially guilty of murder, and would face no further prosecution or punishment. When a Crown prosecutor sought to establish disturbance of mind as part of the *mens rea* of the crime and failed, the accused would go free. Prior to 1976, there was also the additional problem of determining the age at which a child was no longer considered newly born. The original statute did not define an age limit after which a child could no longer be considered newly born.

EARLY PROSECUTORIAL CHALLENGES

Both of these problems arose in the early 1950s in *R v. Marchello* (1951) and *R. v. Jacobs* (1952) (see Table 4–1). In *Marchello*, the accused was tried for murder (in a scenario that met the requirements for an infanticide charge) and acquitted by a jury on account of insanity (Kramar 2005). The deceased infant had been 4.5 months old. Thus, the judge, McRuer, instructed the jury that they could not consider the lesser offense of infanticide because the baby was not newly born. With no legal definition of *newly born* for guidance, he determined it to mean a child that had only been very recently born and therefore did not fit the *actus reus* for a substituted infanticide verdict. McRuer's interpretation of *newly born* was strict in his identification of the age threshold. Because the charge was murder, the defense instead sought an acquittal using a plea of insanity. The jury, who was sympathetic to the mother's plight, accepted the insanity defense despite very little evidence of a mental disorder, and in doing so avoided seeing a young woman sentenced to death for murder (Kramar 2005). Juries were often unwilling to convict for murder and impose a mandatory sentence of death in these cases. Had the Crown opted to prosecute using the infanticide charge, there might well have been a conviction in *R. v. Marchello* (1951).

The following year, in *R. v. Jacobs* (1952), the Crown opted to proceed with an infanticide charge and introduced expert psychiatric testimony that Annie Jacobs had been in good mental health shortly after the birth of her baby, seeking to prove willful intent to commit murder in order to secure a conviction within the homicide framework. The Crown believed that a conviction for infanticide required proof of mental health instead of proof of a disturbed mind related to childbirth and/or lactation and thought that expert evidence of a disturbed mind would lead to acquittal (Kramar 2005, p. 107). However, the jury acquitted Jacobs on the charge of infanticide, and a murder conviction could not be sought due to prosecutorial double jeopardy.[3] If the Crown had sought to establish that Jacobs *was* suffering from a disturbance of the mind as a consequence of childbirth and/or lactation, a conviction on the lesser charge of infanti-

---

[3]The procedural defense of double jeopardy found in s. 11(h) of the *Canadian Charter of Rights and Freedoms* (1982) prevents an accused from being retried on similar charges for the same offense following an acquittal (or conviction).

cide would have been the likely outcome. Instead, the Crown sought to prove a positive (good mental health) rather than a negative (disturbed mind connected to childbirth and/or lactation) because they misunderstood the nature of the infanticide defense (Kramar 2005).

MID-TWENTIETH CENTURY CRIMINAL LAW AMENDMENTS

The issues raised in *Marchello* and *Jacobs* led the Canadian Parliament to rework and revise the infanticide framework through the *Criminal Code Amendment Act* (1953–1954), which was debated in the House of Commons in March 1954 (Kramar 2005). Section 570, no acquittal unless act or omission not willful (as it then was), came into force following the adoption of this Act. Today this provision reads as it was then adopted:

> 663. Where a female person is charged with infanticide and the evidence establishes that she caused the death of her child but does not establish that, at the time of the act or omission by which she caused the death of the child,
>
> > (a) she was not fully recovered from the effects of giving birth to the child or from the effect of lactation consequent…birth of the child, and
> > (b) the balance of her mind was, at that time, disturbed by reason of the effect of giving birth to the child or of the effect of lactation consequent …birth of the child, she may be convicted unless the evidence establishes that the act or omission was not wilful [sic]. (*Criminal Code of Canada* R.S.C. 1985, c. C-46)

The amendment was designed to capture cases in which a "slightly deranged, distressed mother" who would otherwise be guilty of murder could be found guilty and punished for infanticide, which by 1955 carried a maximum penalty of 5 years' imprisonment (Garson 1954, p. 5187). The provision removed the need to prove (or disprove) the mental element and clearly defined the *actus reus* required for a verdict of guilt for infanticide. All that is required for a conviction is that the Crown prove each of the combined *actus reus* elements outlined therein, along with the *mens rea* element: that the act or omission was willful. For a verdict of guilt for infanticide, the *actus reus* elements of the charge are determined in combination with the required *mens rea* element. Of course, if the act or omission was not willful, it would not be a crime.

The 1954 amendment effectively removed any requirement to prove a reproductive mental disorder or a disease of the mind by clearly defining the *actus reus* elements required for an infanticide charge (Garson 1954). Unlike the insanity defense or mental disorder defense, which is put forth when a person has a mental disorder that renders him or her incapable of appreciating the nature and quality of the act or knowing that it is wrong, the infanticide law requires proof of a disturbance of the mind connected to childbirth and/or lactation in order to secure a conviction on the lesser included offense. The only instance in which evidence of a mental disorder would be required would be to establish that the act or omission was not willful.

The burden of proving mental disorder is on the accused in order to be found exempt from criminal responsibility (*Criminal Code of Canada* R.S.C. 1985, c. C-46, s. 16[1][2] and [3]). Proof of a disturbance of mind consequent to childbirth and/or lactation in circumstances in which a biological mother kills her own child of younger than 12 months of age allows for a verdict of infanticide. With the passage of section 633, expert medical testimony to establish the accused's state of mind at the time of the killing effectively became irrelevant on a charge of infanticide. All that is now required for an infanticide conviction is to establish that a child's life was taken, before its first birthday, in the context of recent childbirth and/or lactation. Mental disturbance is merely read in as one element of the *actus reus* framework of the infanticide offense. Nevertheless, forensic psychiatric assessments are often conducted when women are accused of killing children older than 1 year of age; in these cases, an assessment for possible postpartum psychosis is necessary to assist with a "not criminally responsible on account of mental disorder" (NCRMD) defense.

Following a landmark decision in *R. v. Swain* (1991) (see Table 4–1), a provision was added in s. 672.11(c) of Part XX.1 of the *Criminal Code* (1985) addressing the rights of mentally ill persons in their criminal defense. This provision, which provided an assessment order in cases of infanticide, substantially confused matters for Canadian courts. Trial court judges sometimes sought assessment orders under s. 672.11(c) to establish disturbance of the mind through expert forensic medical testimony in order to sustain an infanticide conviction. Under Section 672.11(c), a court can order an assessment of the accused's mental condition if it has reason to believe that expert evidence is necessary to determine "whether the balance of the mind of the accused was disturbed at the time of the commission of the alleged offense, where the accused is a female person charged with an offense arising out of the death of her newly born child" (*Criminal Code of Canada* R.S.C. 1985, c. C-46, 1991, c. 43. S. 4; 2005, c. 22, s. 1; 2014 c. 6, s. 3).

This provision may have led to the common misunderstanding that the legal element of the infanticide provision—disturbance of the mind—formed a part of the *mens rea* of the offense and required expert psychological testimony to establish. All that is required, however, is confirmation of the sequence of events. In many cases, as long as the sequence of events was also established, any expert criminological testimony regarding socioeconomic or cultural conditions that gave rise to maternal neonaticide, thus justifying the reduced punishment framework, would have been much more in line with the Canadian Parliament's intentions when it passed the law in 1948. Courts may rely on expert medical testimony to confirm recent childbirth and/or lactation, the physiological presence of which is required to establish a disturbance of the mind.

Quantifying Maternal Neonaticide in Canada

Daly and Wilson (1988) examined the victim/perpetrator relationship in homicide data across the United States and Canada. Their research predicted the risk of fatal violence faced at birth by an infant from its biological mother to be exceedingly low. Homicide data in both countries reveal that "genetic posterities of blood relatives co-vary," or that biological parents seek to ensure their own genetic survival (Daly and Wilson 1988, p. 519). However, the rates of maternal neonaticide are much higher in young mothers (age <20 years), married or unmarried, who are genetically related to the victim (age <1 year). Accepting that parental inclinations can be shaped by genetic relationships that predict mitigation of conflict, we may also expect that maternal psychology exhibits sensitivity to residual reproductive value, thus offering an explanation for why younger mothers (who presumably have more time to reproduce) are inclined to kill newborn babies (Daly and Wilson 1988). In the case of parent/offspring conflict, evolutionary models of social motives can predict variations in the risk of violence faced by infants as a function of the age, sex, and other characteristics of the perpetrators (Daly and Wilson 1988). That is, as a mother ages, the likelihood of maternal filicide decreases. Homicide data in Canada from 1974 to 1983 examined by Daly and Wilson (1988) supported this hypothesis, as did their cross-cultural comparison of other homicide data.

Overall, biological kinship *substantially mitigates* fatal conflict. Infants raised in stepfamilies are vastly overrepresented in fatal child abuse samples "independent of risk attributable to low socioeconomic status, maternal youth, family size, or personality characteristics of the abusers" (Daly and Wilson 1988, p. 520). Regardless of whether one accepts or rejects the predictive utility of parental inclinations using the evolutionary model of social psychology framework, stepchildren "are several dozen more times likely" to be killed by a nongenetic parent (Daly and Wilson 1989, p. 463). Homicide data demonstrate that although infants may be at a higher risk in their first year of life, that risk is not from the biological mother unless she is very young (age <20 years). The infanticide law therefore addresses a very tiny subset of all homicides of children and youth.

Determining the rates of maternal neonaticide that would qualify for an infanticide charge (or verdict) is exceedingly difficult. First, homicide is a relatively rare occurrence in Canada and has been declining steadily since the early 1990s. The statistical profile of family violence in Canada allows a parsing of victimization by age group of the victim and type of motive (Burczycka et al. 2018). Relying upon the aggregate data (2007–2017) provided by the Canadian Centre for Justice Statistics, the total number of child (age <5 years) homicides motived by concealment (i.e., to hide evidence of a pregnancy or birth of a child) was 13, or 5% of total victims ages 0–17 years over that 10-year period (Burczycka et al. 2018), whereas non-family-related homicide data that combined age and motive for victims of child (age <5 years) homicide were 0 (Burczycka et al. 2018). From these data, we can infer that at least some, if not all, of the 13 homicides reported to police over that 10-year period would meet the legal requirements for an infanticide charge.

The total number of all homicides reported to police in Canada between 2007 and 2017 was 6,458 (Statistics Canada, n.d.). Therefore, taken as a fraction of all homicides reported to police, the 13 cases motivated by concealment (for which an infanticide charge or verdict is appropriate) accounted for 0.002 of the total number of reported homicides. Infanticide cases therefore made up one-fifth of 1% (or 0.2%) of all homicides reported to police in Canada between 2007 and 2017. In short, maternal neonaticide is an *exceedingly* rare crime in Canada as measured by police reports.

Of course, a small number of cases are not documented as a result of undetected disposals shortly after birth or misdiagnoses as to the infant's cause of death at autopsy. Some evidence suggests that sudden infant death syndrome (SIDS) or sudden unexplained death in infants (SUDS) may mask intentional child homicide by mothers. However, this anxiety over undetected cases has also led to an overdiagnosis of intentional homicide (suspected infanticide) as the motivating cause of death, resulting in a significant number of wrongful prosecutions and convictions of mothers and other caregivers for murder, manslaughter, and infanticide in Canada (Kramar 2005, 2006). An internal review of pediatric autopsy reports produced by Dr. Charles Smith by the Office of the Chief Coroner for Ontario found that 14 women had been wrongfully prosecuted, and some convicted, for the deaths of infants and children.

These reports were found to be wholly fraudulent and pointed the finger at young mothers and other caregivers who were later found innocent of murder (Kramar 2006).

The discovery of the fraudulent pediatric autopsy conclusions led the provincial government of Ontario to convene the Goudge Inquiry Into Pediatric Forensic Pathology in Ontario in 2007. The inquiry sought to investigate the systematic failings that took place in the coroner's service in Ontario over many years and to make recommendations to restore public confidence in pediatric forensic pathology and its use in the criminal justice system. The Ontario prosecution service had been working hand-in-glove with the provincial coroners' offices to aggressively prosecute mothers for murder, believing a significant number of undetected child homicide crimes had been masked by inaccurate pediatric forensic pathology that sometimes ruled SIDS (or SUDS) as the cause of death. Dr. Smith had provided much-needed forensic diagnoses of infanticide or shaken baby syndrome as cause of death, which allowed the police to lay murder charges and the Crown to aggressively prosecute mothers they quite illogically suspected of murdering their babies and children (Kramar 2006).

CONTEMPORARY MEDICOLEGAL CHALLENGES

The issues brought before the Supreme Court by the attorney general for Alberta in 2016 with regard to individual homicide cases had been brewing in Canada for some time. Provincial governments in both Ontario and Alberta had adopted a punitive prosecutorial approach, evidenced by the Crown's election to proceed to trial in murder cases and then file appeals when the cases resulted in verdicts of guilt for the lesser offense of infanticide. The practice of seeking to secure murder convictions in cases of maternal neonaticide and to impose the much harsher punishment framework on the accused women nevertheless continued to lead to substituted infanticide convictions by judges and juries, thereby frustrating prosecutors' attempts at securing harsher punishment. The more punitive law-and-order approaches that sought to deter infant homicide through harsh punishment were regularly thwarted by the availability of the infanticide defense.

In response, prosecutors sought to shift the disturbance of mind element of the offense into the *mens rea* category to make it more difficult for women to rely upon the infanticide defense. The prosecution sought to have the courts define *disturbance of mind* as a different and perhaps lower *mens rea* requirement standard to be established through expert psychiatric testimony. The 1954 *Criminal Code* amendment, however, was clearly intended by Parliament to ensure that women did not have to be diagnosed with a full-blown mental disorder to be convicted of infanticide. If expert testimony establishes a mental disorder, the law requires an acquittal on any criminal charge, because the act or omission would not be willful. The amendment required only that the sequence of events had occurred in order to convict on the charge of infanticide or to substitute infanticide on a charge of murder.

Two cases, one in Guelph, Ontario, and the other in Calgary, Alberta, frustrated prosecutors' attempts to secure convictions for murder and apply the harsher punishment framework. Both resulted in substituted guilty verdicts for infanticide that were upheld by the higher courts on appeal. In *R. v. L.B.* (2008, 2011) and *R. v. Borowiec* (2015, 2016) (see Table 4–1), the accused women each confessed to killing infants born prior to the discovery of their subsequent attempted homicides of newly born babies, which had each been found in dumpsters. In each case, the deaths of the previous infants had gone either undetected or had been ruled SIDS and SUDS at autopsy. L.B.[4] was initially charged by police with two counts of first-degree murder, but she was convicted on the lesser offense of infanticide. Similarly, Borowiec was initially charged by police with two counts of second-degree murder but was convicted on the lesser offense of infanticide. Each of these cases raised old questions about the contemporary validity of the underlying medicolegal assumptions related to the effects of childbirth and/or lactation on the mental state of women.

R. v. L. B.: First-Degree Murder for Two Infant Deaths

In 1998, L.B., who was 17 years old at the time, killed her 48-day-old firstborn child. Four years later, she killed her 69-day-old child. Between the deaths of these two infants, L.B. had given birth to a child who survived. The first death had been ruled SIDS, and the second death ruled SUDS. L.B. confessed to these killings while undergoing psychiatric treatment at the Homewood Health Centre in Guelph, Ontario, in 2004. By that time, she had two surviving children (*R. v. L.B.* 2008). Among other questions, the trial court considered the following: "Can there be

---

[4]Because L.B. was a young offender at the time of the first offense, a publication ban required under the *Youth Criminal Justice Act* (2003, c. 1) prevents the use of her full name.

a conviction for infanticide if murder is proven?" and "What is the degree of the mind disturbance, or departure from the norm, which is contemplated by section 233?" (*R. v. L.B.* 2008, para 14).

The Crown argued that the phrase "but does not prove murder" contained within section 662(3) of the *Criminal Code* prevents a finding of an included offense and a substituted verdict for infanticide when the Crown establishes murder beyond a reasonable doubt, as the judge did in this case (*R. v. L.B.* 2008, para 30). The Crown's position was that because they had proven first-degree murder on the basis of L.B.'s confession, no defense of infanticide was thus allowable in law, and she should be convicted of first-degree murder and sentenced to life imprisonment without the possibility of parole for 25 years. Relying upon previous case law, however, the trial court judge ruled that, under the appropriate circumstances, infanticide is a defense where the Crown establishes murder.

On the issue of the degree of disorder required for the defense of infanticide, the court found that no causal connection was required between the act or omission and the mother's mental state, but rather that a *temporal* one was required for a defense of infanticide under the law (*R. v. L.B.* 2008). It must be established by way of evidence that each of the *actus reus* elements of the infanticide law occurred at the same time. As a result, expert testimony as to any of the three identified categories of postpartum disturbances—postpartum blues, postpartum depression, and postpartum psychosis—is unnecessary for a mother to be found guilty of infanticide, even when murder is proved beyond a reasonable doubt (*R. v. L.B.* 2008).

The Canadian Parliament intentionally provided for an *actus reus* defense to murder in passing the infanticide law in 1948 as a means of recognizing the unique and rare circumstances under which a mother kills her newly born child. In these cases, a mother must possess the *mens rea* for murder yet be convicted for infanticide if the circumstances meet each of the *actus reus* elements set out in the law. The only circumstance in which an acquittal of infanticide may be found is when the act or omission is not willful. The Crown's appeal of the trial court's finding of guilt for infanticide for L.B. was later dismissed by the Alberta Court of Appeal, who affirmed the trial judge's interpretation of the proper application of the infanticide defense when he allowed a substituted verdict of guilty for infanticide (*R. v. L.B.* 2011).

The Alberta Court of Appeal confirmed that infanticide is a mitigating defense to murder because the conduct is different and less culpable than murder, justifying the lesser maximum 5-year punishment framework. The law requires that a trial judge may determine, on the balance of probabilities, whether an accused meets the criteria for infanticide in order to justify a reduced punishment under the infanticide framework (*R. v. L. B.* 2011, para 140). In this regard, expert medical testimony may be called to establish the physiological temporal elements of the legal requirements for an infanticide verdict: to determine whether at the time of the act or omission the accused was in a disturbed mental state consequent to childbirth and/or lactation. This medical evaluation may be necessary, but only for the court to establish the temporal *actus reus* element of the infanticide defense; it is wholly unconnected to the *mens rea* required to prove willfulness beyond a reasonable doubt. If expert testimony establishes that the accused had a mental disorder, then she may be acquitted on the grounds that she was NCRMD. Under those circumstances, she lacks the requisite *mens rea* required for a murder, manslaughter, or an infanticide conviction.

If the accused had a mental disorder at the time, then an acquittal is required because the act or omission was not willful and NCRMD applies. The key evidence required for an infanticide conviction is medical: if psychiatric or psychological testimony of the presence of disease of the mind (to establish NCRMD) indicates that the accused failed to appreciate the nature and quality of her act or did not know that the act was wrong, she may be acquitted on any of the verdicts available within the homicide framework. It should also be noted that in those cases in which a mother is interviewed many years after an alleged homicide, she may be prone to retrospectively *underestimate* the extent of her own mental distress at the time of the death of the child. This could result in an unsafe verdict of infanticide rather than an acquittal on the grounds of NCRMD, if appropriate in the circumstances. Interviewing the defendant's friends and family as to their observations of her mental state at the time of the child's death becomes rather more important. All that is required is for the court to establish that the accused mother had recently given birth and/or was lactating and that the child's death occurred prior to its first birthday. Causing the child's death is evidence of a disturbed mind consequent to childbirth and/or lactation and therefore forms part of the overall mitigating external elements recognized in Canadian law.

These external elements of the infanticide offense establish the statutorily defined context for this type of homicide as the legal definition of infanticide in Canadian law. The Crown must then also prove the criminal act to be both conscious and voluntary. Because many cases of maternal neonaticide involve confessions of guilt, maternal mental health expert testimony is rarely needed in Canada in order to establish *mens rea*; the confession alone establishes the blameworthy state of mind (willful act or omission).

R. v. Borowiec: Second-Degree Murder for Two Infant Deaths

Between 2008 and 2010, Meredith Borowiec,[5] then 26–29 years of age, gave birth at home without assistance three times while living alone. After each delivery, she placed the newborns in a garbage bags and disposed of them in a dumpster near her apartment. The third baby was found alive (Factum of the Appellant, Attorney General of Alberta 2016). Upon being interviewed by police after discovery of the third child, Borowiec admitted to the live births and disposal of the previous two babies as well as the third. She was then charged with two counts of second-degree murder for the first two newborns. At trial, the Crown relied on expert medical opinion evidence under section 672.11(c) of the *Criminal Code* (1985, c. C-46) to disprove infanticide by establishing that at the time of the act or omission her mind was not disturbed. They sought to secure convictions for second-degree murder (Factum of the Appellant, Attorney General of Alberta 2016)—in other words, to establish that the accused did not have a mental disorder at the time and thus the act was willful. Such a conviction would fall under the harsher punishment framework for second-degree murder.

In the opinion of the court-appointed expert, Dr. Hashman, the accused had not had a mental disorder at the time she abandoned her three newborns in the dumpster (Factum of the Appellant, Attorney General of Alberta 2016); rather, in his opinion, Borowiec was concerned about her ability to cope, feared losing her boyfriend, and felt unprepared for motherhood (Factum of the Appellant, Attorney General of Alberta 2016). Expert testimony by Dr. Smith, retained by the defense, confirmed pregnancy denial as a coping mechanism that led to dissociative symptoms and depersonalization in the aftermath of giving birth to an unwanted child (Factum of the Appellant, Attorney General of Alberta 2016). Dr. Smith was of the opinion that the accused's mind had been disturbed at the time of the acts as a result of her pregnancy denial and that the births had produced high levels of panic and anxiety, which led the accused to dispose of the infants in the dumpster (Factum of the Appellant, Attorney General of Alberta 2016).

---

[5]This case was subject to a publication ban until 2016 when the case was heard by the Supreme Court of Canada. The accused's name appears here because that ban was lifted.

During a psychiatric assessment in 2012, Borowiec revealed that she was pregnant with her fourth child, which she delivered while in custody (Factum of the Appellant, Attorney General of Alberta 2016). The case illustrated what had been a longstanding practice in these cases: prosecutors and defense both sought to prove (or disprove) greater or lesser degrees of mental disorder to secure their desired outcomes. Prosecutors used expert psychiatric testimony to disprove mental disorder (the wrong standard), whereas defense attorneys attempted to prove some form of mental disturbance that did not rise to the level of mental disorder. In this case and others like it, all that is required according to the Canadian infanticide provisions is for the defense to establish the successive *actus reus* elements of infanticide law and connect them to the death of the newly born child.

At trial, the judge found that Borowiec's confession was reliable in describing each of the three circumstances such that she had willfully caused, or intended to cause, the death of her newborn children (Factum of the Appellant, Attorney General of Alberta 2016). Furthermore, on the issue of whether the Crown had disproven infanticide, the judge found that Dr. Hashman erred when he equated a mental disorder with the lower standard of disturbance of mind and that he had used the wrong test for infanticide. In finding that the balance of Borowiec's mind was not disturbed (to disprove mental disorder for the NCRMD defense), the trial judge noted that a verdict of infanticide did not require evidence of acute mental disturbance, mental disorder, or significant mental illness (Factum of the Appellant, Attorney General of Alberta 2016). Here the trial judge recognized and properly understood the intention of the Canadian Parliament in passing the law and its amendments and creating the infanticide offense/defense to murder.

On appeal, the attorney general for Alberta sought a new trial on the two counts of second-degree murder, but the appellant court dismissed the application, affirming that the trial judge had correctly interpreted the expert testimony when convicting for two counts of infanticide (*R. v. Borowiec* 2015). The majority found that the *actus reus* elements of the infanticide defense had been made out at trial, justifying the substituted verdict for infanticide on both counts of murder. They also affirmed the reasoning of the lower court trial judge (and the defense) that the Crown had sought to set the bar too high for establishing a disturbance of the mind for an infanticide verdict (*R. v. Borowiec* 2015).

However, Justice Wakeling dissented on the question of the legal standard used to evaluate expert testimony, arguing that there was a dearth of guidance on what "disturbed" means in law (Factum of the Appellant, Attorney General of Alberta 2016). Wakeling concluded that an infanticide defense requires that the mother's "psychological health must be substantially compromised so that it can be classified as an abnormal mental health state" arising as a result of childbirth and the new responsibilities of motherhood (*R. v. Borowiec* 2015, para 150). In his view, "Parliament would not have reduced the consequences for the commission of a serious crime committed in the context of a minor diminution of the mother's psychological health" (*R. v. Borowiec* 2015, para 150). Furthermore, Wakeling rejected the notion that "baby blues" met the standard for a "disturbed mind," given that this mild form of depression experienced by many women during the postpartum period was a normal occurrence and would therefore not meet the standard required for an infanticide verdict.

In an effort to reframe the definition of *disturbed mind* as *postpartum psychosis*, Wakeling relied on the DSM-IV (American Psychiatric Association 1994) definition of infanticide:

> Infanticide is most often associated with postpartum psychotic episodes that are characterized by command hallucinations to kill the infant or delusions that the infant is possessed, but it can also occur in severe postpartum mood episodes without such specific delusions or hallucinations. (p. 386)

Wakeling noted "a mother with postpartum psychosis certainly would" meet the test because she would be "grossly impaired in [her] ability to function, usually because of hallucinations or delusions" (*R. v. Borowiec* 2015, para 153). Finally, he concluded that women experiencing "a more severe form of postpartum depression than the baby blues but less debilitating than a psychotic state" may also meet the test for a disturbed mind (para 154).

The majority of the Alberta Court of Appeal rejected this reasoning, finding instead that "one aim of Parliament was to let the Crown get a conviction for something in such cases" because "[m]urder has always had a very high minimum sentence" and "few juries and likely not a large number of trial judges (if there is no jury) are very willing to convict such new mothers of murder or even manslaughter" (*R. v. Borowiec* 2015, para 32). They concluded that "[m]aking it hard to convict of infanticide would simply produce more outright acquittals, either directly or via fewer charges of infanticides. That result would be as paradoxical as the pre-1948 situations and following much the same route" (para 89).

The attorney general for Alberta relied upon the reasoning given in the dissent in its appeal to the Supreme Court of Canada. The Crown sought the higher court's direction on the mental element standard required for a conviction as well as a declaration that the infanticide law was based on outdated social policy with respect to the conditions affecting women during pregnancy, childbirth, and childrearing and that Parliament's original intent in creating the mitigating framework for the infanticide defense was no longer apposite. The Crown sought to have the Supreme Court of Canada create a new *psychological* standard for disturbance of mind and replace the common-law test that looked to the circumstances of these cases to draw a connection between childbirth and/or lactation and the mother's mental state at the time of the offense. In essence, the Crown sought to have the highest court in Canada effectively rewrite the law and undermine Parliament's intent in creating the infanticide framework.

INFANTICIDE LAW RECOGNIZES SUBSTANTIVE EQUALITY

The Supreme Court of Canada agreed to hear the appeal from the attorney general and authorized intervenor arguments from the Women's LEAF, the Attorney General for Ontario, the Criminal Lawyers' Association for Ontario, and the respondent, Borowiec. LEAF argued that Parliament's intent "[i]n defining the class of cases to which the new mitigating framework of infanticide would be available…[was] to adopt the concept of disturbance of the mind" to create a non-medical category distinguished from the rigorous requirements for an insanity defense (Factum of the Intervenor, Women's Legal and Education Action Fund Inc. 2016, para 7). LEAF pointed out that "the concerns that motivated legislators in creating the mitigating framework of infanticide were not medical" (para 8). Rather, in adopting the mitigation framework of infanticide, Parliament "[chose] to recognize the unique stressors accompanying the reproductive and caregiving roles ascribed to women" and that these "remain pressing social concerns" (paras 8 and 9). LEAF argued further that the mental disturbance contemplated by section 233 of the *Criminal Code* was intended to recognize that

> Women continue to disproportionately experience the negative effects of continuing inequality in relation to childbirth and child-rearing. Social, economic, cultural, psychological and biological factors intersect to cause some mothers of newly born children to experience a disturbance of the mind. Single mothers still experience discrimination and social stigma related to family status. Women continue to be disproportionately responsible for the care of young children. Access to safe abortions, birth control and adequate health care is by no means a guarantee, particularly for impoverished women and those in remote areas. (Factum

of the Intervenor, Women's Legal and Education Action Fund Inc. 2016, para 9)

The Supreme Court of Canada agreed with this analysis. In its unanimous 7–0 decision, the Court determined that the intent of the Canadian Parliament was to draw a conceptual distinction between a disturbed mind that is "different from a 'mental disorder,'" and "different from non-insane automatism" (*R. v. Borowiec* 2016, para 23). Accordingly, the Court stated:

> From this we may infer that the disturbance addressed in the infanticide provisions need not reach the level required to provide a defence under s. 16 of the *Criminal Code*, that is, to be the result of a mental disorder (which is defined as a "disease of the mind" under s. 2 of the *Criminal Code*) that renders the accused incapable of appreciating the nature and quality of the act or omission or of knowing that it was wrong. We can also infer that the disturbance aspect of the infanticide need not rend the accused's acts or omissions involuntary as is required for automatism. (para 24)

The Court went on to note that "Canadian jurisprudence establishes that there is a 'very low' or 'fairly low' threshold for a finding of mental disturbance and that it does not require evidence that the accused has a mental disorder" (para 34). The Supreme Court thus rejected "the conclusion from the dissenting judge in the Alberta Court of Appeal decision that Parliament intended to restrict the concept of a disturbed mind to those who have 'a substantial psychological problem'" (para 35). The Supreme Court then provided a definition for the phrase "mind is then disturbed" as found in the text of the infanticide law:

> Rather, I conclude that the phrase "mind is then disturbed" should be applied as follows:
> (a) The word "disturbed" is not a legal or medical term of art, but should be applied in its grammatical and ordinary sense.
> (b) In the context of whether a mind is disturbed, the term can mean "mentally agitated," "mentally unstable" or "mental discomposure."
> (c) The disturbance need not constitute a defined mental or psychological condition or mental illness. It need not constitute a mental disorder under s. 16 of the *Criminal Code* or amount to a significant impairment of the accused's reasoning faculties.
> (d) The disturbance must be present at the time of the act or omission causing the newly born child's death and the act or omission must occur at a time when the accused is not fully recovered from the effects of giving birth or lactation.

(e) There is no requirement to prove that the act or omission was caused by the disturbance. The disturbance is part of the *actus reus* of infanticide, not the *mens rea*.

(f) The disturbance must be "by reason of" the fact that the accused was not fully recovered from the effects of giving birth or from the effect of lactation consequent on the birth of the child. (para 35)

On these grounds, the Supreme Court of Canada dismissed the Crown's appeal, upheld the substituted conviction for infanticide, and provided considerable clarity on the meaning of *disturbance of mind*.

LEGAL DISTINCTION BETWEEN A MENTAL DISORDER AND A DISTURBANCE OF MIND

Maternal mental health experts will note that assessment as to whether the accused has a mental disorder is not required in these cases. Arguments as to the nature and extent of mental disorder confuse the legal issues under consideration in these cases. The decision of the Supreme Court of Canada makes it clear that a disturbance of mind is not a mental or psychological condition to be assessed and that the act or omission need not have been *caused* by the mental disturbance itself. All that is required for an infanticide defense is to establish that the disturbance is connected to childbirth and/or lactation consequent to the birth of the child who lost its life. This has always been the legal standard required in Canada since the time of the infanticide law's inclusion in the *Criminal Code* in 1948. The Court also affirmed the principle of substantive equality as the lens through which Canadian law should be interpreted when considering criminal law defenses such as infanticide.

The purpose of s. 233 was to recognize the range of medical, social, and economic factors that may arise in the context of childbirth and/or lactation. The provision requires proof of a connection between childbirth and/or lactation and a mental disturbance but does not require proof of a causal link between the mental disturbance and the act that causes the death of the biological child (*R. v. Borowiec* 2015). The infanticide offense/defense is intended to allow for a lesser punishment framework to be applied in these exceedingly rare cases by recognizing the social inequalities that *some* women continue to experience in the context of reproduction and mothering. The statutory language in s. 233 thus recognizes the complex interaction of a diverse array of factors (social, economic, psychological, biological, and cultural) that play a role in justifiably mitigating punishment in these rare cases.

Concluding Comments

Critics of the infanticide defense are concerned about the differential treatment that women receive from these laws in the context of a constitutional framework guaranteeing equal treatment of the sexes (Anand 2010). The availability of the infanticide defense for women who kill a newly born child challenges some interpretations of equality before the law (formal equality) but fails to account for reproductive differences, the exceedingly rare occurrence of maternal neonaticide, and the circumstances in which women commit the act (substantive equality).

Some Canadian prosecutors nevertheless assert that the infanticide law allows a mitigated punishment framework for a crime that amounts to 9 months' premeditated murder (in the context of pregnancy denial) and thus allows women to get away with the most heinous form of culpable homicide. The Supreme Court of Canada has put this unfounded argument to rest now that it has provided a clear articulation of the legal meaning of "mind is then disturbed," placing it firmly within the *actus reus* for an infanticide verdict.

MAIN CLINICAL/LEGAL POINTS AND CULTURAL PERSPECTIVES

- An accused has the benefit of the infanticide law only when
    - The Crown can prove the infant was born alive via accurate forensic pathology that is subject to verification by an independent third-party expert. Faulty forensic conclusions based on substandard pediatric autopsy procedures and inferences have produced numerous unsafe convictions in Canada.
    - The baby is the biological child of the mother. Only the biological mother of the deceased child can be charged with the crime of infanticide or have the benefit of a substituted verdict for infanticide when murder is made out at trial.
    - Evidence shows that, at the time of the alleged killing, the mother had recently given birth or was experiencing the effects of childbirth and, as a consequence, her mind was disturbed. These elements are together the *actus reus* elements of the infanticide law.

- The Crown must *disprove* the *actus reus* elements of the crime and prove that the act or omission was willful (*mens rea*).
- A *newly born* baby is defined as a child who is 12 months of age or younger.
- The term *disturbed mind* is not a legal or medical term of art but must be used in its grammatical or ordinary sense:

    1. The mental disturbance need not be a preexisting mental or psychological condition or a mental illness.

    2. The mental *actus reus* element need not amount to a significant impairment of the accused's capacity for reasoning.

    3. The disturbance along with recent childbirth and/or lactation must be present at the time of the act or omission that caused the newly born child's death.

    4. At the time of the act or omission, the accused is not fully recovered from the effects of childbirth and/or lactation.

    5. There is no requirement to prove that the act or omission was caused by the mental disturbance. The mental element forms part of the *actus reus* of infanticide, not the *mens rea*.

    6. The disturbance must be "by reason of" the fact that the accused was not fully recovered from the effects of childbirth and/or lactation.

    7. The Crown must prove the *mens rea* element as they would with any other crime and disprove the *actus reus* elements for a verdict of guilt.

    8. A judge (or jury) is only required to determine, on a balance of probabilities, whether an accused meets the criteria for an infanticide verdict once willful murder is proven beyond a reasonable doubt.

Practice and Discussion Questions

1. What distinguishes the mental element in Canadian infanticide law from a preexisting psychological impairment or mental disorder?
2. What connection must be made between childbirth and/or lactation and disturbance of mind to sustain a verdict of guilt for infanticide?

3. Where does the disturbance of mind requirement stand in relation to the *mens rea* and *actus reus* of the infanticide framework?
4. Is an assessment under s. 16 of the *Criminal Code* required for an infanticide verdict?
5. As a forensic expert witness in Canada, what do you see or not see as your role in maternal infanticide (maternal neonaticide) cases?

References

American Psychiatric Association: Diagnostic and Statistical Manual of Mental Disorders, 4th Edition. Washington, DC, American Psychiatric Association, 1994

Anand S: Rationalizing infanticide: a medico-legal assessment of the Criminal Code's child homicide offence. Alberta Law Review 47(3):705–728, 2010

Burczycka M, Conroy S, Savage L: Family violence in Canada: a statistical profile, 2017. Juristat, December 5, 2018

Canadian Charter of Rights and Freedoms, Part I of the Constitution Act, 1982, being Schedule B to the Canada Act 1982 (UK), 1982, c 11

Criminal Code of Canada, R.S.C. 1985, c C-46

Daly M, Wilson M: Evolutionary social psychology and family homicide. Science 242:519–524, 1988

Daly M, Wilson M: Response: evolution and family homicide. Science 243:463–464, 1989

Factum of the Appellant, Attorney General for Alberta (R. v Borowiec, S.C.C. 11), 2016. Available at: https://www.scc-csc.ca/WebDocuments-DocumentsWeb/36585/FM010_Appellant_Her-Majesty-the-Queen.pdf. Accessed February 2020.

Factum of the Intervenor, Attorney General for Ontario (R. v. M.K.B. , S.C.C. 11), 2016. Available at: https://www.scc-csc.ca/WebDocuments-DocumentsWeb/36585/FM050_Intervener_Attorney-General-of-Ontario.pdf. Accessed February 2020.

Factum of the Intervenor, Criminal Lawyers' Association of Ontario (R. v Borowiec, S.C.C. 11), 2016. Available at: https://www.scc-csc.ca/WebDocuments-DocumentsWeb/36585/FM030_Intervener_Criminal-Lawyers-Association-Ontario.pdf. Accessed February 2020.

Factum of the Intervenor, Women's Legal and Education Action Fund Inc. (R. v Borowiec, S.C.C. 11), 2016. Available at: https://www.scc-csc.ca/WebDocuments-DocumentsWeb/36585/FM040_Intervener_Womens-Legal-Education-Action-Fund.pdf. Accessed February 2020.

Garson S: Criminal Code: Revision and amendment of existing statute. Canada. House of Commons. 22nd Parliament, 1st session. Vol 3, February 24, 1954. Available at: http://parl.canadiana.ca/view/oop.debates_HOC2201_03/252?r=0ands=1. Accessed February 2020.

Ilsley J: Criminal Code: Amendments with respect to defamatory libel, culpable homicide et cetera. Canada. House of Commons. 20th Parliament, 4th session, Vol 5, June 14, 1948. Available at: http://parl.canadiana.ca/view/oop.debates_HOC2004_05/1003?r=0ands=1. Accessed February 2020.

Kramar K: Unwilling Mothers, Unwanted Babies: Infanticide in Canada. Vancouver, BC, UBC Press, 2005

Kramar K: Coroner's interested advocacy: understanding wrongful convictions and accusations. Canadian Journal of Criminology and Criminal Justice 48:803–822, 2006

Lacqueur T: Bodies, details, and the humanitarian narrative, in The New Cultural History. Edited by Hunt L. Berkeley, CA, University of California Press, 1989

National Defence Act, R.S.C. 1985, c. N-5

R. v. Borowiec, A.B.C.A. 232 (2015)

R. v. Borowiec, S.C.C. 11 (2016)

R. v. Jacobs, 105 C.C.C. 291 (1952)

R. v. L.B., 2008 CanLII 45550 (ON SC)

R. v. L.B., 2011 ONCA 153 (CanLII)

R. v. Marchello, 100 C.C.C. 137 (1951)

R. v. Swain, 1 S.C.R. 993 (1991)

Statistics Canada: Number, rate and percentage changes in rates of homicide victims (Table 35-10-0068-01), n.d. Available at: https://doi.org/10.25318/3510006801-eng. Accessed February 2020.

Youth Criminal Justice Act, S.C. 2003, c 1

CHAPTER 5

Fathers and Filicide

MENTAL ILLNESS AND OUTCOMES

Susan Hatters Friedman, M.D., DFAPA

In this chapter, the research literature regarding paternal filicide is reviewed and compared with what is known about maternal filicide and neonaticide. Unlike other types of murder of which men are much more commonly the perpetrator than women, only approximately half of filicides are committed by fathers. However, much less is known about fathers who kill than about their counterpart mothers. In fact, most extant research literature focuses on maternal perpetrators. A chapter elucidating paternal filicide in a book about maternal mental health forensics may seem out of place, but it is imperative to understand the experiences of fathers and recognize that they too may commit filicide due to mental illness and deserve fair treatment. This chapter highlights similarities and differences between maternal and paternal filicide and explores suicide risk, gender disparities, legal outcomes for paternal filicide cases, and prevention strategies. Increasing one's breadth of knowledge in maternal filicide involves recognizing and understanding paternal filicide.

As a maternal mental health and forensic psychiatrist who researches filicide, I have evaluated perpetrators (both mothers and fathers) for courts, in forensic hospitals, and in correctional facilities both in the United States and in New Zealand. Through this work, I see firsthand the need for caution regarding gender bias in the examination of filicide cases, partially because of societal norms and assumptions about culpability. Mothers and fathers should be considered with similar compassion when an underlying mental health issue was active during the filicide. Emerging research about paternal postnatal depression and stress can help us further conceptualize the mental state of some fathers. Furthermore, understanding the characteristics of fathers who kill their children can help us target preventive efforts, including providing support to decrease parenting and family stress and improving early identification of paternal mental illness.

Societal Perceptions of Fathers Compared With Mothers Who Kill

Women are societally constructed as the nurturer, yet when women are violent, it happens most commonly within the home. Society tends to view those who perpetrate filicide as evil, with few exceptions. Men are more violent in the general population than women. The vast majority of murders—other than child murder—are perpetrated by men. Filicide is unique in that mothers and fathers commit filicide at similar rates, but fathers who kill are almost always considered "monsters."

Maternal and Paternal Filicide in the Media

Wiest and Duffy (2013) noted that although mothers and fathers kill children at similar rates, it is the maternal filicide cases that usually lead to more media coverage and community outrage. Kaladelfos (2013) noted that the violent acts of fathers, in comparison to mothers, appear to occur in light of different social pressures. Easteal et al. (2015) found that mothers who killed their children were framed in media stories as having either innate *bad*-ness or psychiatric (mad or sad) reasons rather than considered within a wider societal context and the individual situation.

Easteal et al. (2015) echoed Wiest and Duffy (2013) by noting that "female killers' degree of femininity has been found to correlate with how they are portrayed in the media, which may affect charging, prosecution, and sentencing" (Easteal et al. 2015, p. 38). Collosso and Buchanan (2018) identified that mothers who killed their children were much more likely to be featured in national American media than fathers who killed. Likewise, name recognition surveys among college students revealed that maternal filicide perpetrators' names were recognized much more often than paternal perpetrators.

Other studies reveal additional bias in media reporting, such as Israeli news reports that emphasized the mental illness of Jewish married mothers who committed filicide but did not do so for ethnic minority women or for women who did not fulfill their traditional roles (e.g., unmarried or young women) (Cavaglion 2008, 2009). Cavaglion (2008, 2009) noted that among fathers who killed, the press described paternal filicides as rationally motivated and premeditated and did not include descriptions of mental health or social distress. Cavaglion also stated that "there was a process of oversimplification and polarisation that emphasised the fathers' negative traits and actions, and mitigated the positive ones" (Cavaglion 2009, p. 131). Rather than portraying events of paternal filicide ambiguously, and rather than considering the diversity of contexts, filicides in media narratives were "reduced as much as possible to a common denominator" (p. 131) and "an atrocity" (p. 132). Finally, Cavaglion noted, "the portrayal of men who kill [their children] usually adheres to traditional, stereotypical roles of masculinity. Among fathers, there is more room for will, intention, volition, and rationality ....They have more space for both decision making and for rage and anger" (p. 139). These studies indicate that fathers, and certain groups of mothers, are portrayed more harshly in the media after a filicide.

Paternal Depression in Pregnancy and the Postpartum

Similar to new mothers, new fathers may experience biological stress and hormonal changes that increase their risk of depression (Underwood et al. 2017). A meta-analysis (Cameron et al. 2016) considered studies of paternal depression throughout pregnancy and the first year postpartum. Of 74 studies published between 1980 and 2015 with more than 40,000 participants, the meta-estimate was that paternal depression occurred in 8.4% of the population (95% CI 7.2%–9.6%). Studies differed regarding whether the mother was also depressed. When studies differed on the rates of paternal depression, it may have been due to differences in the year, location, or culture or in how depression was measured.

Paulson et al. (2016) noted that each article in a meta-analysis that considered the correlation of paternal and maternal depression found that increased depressive symptoms in one partner were significantly associated with increased depression in the other partner. Another review (Edward et al. 2015) found that depression in fathers in the postpartum period was associated with a personal history of depression and with depression in their partner (the mother) during pregnancy or soon after delivery. However, Cameron et al. (2016) found that the prevalence of paternal depression was not conditional on previous history of paternal depression, paternal age or education, or timing. Further studies may aid in understanding the complex interactions of variables regarding postpartum depression in fathers.

In the Growing Up in New Zealand study, Underwood et al. (2017) found that *antenatal* paternal depression symptoms were present in 2% of fathers and associated with perceived stress levels and decreased physical health during their partner's pregnancy. They also identified that *postpartum* paternal depression symptoms affected 4% of fathers and were associated with stress during the pregnancy, the ending of the relationship with the mother, health issues, unemployment, and a personal history of depression. Additional postpartum paternal depression risk factors may include lower income, maternal depression, and marital conflict, as well as lack of social support (Underwood et al. 2017). Paternal depression was experienced by fathers across various ethnicities and educational backgrounds.

Examining the relationship of sex hormones to postpartum depression, Saxbe et al. (2017) found that testosterone levels in new fathers may be related to both paternal and maternal depression. Specifically, higher levels of paternal testosterone potentially protected fathers from developing postpartum depression but were related to elevated maternal distress. Fathers with lower testosterone levels, on the other hand, reported more depressive symptoms. However, high testosterone may be related to other risks to the family, such as fathering stress and intimate partner aggression (Saxbe et al. 2017).

PATERNAL FILICIDE

As discussed, most of the literature about child murder has focused on maternal filicide. More than a decade ago, West et al. (2009) analyzed the extant international literature regarding fathers who killed their children, which included 12 studies. West and colleagues found that fathers who ended the lives of their children had an average age in their thirties, and the average age of their victims was 5 years. Fathers sometimes had multiple victims and tended to kill sons and daughters in equal numbers. The methods utilized often included wounding violence, such as stabbing, shooting, and beating. Fathers often also committed suicide at the time of the filicide.

West et al. (2009) noted that although mental illness was identified in some fathers, the fathers often did not seek help for psychiatric symptoms prior to the filicide. They were often either unemployed or working in low-paying jobs. Approximately one-third were separated from their partners. The authors noted that some had experienced significant stressors in their own childhoods and seemed to have difficulties building their own support systems. They also noted that approximately one-fifth of the child homicides committed by fathers involved the killing of infants. West et al. (2009) explained that "this may be related to the stress of being a new parent" (p. 466). However, as opposed to mothers, paternal neonaticide (murder in the first day of life by the father) was quite rare, which is consistent with other findings that neonaticide is almost always perpetrated by a mother acting alone (Hunter et al. 2019; Kauppi et al. 2010).

MOTIVES FOR CHILD MURDER BY FATHERS

Fathers have been found to commit filicides for the same five motives as mothers, previously defined by Resnick (1969) and further described in Friedman and Resnick (2007): *altruistic, acutely psychotic, unwanted child, fatal maltreatment* (previously known as *accidental*), and *partner revenge* (described more fully in Chapters 9 and 11). West et al. (2009) noted that the precipitants for paternal filicide included fatal maltreatment; factors related to mental illness, including severe depression or acute psychosis; and revenge against a partner. Fathers may also have *extended suicide* cases in which they kill their children and themselves with altruistic motives. Lastly, fathers are more likely to kill their partner (the mother) at the same time as the children and themselves, known as *uxoricide*; whereas mothers are unlikely to commit *mariticide* (killing their partner, the father) when committing filicide-suicide.

Regarding motive, Liem and Koenraadt (2008) reviewed forensic psychiatric records in the Netherlands. They determined that "accidental" filicides and retaliating filicides were most commonly committed by fathers, whereas "pathological" filicide and neonaticide were perpetrated by mothers. These researchers noted that for some fathers, "the primary target is his (estranged) spouse, and the children only pawns in this process" (p. 172). Regarding their filicidal act, Putkonen et al. (2011) reported that in Austria and Finland, fathers tended to be more impulsive than mothers. In Canada, Dawson (2015) noted "the likelihood that fathers are more likely to be motivated by jealousy, revenge, or retaliation" (p. 170). A small Australian study of five mothers and nine fathers found that fathers were more likely to perpetrate an "accidental" filicide (Eriksson et al. 2014).

Although multiple studies in the past decade have reported demographic characteristics of fathers who committed filicide, determining the motive requires more in-depth examination. Researchers assigning motives are not blinded to the gender of the parent who killed, and thus gender bias may still be an issue. In other words, gender bias may be so entrenched that the lens through which these cases are examined impacts the assignment of intent and motive for the filicide.

RECENT ILLUSTRATIVE CASES IN THE MEDIA

A 38-year-old father stabbed his 5-year-old son to death in Sydney, Australia. He had a lengthy history of schizophrenia, was acutely psychotic, and believed that he could "save the world" by killing his son. He was adjudicated not criminally responsible (insane) (McKinnell 2019). In another case, in Canada, a father killed his three children, ages 5, 8, and 10, as they slept. He was psychotic at the time and was found not criminally responsible due to his mental illness (Omand 2017). Although fatal maltreatment may be a more common motive overall for child murder than is a psychotic motive (Friedman and Resnick 2007), fathers as well as mothers may be psychotic at the time of the killing and may have altruistic motives.

Other cases involve filicide-suicide, such as in Montreal, Canada, where a 40-year-old father violently took the lives of his two children, ages 5 and 7, and then his own (Henriques 2019). As discussed, paternal filicide-suicide is more common than maternal filicide-suicide. However, less detail is available after a filicide-suicide because the perpetrating parent cannot be interviewed, as they could be after a filicide alone. These cases appear to quickly fade from the media; there is no trial because both victim and perpetrator are deceased.

Another Australian father, age 24, was referred to as the "Facebook killer" after posting online that he was going to kill his 2-year-old daughter. He called her mother and asked if she had any last words for her daughter. He was intoxicated at the time of the killing and had been separated for most of the toddler's life after a volatile relationship. He also posted on Facebook that this was payback to her mother. The father was diagnosed with a personality disorder with borderline, antisocial, and narcissistic traits. The judge described that he killed out of revenge against the girl's mother (Lambert 2015).

A father in Texas was executed 17 years after the murder of his two daughters, ages 6 and 9. He was an accountant who had been on probation for intimate partner violence and had been in violation at the time. He shot the girls while their mother was listening on the phone. Years later, on death row, he used the prison library to research competency and also discussed how to avoid execution, such as by having a mental illness. However, courts found that he was malingering mental illness to avoid being executed (Tsiaperas 2018).

Media coverage from the second Australian case and the Texas case suggested motives of partner revenge. However, these cases require psychiatric assessment, whether regarding diagnosis at trial or at the execution stage, and knowledge of paternal mental health is critical. As these five cases demonstrate, prevention of paternal filicide (like maternal filicide) requires different strategies for different motives. Some parents are psychotic at the time of the killing, whereas others have a history of partner violence or restraining orders and may act out of vengeance toward their former partner.

RECENT RESEARCH COMPARING FATHERS WHO KILL WITH MOTHERS WHO KILL

In more recent years, research has focused somewhat more on fathers who kill than it had done previously. Still, only rarely have studies systematically compared maternal and paternal filicides (see Table 5–1 for a description of the nations, sample sizes, and data sources of the recent literature).

In this section, commonalities and differences between mothers and fathers who kill are discussed. Remember that although there may be characteristics in common between paternal filicide and maternal filicide perpetrators, it is critical that each person's motive be considered, regardless of gender. For example, fathers and mothers who commit a partner revenge filicide may have more in common with each other than would a mother who commits a partner revenge filicide with a mother who commits an altruistic filicide. Fathers, like mothers, may experience various socioeconomic disadvantages before the filicide. Table 5–2 summarizes data from various recent studies regarding age of the perpetrator, age of the child victim, partner and relationship status, additional victims (e.g., the partner), previous perpetration of abuse of the child killed or intimate partner, substance abuse, suicidality, mental illness in the parent, and the method of killing. In general, data support that the father who kills is usually older than the mother who kills and that the father may have older victims.

Fathers may be more likely to be experiencing discord in their intimate relationships and more likely to also commit partner homicide. They are overall more likely to commit filicide-suicide and to use firearms. While either parent should be evaluated for mental illness, mothers have been more likely to be diagnosed with mental illness, which may capture a reality or be related to gender bias.

Léveillée et al. (2007) studied all registered filicides in Quebec, Canada, from 1986 to 1994. They found that fathers (compared with mothers) who killed were more likely to also commit partner homicide. Further

TABLE 5–1.   Recent studies including fathers who kill

Nation	Author (year)	N	Sample
Australia	Eriksson et al. (2014)	14 filicides	Australian Homicide Project
Australia	Brown et al. (2019)	238 filicides by 260 offenders	Australian Institute of Criminology's National Homicide Monitoring Program
Canada	Harris et al. (2007)	378 filicides (including by step-parents)	Violent Crime Linkage Analysis System (national police database)
Canada	Léveillée et al. (2007)	75 filicides	Officially registered filicides
Canada	Dawson (2015)	1,612 filicides	Statistics Canada annual Homicide Survey
Finland	Kauppi et al. (2010)	200 filicides	Statistics Finland
Finland and Austria	Putkonen et al. (2011)	120 filicides	Coroner Institutions of Austria and Statistics Finland
Netherlands	Liem and Koenraadt (2008)	161 filicides and attempted filicides	Forensic psychiatric hospital records
United Kingdom	Flynn et al. (2013)	297 filicides (45 filicide-suicides)	National Confidential Inquiry Into Suicide and Homicide by People With Mental Illness
United Kingdom	Sidebotham and Retzer (2019)	86 deaths by immediate family	English Serious Case Reviews
United States	Logan et al. (2013)	129 incidents of homicide-suicide with child victims	National Violent Death Reporting System
United States	Dixon et al. (2014)	787 filicides	National Incident Based Reporting System
United States	Mariano et al. (2014)	94,146 arrests for filicide	U.S. Federal Bureau of Investigation's Supplementary Homicide Reports
United States	Hunter et al. (2019)	1,023 child maltreatment deaths by all perpetrators	National Violent Death Reporting System

TABLE 5–2. Findings of recent studies comparing paternal filicide and maternal filicide

Factor	Fathers vs. mothers	Studies
Age of perpetrator	Fathers older than mothers	Dawson 2015; Dixon et al. 2014; Harris et al. 2007; Liem and Koenraadt 2008; Mariano et al. 2014
Age of child victim(s)	Child victims of fathers older	Dawson 2015; Harris et al. 2007; Kauppi et al. 2010; Liem and Koenraadt 2008; Putkonen et al. 2011
	Similar rates of killing infants	Brown et al. 2019; Mariano et al. 2014
	No significant difference in victim age	Dixon et al. 2014
Partner/Relationship status	Fathers more likely separated or experiencing marital discord	Harris et al. 2007; Léveillée et al. 2007; Putkonen et al. 2011
	Mothers more likely separated in fatal maltreatment cases	Sidebotham and Retzer 2019
Additional victims	Fathers more often kill partner	Harris et al. 2007; Léveillée et al. 2007; Liem and Koenraadt 2008; Putkonen et al. 2011
Previous perpetrator of child abuse	Fathers more often	Putkonen et al. 2011
	No significant difference in prior child abuse	Harris et al. 2007
	Fathers more likely to use tyrannical discipline	Léveillée et al. 2007
Intimate partner violence	Fathers more often had history	Brown et al. 2019; Kauppi et al. 2010; Léveillée et al. 2007; Sidebotham and Retzer 2019

TABLE 5–2. Findings of recent studies comparing paternal filicide and maternal filicide (*continued*)

Factor	Fathers vs. mothers	Studies
Substance abuse	Fathers more often had history	Flynn et al. 2013; Kauppi et al. 2010
	No significant difference	Mariano et al. 2014
Suicide	Fathers more often	Harris et al. 2007; Léveillée et al. 2007; Putkonen et al. 2011
	Similar rates	Brown et al. 2019
Method of killing		
Fathers	Violent methods (e.g., firearms or banging more commonly)	Dawson 2015; Flynn et al. 2013; Kauppi et al. 2010; Mariano et al. 2014; Putkonen et al. 2011
Mothers	Passive means (e.g., drowning, poisoning, suffocating) more commonly	Flynn et al. 2013; Kauppi et al. 2010; Putkonen et al. 2011
Mental illness	Mothers more often diagnosed, although fathers also suffer	Flynn et al. 2013; Kauppi et al. 2010
	Fathers more often diagnosed with personality disorder	Kauppi et al. 2010

comparisons are described in Table 5–2. Some fathers were also noted to have a history of "tyrannical discipline" (p. 287), a term not commonly applied to mothers in the literature. Fathers who did not attempt suicide (along with filicide) were frequently noted as having previously abused their child. When they compared fathers who committed filicide alone with those who committed filicide-suicide, fathers who committed filicide alone were younger and had not threatened to kill themselves. They were less likely to be depressed, to kill multiple victims, and to be motivated by revenge against their partner.

Harris et al. (2007) examined a Canadian national register that included 378 cases of parents and stepparents who had killed their children. Infants were found to be at greatest risk of filicide. When biological fathers committed filicide, marital discord, suicide, and uxoricide were more often noted. As well as the differences noted in Table 5–2, 40% of fathers committed filicide-suicide compared with 11% of mothers. Fathers' criminal history and marital conflicts and problems were noted to be significantly greater than those of mothers. Although fathers were more likely to be intoxicated (8%) compared with mothers (2%), they were still rarely intoxicated at the time of the filicide. No significant difference was noted in whether the biological parental perpetrator used a weapon or instrument or had previously injured the victim.

Records from a forensic psychiatric hospital in The Netherlands, which would only include a subgroup of parents who killed, found that half of the women and one-third of the men had been mentally ill at the time of the homicide (Liem and Koenraadt 2008). In a study in Finland, Kauppi et al. (2010) investigated filicides over 25 years, including victims younger than 15 years of age. They found that 59% of filicides were perpetrated by mothers, 39% by fathers, and 2% by stepfathers. Consistent with other findings, all known neonaticide perpetrators were mothers. Emotional abuse was commonly noted in the childhoods of both mother and father perpetrators. Of note, in 30% of paternal filicides (and 10% of maternal filicides), the infant had been separated early from the perpetrating parent because of prematurity or been taken into foster care. Fathers were noted to be "jealous" in half of the cases. Whereas three-quarters of mothers had reported mental health distress before the filicide, only 10% of fathers had.

Consistent with these findings, Putkonen et al. (2011) reported on a register-based study of Finland and Austria that included perpetrators of filicide. Compared with mothers, fathers were more likely to have previously committed violent offenses (28% vs. 5%); more often employed, although only half (49%) were working; and more likely to be intoxicated at the time of the murder (42% vs. 11%). Researchers found that fathers' motives were more likely to be impulsive (41% vs. 13%); however, mothers were more likely to attempt to hide the child's body or "clean to cover tracks" after the homicide than fathers. Fathers and mothers both experienced significant economic, occupational, and social support group issues fairly commonly. "Constant quarrels" were noted prior to the filicide for 23% of fathers compared with 7% of mothers. Furthermore, fathers were more likely to be experiencing a current threat of separation at the time of the murder (42% vs. 12%). They were also more likely to commit suicide along with the filicide (38% vs. 15%). Putkonen et al. (2011) concluded that there may be at least two subgroups of fathers who kill: the "common homicide offender" and the "overloaded, working and suicidal father."

Flynn et al. (2013) completed a study of filicide and filicide-suicide cases in England and Wales utilizing the National Confidential Inquiry Into Suicide and Homicide by People With Mental Illness. Data were also collected from psychiatric reports and mental health teams. Fathers were less likely than mothers to have a history of mental disorder (27% vs. 66%) and to have mental health symptoms at the time of the offense (23% vs. 53%). More than one-third (37%) of the sample, including 23% of fathers, were mentally ill at the time of the murder. In most cases, mental illness was determined to be unrelated to the filicide. Biological fathers compared with stepfathers were more likely to have been mentally ill, including having depressive symptoms, at the time of the offense. Stepfathers in particular were more likely to have a history of illicit substance use, to kill preschool-age victims, and to perpetrate the killing by hitting or kicking, but they were less likely to kill infants.

Mariano et al. (2014) analyzed the U.S. Federal Bureau of Investigation's Supplementary Homicide Reports data from 94,146 arrests over a period from 1976 to 2007. They determined that 15% of all murders were filicides and that fathers and mothers were similarly likely to kill infants. Both male and female offenders killed victims with a modal (most common) age of younger than 1 year (representing infanticide cases). They also found that just over half of the offenders were male, but as the ages of the victims decreased, the rates of female perpetration increased. The most common type of filicide was a father killing a son.

With some contrasting results, Dixon et al. (2014) examined 15 years of National Incident-Based Reporting System data, from 1995 to 2009. Filicides made up 3% of all homicides, with fathers being the primary offender in 432 cases (55% of all cases). No significant differences were found in analysis of victim age. Notably, 39% of victims of fathers and 33% of victims of mothers were younger than 1 year of age. No significant differences were found in alcohol or drug use when parent gender was considered. Although males were more likely to use firearms than females, 15% of fathers compared with 11% of mothers did so. In fact, Dixon et al. (2014) noted that "one of the most significant findings is the lack of statistical significance between maternal and paternal filicides. Strikingly similar profiles exist by offender gender" (p. 351). They further noted that "for both genders, offenses typically occurred within the home and involved personal weapons, such as beating with hands and feet or strangulation" and that "incident characteristics revealed few gender differences" (p. 352), concluding that "mothers and fathers have similar offending profiles" (p. 353).

Subsequently, Dawson (2015) studied the trends in Canadian filicide, finding significant differences in filicide by the gender of the perpetrator. These included a relationship breakdown as a possible emerging trend, a growing number of stepfather-perpetrated cases, an increasing gender gap of fathers committing filicide, family violence predating the filicide, and a decrease in suicide attempts by the parent perpetrator. Dawson also found that, in Canada, fathers outnumbered mothers as filicide perpetrators, with an increasing gender gap over time.

Hunter et al. (2019) examined child maltreatment deaths in America from 2011 to 2015 using the National Violent Death Reporting System and found that males were the most likely perpetrator of child deaths in victims 10 years of age and younger (58%) except in neonaticides. In addition to parents, other intimate partners acted as perpetrators. One in five (19%) perpetrators had a history of abusing the child prior to the death. Their results support previous studies that found children ages 5 years and younger are at greatest risk of fatality from maltreatment and have an increased risk in fatalities from maltreatment when an unrelated male adult is living with the family, specifically the partner of the mother. They underscored the need for interventions focused on fathers (Hunter et al. 2019).

Sidebotham and Retzer (2019) studied English Serious Case Reviews from 2011 to 2014 of child deaths attributed to maltreatment. They found that "those deaths resulting from impulsive violence or severe persistent cruelty are almost exclusively perpetrated by males, while those with an apparent intent to kill the child are slightly more likely to be perpetrated by mothers" (p. 139). Most cases occurred in the context of known family domestic violence, but fathers were more likely to participate in fatal physical abuse and severe and persistent cruelty, whereas mothers were more likely to participate in extreme neglect or deprivational abuse. In distinction to other research, parental separation was much more likely in cases of maternal filicide (72% vs. 29%). It was suggested that in paternal cases, violence and impulsivity were both prevalent.

Brown et al. (2019), utilizing data from the Australian Institute of Criminology's National Homicide Monitoring Program, found similar rates of maternal and paternal perpetrators. They found that similar numbers of male and female offenders had used drugs, whereas male offenders were more likely to have consumed alcohol prior to the offense (23% vs. 6%). Regarding previous offending, fathers were more likely than mothers to have had a previous conviction (54% vs. 30%). If evidence was presented by medical professionals during the court proceedings or was agreed upon in court, mental illness was considered to be present in 13% of fathers and 51% of mothers. In contrast to other studies, rates of suicide by the parent were similar for both genders: 53% of the suicide cases occurred in fathers, compared with 47% of the suicide cases occurring in mothers.

FILICIDE-SUICIDE BY FATHERS COMPARED WITH MOTHERS

Around the world, fathers are approximately twice as likely to kill themselves when they kill their children compared with mothers who kill. This may be related to the means used, similar to higher rates of suicide deaths among men in general. Approximately 16%–29% of mothers who commit filicide also commit suicide, compared with 40%–60% of fathers, "consistent with the fact that men more often complete suicide than women, and men tend to use more lethal means (i.e., guns) rather than overdose" (Friedman et al. 2012, p. 788). However, high rates of suicide may also imply that a relatively high proportion of fathers were mentally ill at the time.

Friedman et al. (2005b) evaluated records from the coroner's office of a major American metropolitan area for 30 cases of filicide-suicide. They found that twice as many fathers committed filicide-suicide than mothers. Two-thirds of these fathers also attempted to kill their partners, whereas no mother attempted to do so. The motives of both mothers and fathers who committed filicide-suicide were primarily altruistic; evidence of fatal maltreatment, unwanted child, or revenge motives in these cases was lacking. More than three-quarters of parents had evidence of mental illness, yet less than two-thirds of them had been in treatment. In this American study, the most frequent method of the filicide-suicide involved firearms. Fathers were significantly older than mothers, and children who were killed were on average 6.8 years old.

In Léveillée et al.'s (2007) Canadian study, fathers who committed filicide-suicide often were angry at their partner. These paternal perpetrators were more likely to have been living without their children and to kill more victims, as well as committing their offenses in the context of a separation. The authors suggested that this subgroup of men had a poor reaction to separation and, in some situations, saw the child as part of the ex-partner. Similarly, in the subsample of filicide-suicide cases in Finland, Kauppi et al. (2010) found that fathers were the more likely perpetrators and had older victims. Shooting was the most common cause of death by a father, whereas mothers killed by poisoning, drowning, and stabbing. Likewise, in Flynn et al.'s (2013) U.K. study of the filicide-suicide cases, 62% were committed by fathers. The median age of the children killed in a filicide-suicide was 6 years, similar to the findings of Friedman et al. (2005b) in America.

Finally, Logan et al. (2013) considered American filicide-suicide cases using National Violent Death Reporting System data from 2003 to 2009. Approximately one-third of the 97 filicide-suicides occurred when the offending parent was experiencing mental health symptoms. Although mothers were twice as likely as fathers to have been experiencing psychosis, this finding means that some fathers still experienced psychosis. Regarding mental health, 21% of father perpetrators were noted to have had a mental health issue at the time of the killing compared with 52% of mothers. Women generally are more likely to seek help for mental health concerns than are men, which could influence the perception of men with no documented history of mental illness. Notably, Logan and colleagues reported that parental discord preceded four-fifths (81%) of the paternal filicide-suicides and three-fifths (59%) of the maternal filicide-suicides.

GENDER BIAS

It is imperative to be cognizant of gender bias in the courts and also in our own thinking, whether we are acting as researchers or evaluators. Researchers have recently begun examining the perceptions of mock jurors and of attorneys regarding parents who kill, with concerns of gender bias in mind. For example, Dunn et al. (2006) utilized a sample of college student mock jurors and found that when white women used a gun to kill rather than smothering the child, they were judged more harshly. However, when white men smothered the child rather than using a gun, they were judged more severely. Black fathers who used a gun had the most severe judgments from the mock jurors. These findings imply both racial and gendered narratives of acceptability.

Orthwein et al. (2010) studied attorneys' perception of both motive and strategies for the defense regarding a fictional vignette. The vignette described a filicide case, the only difference being the gender of the parent who killed. When the perpetrator was a father in a filicide case, participants were more likely to believe that retaliation and jealousy were the motivating factors. However, when a mother was the perpetrator of the filicide, participants were more likely to believe that mental illness was the motivation. Regarding defense strategy, fathers who killed their children were more likely to be encouraged to accept a prison term of 15 years, whereas insanity and other mitigating defenses were more likely to be recommended to mothers (Orthwein et al. 2010). These results may be based upon the attorneys' own biases or on their perception of the criminal justice system outcomes (discussed later).

Finally, Collosso and Buchanan (2018) studied a sample of college students using a fictional vignette in which the same story about a filicide case was told, but the parent's gender was altered. Respondents disproportionately believed the mother was mentally ill and should receive psychiatric treatment, even though the scenario involved the exact same symptoms in both mothers and fathers. This showed a clear gender bias among educated people potentially in a jury pool in the future. These authors also suggested that "mothers who killed their children would be seen as mentally unstable because their actions conflict drastically with traditional maternal roles" (p. 5), which coincides with the findings of Wiest and Duffy (2013) and Cavaglion (2008, 2009) that mothers perceived as being more in the traditional female role were regarded more compassionately by media. Expert witnesses should similarly consider and examine their own potential for gender bias.

LEGAL OUTCOMES FOR FATHERS COMPARED WITH MOTHERS

Friedman et al. (2012) noted that, in the first week of life, the mother is the most common perpetrator of filicide. They also noted that fathers who killed their children often have many commonalities with mothers who kill their children. Mothers and fathers may each individually be in the throes of mental illness when they kill their child. Alternatively, either a mother or a father may not be experiencing mental illness at the time. Either parent who has killed merits a thoughtful mental health evaluation for legal determination of insanity.

Evolutionary psychology helps conceptualize rational and irrational (i.e., potentially psychotic or depressive) reasons for filicide, offering an explanatory model that helps people understand the murders of children and can help guide evaluations and courtroom testimony. The various evolutionary reasons, from across the animal kingdom, include scarce resources, poor-quality child, paternal uncertainty, and coercion

(Daly and Wilson 1988). Mothers' and fathers' motives both may be interpreted through an evolutionary lens. When younger mothers (vs. older mothers) kill, it is more likely that this reflects past adaptive patterns. Younger mothers are more likely to be able to reproduce again. Stepparents kill more often than biological parents, who are passing on their genes (Friedman et al. 2012).

However, Wiest and Duffy (2013) found that both the verdict and sentence vary by gender—that is, fathers tended to be more frequently incarcerated than hospitalized afterward. The treatment of female offenders depended on how well the mother fit traditional gender roles. Although women may be considered *mad* or *sad* when they kill their children, men are often considered *bad*, even when similar mental health issues underlie the incident.

Legal experts, forensic practitioners, and others involved in filicide cases should be aware both of their own potential gender biases (Friedman 2015) and potential biases of the legal system. Evidence of gender bias has been seen in studies of mock jurors. If it is difficult for forensic professionals to grasp that fathers may have similar motives to mothers for killing their children (as described in this chapter), it is most certainly difficult for the general population (i.e., the jury) to understand that fathers may be similarly mentally ill as mothers. Fathers are more likely to be incarcerated after killing their child, whereas mothers are more likely to be found insane and hospitalized. In fact, one study of parents found not guilty by reason of insanity (NGRI) for killing their child in two American states found more than 39 mothers yet only 1 father (Friedman et al. 2005a).

Further highlighting the gender difference in outcomes, Flynn et al. (2013) identified through their U.K. study that a significantly higher proportion of fathers than mothers were convicted for their filicide, with a two-to-one ratio. For the paternal filicide cases, 43% had a conviction for murder and 52% for manslaughter. Although the majority of mothers were convicted of manslaughter, 21% had an outcome of infanticide. In the aforementioned Finnish study, 18% of fathers were found NGRI and two-thirds (65%) were found to have diminished responsibility. In contrast, mothers who killed were found NGRI three-quarters (76%) of the time (Kauppi et al. 2010).

As discussed, fathers and mothers each individually could be mentally unwell (or not) when killing their children. Likewise, research reviewed in this chapter has noted that fathers and mothers generally kill infants at similar rates. Yet whereas mothers have an infanticide defense available to them in two dozen nations, no such defense is available to fathers. It has been noted that "[t]his gender bias in the infanticide laws appears to attach reduced significance to the lives of children" (Fried-man 2015, p. 275) killed by their mothers, as well as punishing fathers more punitively for the same crime.

Considerations in Evaluations of Fathers Who Have Killed

For a comprehensive discussion of principles for the forensic mental health evaluation in filicide cases, please see Chapter 11. Here, the focus is on major principles and the differences between evaluation of females and males. Expert witnesses should be careful to guard against their own gender biases in the evaluation (Friedman 2015). Fathers who have killed should be asked about parenting, just as mothers are. A motive based on anger rather than mental illness should not be presumed in paternal filicide cases. In addition, mental health and substance abuse symptoms, as well as other categories of query in the post-filicide foren-sic evaluation, should be examined as carefully in fathers as they are in mothers. To objectively evaluate a parent of either gender, the forensic evaluator should have competency in identifying and diagnosing men-tal health issues in both genders. Evaluators should also guard against bias related to the parent's sex.

Questions about the relationship with the child's mother should be asked, as well as about the motive and any suicidal intent at the time. Careful expert witnesses, aware of common characteristics among fa-thers who kill (as described herein), should not jump to unwarranted conclusions. For example, fathers are more likely to use firearms in kill-ing their children, referred to in some literature as a more violent means. However, this should not lead an evaluator to conclude that the father killed out of anger rather than out of love. Fathers and mothers who kill have many similarities, and expert witnesses should keep an open mind when evaluating any parent, regardless of gender.

Prevention of Paternal Filicide

Prevention efforts must be informed by motives, for fathers as well as for mothers. Family stress and parenting issues, as well as mental health and substance abuse issues, must be considered. Fathers (and mothers) who kill their children in fatal maltreatment ("accidental") cases differ significantly from those parents who kill their children for altruistic or for acutely psychotic reasons; the motive is much more critical than the gender. Dixon et al. (2014) noted the usefulness of empirical research fueling public education campaigns about shaken baby syndrome. They called for continued intervention programs as well as fighting the stereotype of mothers as the most frequent perpetrators, focusing rather on fathers in informing the public and addressing risk factors.

Mental health professionals should think about their male patients in the fathering role just as we think about female patients in the mothering role. In the aforementioned New Zealand study, perceived stress in pregnancy and the father's health status were associated with paternal depression, with other risk factors including history of depression, postnatal unemployment, and relationship issues. Thus, Underwood et al. (2017) recommended that "men who have a history of mental health problems or who are stressed or unwell during their partner's pregnancy should be assessed" (p. 367) for postpartum paternal depression. Edward et al. (2015) similarly suggested routine screening of both parents for depression across pregnancy and the postpartum. Furthermore, because of the correlation between maternal postpartum depression and paternal depression, Paulson et al. (2016) recommended that health care professionals evaluating pregnant and postpartum women make efforts to include fathers in these assessments. Recommendations regarding screening for paternal depression include particularly screening fathers when maternal depression is present.

An Australian study (Eriksson et al. 2014) suggested that mental health support, as well as help with parenting skills, was critical. Similarly, based on their European study, Putkonen et al. (2011) noted that parents and families require support and that health care and social workers should be alert to signs of parental despair, especially in stressful situations. They noted that support is necessary for families when separation has occurred, particularly for the father, and that "since approximately half of the fathers were employed during their [filicide] offense, one cannot but wonder if their desperation was visible at work" (p. 326). Thus, they recommended father-specific family leave as well as family days for employees. Families in distress require particular support, and health care providers should pay attention to parental signs of despair, be aware of depressed parents, ask about suicidal or violent thoughts, and provide social support for families (Kauppi et al. 2010). Fathers with a history of substance misuse, mood disorder, or violence should be targeted for intervention (Flynn et al. 2013).

Studies of filicide-suicide by fathers lead to similar suggestions regarding paternal mental health and the need for services. Based on their filicide-suicide study, Logan et al. (2013) suggested that detection of parental mental health conditions and strategies that help to resolve conflicts between parents may help prevent filicide. They also discussed stressors not being handled effectively and precipitating violence, which highlighted the need for services that help either address or prevent relationship problems and mental health problems, as well as services working together collaboratively to prevent partner and family violence. More research about mental illness in fathers is needed to help with treatment and prevention. Similarly, more gender nonbiased research about the common factors among fathers who kill is needed to embrace a more compassionate lens.

MAIN CLINICAL/LEGAL POINTS AND CULTURAL PERSPECTIVES

- Fathers and mothers kill their children at similar rates, yet fathers are often perceived as *bad* whereas mothers are perceived as *mad* or *sad*.
- Virtually all neonaticides are perpetrated by mothers.
- Rates of filicide are similar for mothers and fathers. However, infanticide laws only include mothers.
- Fathers have a higher suicide rate at the time of killing their child than do mothers. This implies that many fathers may be struggling with mental illness at the time of the homicide yet are not able to subsequently report their mental status.
- Similar to mothers, fathers may or may not have mental illness at the time of the homicide, and this should be considered in evaluations after the filicide.
- Lawyers, forensic experts, and other expert witnesses should have knowledge about paternal mental health and factors related to the perpetration of filicide.
- Expert witnesses should consider gender (and racial/ cultural) bias in completing evaluations of parents who have killed.
- Prevention efforts should include identification and treatment of paternal mental illness and substance use disorders, as well as support for struggling couples and families.

Practice and Discussion Questions

ASSUMPTIONS/BIAS IDENTIFICATION EXERCISE

Read the following case vignette:

> Chris had been experiencing depression at the time of the children's deaths. Chris had been barely functioning at work and had been thinking about divorce due to stress at home. The day of the killings, Chris had left work early after being reprimanded by a manager and had picked Molly (age 3) and Kevin (2 months) up from daycare early. Chris felt at the end of a rope, afraid of financial and relationship ruin, and depressed at the time Molly and Kevin were killed.

1. Discuss or write reflections about what you think of this case, how you would feel as a legal representative or forensic expert witness. Did you assume that Chris was a mother or a father?
2. Now, reread the vignette with the idea that Chris is a father if you initially perceived Chris to be a mother (or a mother if you initially perceived Chris to be a father). How are your reflections different?
3. Review the vignette with the consideration that Chris is in a same-sex relationship. How are your reflections different in this case?
4. How could gender bias, cultural/racial bias, or economic bias (low vs. high socioeconomic status) play a role in your perceptions of paternal filicide? On what basis do you have more compassion or judge more harshly? Is this grounded in data or perception? What if the children had disabilities? How might this impact your approach or assumptions about Chris?
5. Discuss and reflect on what you can do to maintain awareness and keep any biases you hold in check.
6. Discuss and reflect upon what basis you would decide to decline working on a case due to recognized bias.

References

Brown T, Bricknell S, Bryant W, et al: Filicide offenders. Trends and Issues in Crime and Criminal Justice, No 568, February 2019

Cameron EE, Sedov ID, Tomfohr-Madsen LM: Prevalence of paternal depression in pregnancy and the postpartum: an updated meta-analysis. J Affect Disord 206:189–203, 2016

Cavaglion G: Bad, mad or sad? Mothers who kill and press coverage in Israel. Crime, Media, Culture 4(2):271–278, 2008

Cavaglion G: Fathers who kill and press coverage in Israel. Child Abuse Rev 18(2):127–143, 2009

Collosso T, Buchanan B: Media bias in cases of maternal vs. paternal filicide. Metamorphosis, June 19, 2018

Daly M, Wilson M: Killing children: parental homicide in the modern West, in Homicide. New York, Aldine De Gruyter, 1988, pp 61–93

Dawson M: Canadian trends in filicide by gender of the accused, 1961–2011. Child Abuse Negl 47:162–174, 2015

Dixon S, Krienert JL, Walsh J: Filicide: a gendered profile of offender, victim, and event characteristics in a national sample of reported incidents, 1995–2009. J Crime Justice 37(3):339–355, 2014

Dunn KF, Cowan G, Downs D: Effects of sex and race of perpetrator and method of killing on outcome judgments in a mock filicide case. J Appl Soc Psychol 36(10):2395–2416, 2006

Easteal P, Bartels L, Nelson N, et al: How are women who kill portrayed in newspaper media? Connections with social values and the legal system. Womens Stud Int Forum 51:31–41, 2015

Edward KL, Castle D, Mills C, et al: An integrative review of paternal depression. Am J Mens Health 9(1):26–34, 2015

Eriksson L, Mazerolle P, Wortley R, et al: Maternal and paternal filicide: case studies from the Australian Homicide Project. Child Abuse Rev 25(1):17–30, 2014

Flynn SM, Shaw JJ, Abel KM: Filicide: mental illness in those who kill their children. PLoS One 8(4):e58981, 2013

Friedman SH: Realistic consideration of women and violence is critical. J Am Acad Psychiatry Law 43(3):273–276, 2015

Friedman SH, Resnick PJ: Child murder by mothers: patterns and prevention. World Psychiatry 6(3): 137, 2007

Friedman SH, Hrouda DR, Holden CE, et al: Child murder committed by severely mentally ill mothers: an examination of mothers found not guilty by reason of insanity. J Forens Sci 50:132–136, 2005a

Friedman SH, Hrouda DR, Holden CE, et al: Filicide-suicide: common factors in parents who kill their children and themselves. J Am Acad Psychiatry Law 33:496–504, 2005b

Friedman SH, Cavney J, Resnick PJ: Child murder by parents and evolutionary psychology. Psychiatr Clin North Am 35:781–795, 2012

Harris G, Hilton N, Rice M, Eke A: Children killed by genetic parents versus stepparents. Evol Hum Behav 28(2):85–95, 2007

Henriques B: 'I didn't think a guy could do that.' Global News, October 25, 2019

Hunter AA, DiVieto S, Schwab-Reese L, Riffon M: An epidemiologic examination of perpetrators of fatal child maltreatment using the National Violent Death Reporting System (NVDRS). J Interpers Violence 2019 Epub ahead of print

Kaladelfos A: The dark side of the family: paternal child homicide in Australia. Journal of Australian Studies 37(3), 2013

Kauppi A, Kumpulainen K, Karkola K, et al: Maternal and paternal filicides: a retrospective review of filicides in Finland. J Am Acad Psychiatry Law 38:229–238, 2010

Lambert O: Coroner investigates the murder of Yazmina Acar. News.com.au, December 4, 2015. Available at: https://www.news.com.au/national/victoria/courts-law/coroner-investigates-the-murder-of-yazmina-acar/news-story/ecc1c7edf9016f42793afa56074d5ff8. Accessed September 3, 2020.

Léveillée S, Marleau JD, Dubé M: Filicide: a comparison by sex and presence or absence of self-destructive behavior. J Fam Viol 22:287–295, 2007

Liem M, Koenraadt F: Filicide: a comparative study of maternal versus paternal child homicide. Crim Behav Ment Health 18(3):166–176, 2008

Logan JE, Walsh S, Patel N, Hall JE: Homicide-followed-by-suicide incidents involving child victims. Am J Health Behav 37(4):531–542, 2013

Mariano TY, Chan HCO, Myers WC: Toward a more holistic understanding of filicide: a multidisciplinary analysis of 32 years of U.S. arrest data. Forensic Sci Int 236:46–53, 2014

McKinnell J: Man not guilty of five-year-old son's stabbing murder due to mental illness. ABC News, July 24, 2019. Available at: https://www.abc.net.au/news/2019–07–24/man-not-guilty-of-sons-stabbing-murder-due-to-mental-illness/11341796. Accessed September 3, 2020.

Omand G: B.C. judge says father who killed his 3 children doesn't meet high-risk designation. The Canadian Press, August 31, 2017. Available at: https://www.thestar.com/news/canada/2017/08/31/bc-judge-says-father-who-killed-his-3-children-doesnt-meet-high-risk-designation.html. Accessed September 3, 2020.

Orthwein J, Packman W, Jackson R, et al: Filicide: gender bias in California defense attorneys' perception of motive and defense strategies. Psychiatry, Psychology, and the Law 17(4):523–537, 2010

Paulson JF, Bazemore SD, Goodman JH, et al: The course and interrelationship of maternal and paternal perinatal depression. Arch Womens Ment Health 19(4):655–663, 2016

Putkonen H, Amon S, Eronen M, et al: Gender differences in filicide offense characteristics: a comprehensive register-based study of child murder in two European countries. Child Abuse Negl 35(5):319–328, 2011

Resnick PJ: Child murder by parents: a psychiatric review of filicide. Am J Psychiatry 126(3):73–82, 1969

Saxbe DE, Schetter CD, Simon CD, et al: High paternal testosterone may protect against postpartum depressive symptoms in fathers, but confer risk to mothers and children. Horm Behav 95:103–112, 2017

Sidebotham P, Retzer A: Maternal filicide in a cohort of English Serious Case Reviews. Arch Womens Ment Health 22(1):139–149, 2019

Tsiaperas T: John Battaglia taunts ex-wife before being executed for killing their girls while she listened in horror. The Dallas News, February 2, 2018. Available at: https://www.dallasnews.com/news/courts/2018/02/02/john-battaglia-taunts-ex-wife-before-being-executed-for-killing-their-girls-while-she-listened-in-horror. Accessed September 3, 2020.

Underwood L, Waldie KE, Peterson E, et al: Paternal depression symptoms during pregnancy and after childbirth among participants in the Growing Up in New Zealand Study. JAMA Psychiatry 74(4):360–369, 2017

West SG, Friedman SH, Resnick PJ: Fathers who kill their children: an analysis of the literature. J Forensic Sci 54(2):463–468, 2009

Wiest JB, Duffy M: The impact of gender roles on verdicts and sentences in cases of filicide. Criminal Just Stud 26(3):347–365, 2013

FOUNDATION II

The Impact of Perinatal Psychiatric Complications in Maternal Infanticide and Filicide

CHAPTER 6

Role of Perinatal Psychiatric Complications in Infanticide and Filicide

Kimberly Brandt, D.O., PMH-C

Amanda Kingston, M.D.

This chapter presents the impact and prevalence of psychiatric complications in cases of infanticide and filicide in the United States. Different parts of the world approach these cases from a wide variety of perspectives and cultural lenses, some of which are addressed in other chapters. Recognition of psychiatric complications in these cases is important to help expert witnesses become familiar with their presentation and risk as well as differentiate between psychiatric disorders. Dr. Kimberly Brandt, at the University of Missouri, is a perinatal psychiatrist who specializes in the identification and treatment of and advocacy for pregnant and postpartum women with psychiatric illness in both a clinical and judicial setting. Dr. Amanda Kingston, also at the University of Missouri, is a forensic psychiatrist who performs evaluations for justice-involved individuals in a variety of settings and for a variety of cases, including those involving perinatal psychiatric complications.

In a judicial setting, expert witnesses with experience in perinatal psychiatry and forensic work are invaluable to accurately identify mental illness, communicate this to the court, and connect the symptoms to the alleged crime. Such representation can make a meaningful change in the lives of mothers who have killed their child(ren) as well as in the mothers' families and in society by providing treatment for the mothers rather than punishment. The criminal justice system and its penalties are designed to deter future acts; however, perinatal filicide has clear precipitating risk factors such as pregnancy, delivery, and perinatal onset of psychiatric illness. We should seek to identify and prevent the potential tragedy rather than to punish the consequences (Spinelli 2004).

In this chapter, we discuss the most common perinatal psychiatric complications underlying maternal infanticide and filicide and describe commonly confusing presentations. We present three cases to illustrate best practices in forensic assessment and explore outcomes. In the first, we differentiate postpartum psychosis (PPP) from OCD. In the second, we demonstrate key differences between PPP and major depressive disorder (MDD) with psychotic features. In the third and final case, we discuss PPP and the challenges associated with presenting this diagnosis in a courtroom setting. Following these case presentations, we highlight key learning points about clinical, legal, and cultural aspects.

Although cases of infanticide and filicide in the United States are generally rare, many occur in the context of unrecognized and untreated or undertreated perinatal psychiatric illness (Spinelli 2004). The most commonly reported motivations for maternal infanticide in the United States are fatal abuse, unwanted child, or delusional altruistic motives related to acute psychosis (Resnick 1969). In a review of 131 cases of parental child murder and 2 additional maternal filicide cases treated at a hospital in Pennsylvania, Resnick (1969) found that 67% of filicidal women and 17% of neonaticidal women had psychiatric complications.

Among health care providers in the United States, consistent universal screening for psychiatric complications during the perinatal period is lacking, although the prevalence is 10%–20% for depression (Gaynes et al. 2005); 15%–18% for anxiety disorders, including OCD (Fairbrother et al. 2016); 2%–8% for bipolar disorder (Masters et al. 2019); and 0.1%–0.2% for PPP (Robertson et al. 2004). DSM-5 (American Psychiatric Association 2013) is limited in accurately describing perinatal psychiatric conditions, even though these conditions are well described in textbooks and scientific literature, as discussed and cited throughout this chapter.

PPP is not recognized independently as a diagnosis in DSM-5, although it is mentioned as a possible subtype "peripartum onset" specifier of MDD. The length of time specified in DSM-5 for peripartum onset is 4 weeks. This limited time frame is extremely problematic when the literature (Sharma and Mazmanian 2014; Stewart and Vigod 2016; Yawn et al. 2012) and perinatal psychiatry practice use a period of up to 1 year postpartum. It is unlikely that the 4 weeks following pregnancy could encompass all possible psychiatric symptoms that may be exacerbated during or by pregnancy. This lack of a consistent time frame or separate diagnostic label of PPP in DSM-5 can encumber the judicial process.

A lack of clear diagnostic criteria for certain perinatal psychiatric complications in DSM-5 can make it challenging to utilize in a criminal trial. This lack of criteria may also result in these conditions not being recognized or being improperly treated and thus potentially progressing to more severe mental illness, increasing the risk that the mother could harm either herself or her children. Adding PPP as a diagnosis to the next edition of DSM, including diagnostic criteria, timing, and differential diagnoses, is under consideration; proposed criteria include psychotic symptoms, mood instability, and cognitive disorganization (M. Spinelli, personal communication, December 26, 2019). Table 6–1 summarizes the most common perinatal psychiatric complications and their prevalence, symptoms, time of onset, duration, and usual treatment.

Safe and effective treatments, including psychotherapy and psychiatric medications, are available for maternal MDD, bipolar disorder, anxiety disorders, OCD, and other psychotic disorders. Concerns of possible medication risks should be weighed against the risks of untreated maternal illness. For example, untreated bipolar disorder has a 66% risk of relapse in the perinatal period (Wesseloo et al. 2016). In women previously diagnosed with MDD who are taking antidepressants prior to pregnancy, 70% have a relapse of depression during pregnancy when that antidepressant is discontinued (Cohen et al. 2006).

The role, prevalence, and impact of perinatal psychiatric complications in cases of infanticide and filicide are presented in the following sections. It is important to recognize the symptoms of these psychiatric complications in order to differentiate between them, recognize commonalities in their clinical presentation, and evaluate the risk of filicide. Expert witnesses are invaluable in translating this area of medicine for the courts by establishing a diagnosis, articulating the literature base for the disorders, and describing what risks are and are not associated with these perinatal psychiatric complications. We use three cases here to illustrate perinatal psychiatric complications and how they can have an impact on criminal responsibility, competency, and other judicial questions. These cases demonstrate aspects from cases available in the literature and our own clinical experiences.

OCD With Postpartum Onset

CASE DESCRIPTION

Tembia was a 25-year-old woman who was 4 months postpartum. She presented to the psychiatric emergency department with a 3-month history of marked social withdrawal, talking to herself, and suspicious-

TABLE 6–1.   Common perinatal psychiatric complications

Disorder	Prevalence	Symptoms	Onset	Duration	Usual treatment
"Baby blues"	30%–75%[a]	Sadness, emotional lability, irritability	Hours to days following delivery	2 weeks	Reassurance
Major depressive disorder (MDD)	10%–20%[b]	Insomnia, loss of energy, guilt, poor concentration, appetite changes, suicidal ideation	During pregnancy through up to 1 year postpartum	>2 weeks	Psychotherapy and/or psychiatric medications, including antidepressants
Anxiety (including OCD)	15%–18%[c]	Anxiety, worry, intrusive thoughts, obsessions, compulsions	During pregnancy through up to 1 year postpartum	Typically weeks to months	Psychotherapy and/or psychiatric medications, including antidepressants
Bipolar disorder	2%–8%[d]	Features of MDD and mania or hypomania: grandiosity, decreased need for sleep, pressured speech, flight of ideas, distractibility, increase in activity, increased impulsivity	During pregnancy through up to 1 year postpartum	Several days or weeks up to months	Same as MDD; for severe illness (such as mania), hospitalization and/or psychiatric medications are required (e.g., lithium or other mood stabilizers, including antipsychotics)
Postpartum psychosis	0.1%–0.2%[a]	Hallucinations, delusions, disorganized thoughts or speech, fluctuating consciousness, cognitive impairment, severe insomnia, severe mood changes	Usually ≤2 weeks of delivery	Several days to weeks to months	Emergent psychiatric hospitalization; psychiatric medication typically required, such as lithium or other mood stabilizers including antipsychotics

Source.   [a]Robertson et al. 2004. [b]Gavin et al. 2005. [c]Fairbrother et al. 2016. [d]Masters et al. 2019.

ness that began 2 weeks after delivery of her second child. For the past 2 weeks, her symptoms had worsened and included frequent crying spells and a recent suicide attempt by overdose on medications, for which she did not seek medical care. These symptoms were confirmed after psychiatric evaluation, and Tembia was hospitalized on an inpatient psychiatric unit. During the course of her hospitalization, she repeatedly asked other patients, the psychiatrist, and other staff members to forgive her "for a mistake." On further clarification, she stated that she had repeated thoughts that she had harmed her 4-month-old son. She experienced these repetitive, anxiety-provoking thoughts so often that she became concerned that she had actually harmed her infant. To decrease her anxiety, she would seek reassurance from others and speak out loud to herself about the issue. The thoughts were repetitive and distressing, and she felt unable to control them. As the frequency of the thoughts increased, she developed symptoms of depression, including hopelessness, guilt, and increased suicidal thoughts.

DISCUSSION

In-depth discussion of PPP versus OCD is important in order to provide context before offering specific forensic assessment and outcome in this case. First, anxiety disorders are one of the most common psychiatric conditions in pregnancy and the postpartum period, with a prevalence of 15.8% and 17.1%, respectively, and are more prevalent than postpartum depression (PPD; Fairbrother et al. 2016). Pregnancy and childbirth are also associated with the onset of OCD and the worsening of symptoms of preexisting OCD (Forray et al. 2010). A meta-analysis found the prevalence of OCD in pregnancy to be nearly double that of the general population in pregnancy, equal to 2.07%, and more than double that of the general population in the postpartum period, totaling 2.43% (Russell et al. 2013). This compares with the 12-month prevalence in the general population of new onset of anxiety disorders at 2.9% and OCD at 1.2% (Kessler et al. 2012).

Obsessive-Compulsive Disorder

The diagnosis of OCD as defined by DSM-5 involves the presence of obsessions and/or compulsions that are time consuming and cause clinically significant distress or impairment in social, occupational, or other important areas of functioning (Box 6–1; American Psychiatric Association 2013). *Obsessions* are recurrent and persistent thoughts, urges, or images that are intrusive and unwanted. *Compulsions* are repetitive behaviors that the person feels driven to perform in response to an obsession. The criteria in DSM are under constant revision and consultation; the most up-to-date version is necessary for accurate identification and diagnosis as well as for use in testimony.

Box 6–1.   DSM-5 diagnostic criteria for obsessive-compulsive disorder

A. Presence of obsessions, compulsions, or both:

Obsessions are defined by (1) and (2):

1. Recurrent and persistent thoughts, urges, or images that are experienced, at some time during the disturbance, as intrusive and unwanted, and that in most individuals cause marked anxiety or distress.
2. The individual attempts to ignore or suppress such thoughts, urges, or images, or to neutralize them with some other thought or action (i.e., by performing a compulsion).

Compulsions are defined by (1) and (2):

1. Repetitive behaviors (e.g., hand washing, ordering, checking) or mental acts (e.g., praying, counting, repeating words silently) that the individual feels driven to perform in response to an obsession or according to rules that must be applied rigidly.
2. The behaviors or mental acts are aimed at preventing or reducing anxiety or distress, or preventing some dreaded event or situation; however, these behaviors or mental acts are not connected in a realistic way with what they are designed to neutralize or prevent, or are clearly excessive.
    Note: Young children may not be able to articulate the aims of these behaviors or mental acts.

B. The obsessions or compulsions are time consuming (e.g., take more than 1 hour per day) or cause clinically significant distress or impairment in social, occupational, or other important areas of functioning.
C. The obsessive-compulsive symptoms are not attributable to the physiological effects of a substance (e.g., a drug of abuse, a medication) or another medical condition.
D. The disturbance is not better explained by the symptoms of another mental disorder (e.g., excessive worries, as in generalized anxiety disorder; preoccupation with appearance, as in body dysmorphic disorder; difficulty discarding or parting with possessions, as in hoarding disorder; hair pulling, as in trichotillomania [hair-pulling disorder]; skin picking, as in excoriation [skin-picking] disorder; stereotypies, as in stereotypic movement disorder; ritualized eating behavior, as in eating disorders; preoccupation with substances or gambling, as in substance-related and addictive disorders; preoccupation with having an illness, as in illness anxiety disorder; sexual urges or fantasies, as in paraphilic disorders; impulses, as in disruptive, impulse-control, and conduct disorders; guilty ruminations, as in major depressive disorder; thought insertion or delusional preoccupations, as in schizophrenia spectrum and other psychotic disorders; or repetitive patterns of behavior, as in autism spectrum disorder).

Specify if:

With good or fair insight: Individual recognizes that obsessive-compulsive disorder beliefs are definitely or probably not true or that they may or may not be true.
With poor insight: Individual thinks obsessive-compulsive disorder beliefs are probably true.
With absent insight/delusional beliefs: Individual is completely convinced that obsessive-compulsive disorder beliefs are true.

Specify if:
   Tic-related: Individual has a current or past history of a tic disorder.

Source.   Reprinted from American Psychiatric Association: *Diagnostic and Statistical Manual of Mental Disorders*, 5th Edition. Arlington, VA, 2013, p. 237. Copyright © 2013 American Psychiatric Association. Used with permission.

The most common obsessions associated with OCD during the perinatal period include fear of contaminating or causing illness in the infant, need for symmetry, and intrusive thoughts such as accidentally or intentionally causing physical or sexual harm to the child. The most common compulsions associated with OCD in the perinatal period involve cleaning, checking, and avoiding (Namouz-Hadad and Nulman 2014). It is not uncommon for a mother to develop intrusive thoughts that she will sexually abuse her infant (obsession) and to avoid changing the infant's diaper (compulsion) as a result. Postpartum mothers with OCD have insight that their thoughts are intrusive or unwanted and typically represent a fear or worry about something they do not want to happen (Veale et al. 2009). Personal insight that the thoughts are discordant with their desires means the thoughts are *ego-dystonic*—that is, neither consistent with nor acceptable to the mother's typical self-identity (Namouz-Hadad and Nulman 2014).

Women with OCD onset in the postpartum period experience significantly more aggressive obsessions about harming their infants than do women with onset prior to the perinatal period (Brandes et al. 2004). In the literature, there are no documented cases of mothers with OCD as their only diagnosis who have harmed an infant intentionally (Namouz-Hadad and Nulman 2014). However, OCD is commonly associated with other comorbid conditions that may elevate the risk for filicide. For instance, MDD may involve delusions or psychotic features and should also be assessed (Torres et al. 2006). Risk of violence in OCD most often comes from a secondary effect of the compulsions or intervention from a third party attempting to stop the compulsion, which increases the distress and can lead to fatal acts (Veale et al. 2009).

For example, if a mother has concerns about poisoning or contamination involving food, water, or milk, this could lead her to restrict these items for the baby or for herself, which may have downstream consequences including acute dehydration, malnutrition, failure to thrive, and developmental delays (Maina et al. 1999). Concerns about her abilities as a mother or her ability to care for her child could lead to isolation and social withdrawal and potentially to poor or insecure attachment or cognitive and social developmental delays in the child (Veale et al. 2009). Outpatient monitoring and structure are often complex in these scenarios because the recommendation that another adult always be present with the mother and baby can reinforce the mother's feelings of inadequacy and insecurity, thereby potentially worsening the obsessive thoughts.

Postpartum Psychosis

Compared with OCD, PPP is rare, with a most commonly cited prevalence of 0.1%–0.2% (VanderKruik et al. 2017). Although filicide is an uncommon event in PPP, the filicide rate is higher in depressive disorders with psychotic features (4.5%) compared with psychotic disorders without depression (1%) (Brockington 2017). PPP may also present with aggressive or violent thoughts of harming the infant, and when asked, the mother may admit a plan or intent to harm the infant and a justification for doing so, such as believing the child is possessed by a demon or evil spirit or a need to save the child from eternal damnation, as in the Andrea Yates case and many other examples described in this book.

These *delusional thoughts*, or fixed false beliefs, are commonly seen in psychosis. The thoughts are ego-syntonic—consistent with the mother's way of thinking, her goals and needs—and thus are unlikely to be described by the mother as unwanted or intrusive (Lawrence et al. 2017). PPP is theorized to be a subtype of bipolar disorder; its presentation often has the features of a manic or mixed bipolar episode. As such, mental health professionals should closely monitor the care and treatment of women with bipolar disorder in the perinatal and postpartum stages of life. From a treatment perspective, lithium, a mood stabilizer medication, has the most robust evidence for efficacy in PPP, which furthers the theory that PPP falls more within the category of a mood disorder (Bergink et al. 2016; Suppes et al. 2005).

Most women who experience PPP have no previous psychiatric history and are diagnosed with a mood disorder, such as bipolar disorder or MDD, for the first time during or following the postpartum psychotic episode. Approximately 70%–80% of cases of psychosis in the perinatal period are associated with mood episodes, such as mania or depression occurring in bipolar disorder, and 12% of cases are associated with psychosis occurring during an acute episode of schizophrenia (Karakasi et al. 2017). Ninety percent of hospitalizations in cases of PPP happen in the first 4 weeks after delivery.

Symptoms of PPP include inability to function normally, fluctuating consciousness, cognitive impairment, severe mood lability, delusions, hallucinations, severe insomnia, and irritability (Bergink et al. 2015). PPP has a high association with violent behavior and suicide and has a 4% risk of infanticide (Spinelli 2009). Although suicidal thoughts are common in mothers with PPP, completed suicide is rare during an acute episode of psychosis that results in filicide. The rate of suicide increases later in the mother's life, in the years following her recovery from the first episode of PPP. Mothers with PPP also often have a history of suicide among their first-degree relatives, such as their parents or siblings (Brockington 2017). These facts further illustrate the likelihood that PPP is a primary mood disorder and not a primary psychotic disorder, despite having *psychosis* in its name.

FORENSIC ASSESSMENT AND CASE OUTCOME

In Tembia's case, the treating psychiatric team comprised a psychiatrist, social worker, psychologist, and occupational therapist. This team requested a violence risk assessment from a forensic psychiatrist prior to Tembia's discharge from the hospital to determine her risk of harming her child. The consulting forensic psychiatrist assessed the following:

1. Does Tembia have OCD, a psychotic disorder, or both?
2. What is the risk Tembia will act on her thoughts to harm her infant?
3. What are the possible consequences of Tembia performing her compulsions?

The forensic evaluations included a thorough history, which was collected to develop a complete characterization of Tembia's thoughts and behaviors. The history and additional details can help differentiate an obsessive-compulsive process from a psychotic one, which is key to further assessing risk of violence. In cases in which a forensic psychiatric interview and record review are not sufficient to determine risk, forensic psychological testing can help differentiate the diagnosis.

In this case, Tembia experienced intense anxiety when she believed she may have acted on her obsessions, indicating that these beliefs were ego-dystonic. Tembia's perspective of those thoughts were most consistent with an anxiety-driven disorder most closely resembling OCD that had onset following the delivery of her infant. Once the forensic evaluator determined that the thoughts of harming the infant were obsessional in nature rather than psychotic or caused by another phenomenology (e.g., such as another mood or anxiety disorder), the risk assessment of the first consultation question was answered, with a description of OCD and its symptoms. Discussion of the low risk of Tembia acting on these thoughts was included in the report.

For the second question, a much more case-specific assessment was needed. A full detail of Tembia's compulsions was necessary to drive recommendations for her level of risk of violence. She reported that her compulsions involved repeated attempts to seek reassurance that her intrusive thoughts had not occurred, which she did by asking for reassurance and forgiveness from those around her.

With regard to the third question, Tembia's risk of violence as a result of acting on an intrusive thought was very low, and therefore 24-hour supervision was not warranted. Substance use can increase the risk of violence, and assessment for substance use and misuse is an important part of the process. Tembia reported no history of substance use or misuse, and this was confirmed with urine drug analysis and collateral information from friends and family.

Based on this risk assessment, the forensic psychiatry consultant advised the treatment team that Tembia's risk of violence was low based on her diagnosis of OCD, lack of psychotic component in her presentation, and the ego-dystonic nature of her intrusive thoughts. As a result, the treatment team optimized her psychotropic medications and discharged her with ongoing monitoring through outpatient psychiatric treatment and psychotherapy.

Major Depressive Disorder With Psychotic Features and Postpartum Onset

CASE DESCRIPTION

Alice was a 23-year-old married woman who had no previously documented psychiatric history. She delivered a healthy baby via cesarean section due to the baby's breech position. During her pregnancy, Alice had experienced minor anxiety symptoms that worsened over the course of the pregnancy and had reported symptoms of "baby blues" immediately after the delivery. Alice remained home as the infant's primary caregiver for the first 3 months. In anticipation of returning to work, her insomnia and anxiety worsened; after returning to work, she was unable to continue breastfeeding and began using formula. When this happened, Alice began believing that the baby had stopped growing and would appear blue, which she called "developmental issues" that she attributed to the formula. An evaluation by a developmental pediatrician revealed no abnormalities in her infant. Discouraged by this lack of confirmation, Alice did not seek further medical evaluation. Her symptoms worsened, and she increasingly struggled with caring for herself and the baby. As a result, she hardly slept for 5 consecutive days, was thoroughly convinced her baby was having "developmental issues," and became socially withdrawn.

DISCUSSION

Major Depressive Disorder

MDD is one of the most common perinatal psychiatric disorders and one of the most common complications of pregnancy, affecting up to 20% of pregnant and postpartum women (Gaynes et al. 2005). When symptoms of MDD (Box 6–2) become severe, features of psychosis can emerge, including hallucinations, delusions, and paranoia. Although specific rates of MDD with psychotic features in the perinatal population have not been studied, the rate of psychotic features occurring in MDD in the general population is 15%–19% overall, accounting for 25% of patients who are hospitalized in inpatient psychiatric settings (Gaudiano et al. 2009). Perinatal patients diagnosed with MDD can be diagnosed prior to or during pregnancy or postpartum.

Box 6–2.   DSM-5 diagnostic criteria for major depressive disorder

---

A. Five (or more) of the following symptoms have been present during the same 2-week period and represent a change from previous functioning; at least one of the symptoms is either (1) depressed mood or (2) loss of interest or pleasure.
   Note: Do not include symptoms that are clearly attributable to another medical condition.

   1. Depressed mood most of the day, nearly every day, as indicated by either subjective report (e.g., feels sad, empty, hopeless) or observation made by others (e.g., appears tearful). (Note: In children and adolescents, can be irritable mood.)
   2. Markedly diminished interest or pleasure in all, or almost all, activities most of the day, nearly every day (as indicated by either subjective account or observation).
   3. Significant weight loss when not dieting or weight gain (e.g., a change of more than 5% of body weight in a month), or decrease or increase in appetite nearly every day. (Note: In children, consider failure to make expected weight gain.)
   4. Insomnia or hypersomnia nearly every day.
   5. Psychomotor agitation or retardation nearly every day (observable by others, not merely subjective feelings of restlessness or being slowed down).
   6. Fatigue or loss of energy nearly every day.
   7. Feelings of worthlessness or excessive or inappropriate guilt (which may be delusional) nearly every day (not merely self-reproach or guilt about being sick).
   8. Diminished ability to think or concentrate, or indecisiveness, nearly every day (either by subjective account or as observed by others).
   9. Recurrent thoughts of death (not just fear of dying), recurrent suicidal ideation without a specific plan, or a suicide attempt or a specific plan for committing suicide.

B. The symptoms cause clinically significant distress or impairment in social, occupational, or other important areas of functioning.
C. The episode is not attributable to the physiological effects of a substance or another medical condition.
Note: Criteria A–C represent a major depressive episode.
Note: Responses to a significant loss (e.g., bereavement, financial ruin, losses from a natural disaster, a serious medical illness or disability) may include the feelings of intense sadness, rumination about the loss, insomnia, poor appetite, and weight loss noted in Criterion A, which may resemble a depressive episode. Although such symptoms may be understandable or considered appropriate to the loss, the presence of a major depressive episode in addition to the normal response to a significant loss should also be carefully considered. This decision inevitably requires the exercise of clinical judgment based on the individual's history and the cultural norms for the expression of distress in the context of loss.
D. The occurrence of the major depressive episode is not better explained by schizoaffective disorder, schizophrenia, schizophreniform disorder, delusional disorder, or other specified and unspecified schizophrenia spectrum and other psychotic disorders.
E. There has never been a manic episode or a hypomanic episode.
    Note: This exclusion does not apply if all of the manic-like or hypomanic-like episodes are substance-induced or are attributable to the physiological effects of another medical condition.
With peripartum onset: This specifier can be applied to the current or, if full criteria are not currently met for a major depressive episode, most recent episode of major depression if onset of mood symptoms occurs during pregnancy or in the 4 weeks following delivery.
> **Note:** Mood episodes can have their onset either during pregnancy or postpartum. Although the estimates differ according to the period of follow-up after delivery, between 3% and 6% of women will experience the onset of a major depressive episode during pregnancy or in the weeks or months following delivery. Fifty percent of "postpartum" major depressive episodes actually begin prior to delivery. Thus, these episodes are referred to collectively as *peripartum* episodes. Women with peripartum major depressive episodes often have severe anxiety and even panic attacks. Prospective studies have demonstrated that mood and anxiety symptoms during pregnancy, as well as the "baby blues," increase the risk for a postpartum major depressive episode.
>
> Peripartum-onset mood episodes can present either with or without psychotic features. Infanticide is most often associated with postpartum psychotic episodes that are characterized by command hallucinations to kill the infant or delusions that the infant is possessed, but psychotic symptoms can also occur in severe postpartum mood episodes without such specific delusions or hallucinations.
>
> Postpartum mood (major depressive or manic) episodes with psychotic features appear to occur in from 1 in 500 to 1 in 1,000 deliveries and may be more common in primiparous women. The risk of postpartum episodes with psychotic features is particularly increased for women with prior postpartum mood episodes but is also elevated for those with

a prior history of a depressive or bipolar disorder (especially bipolar I disorder) and those with a family history of bipolar disorders.

Once a woman has had a postpartum episode with psychotic features, the risk of recurrence with each subsequent delivery is between 30% and 50%. Postpartum episodes must be differentiated from delirium occurring in the postpartum period, which is distinguished by a fluctuating level of awareness or attention. The postpartum period is unique with respect to the degree of neuroendocrine alterations and psychosocial adjustments, the potential impact of breast-feeding on treatment planning, and the long-term implications of a history of postpartum mood disorder on subsequent family planning.

Source. Reprinted from American Psychiatric Association: *Diagnostic and Statistical Manual of Mental Disorders*, 5th Edition. Arlington, VA, 2013, p6. 160–161, 186–187. Copyright © 2013 American Psychiatric Association. Used with permission.

Researchers examining the onset of depressive symptoms in the perinatal period found that most episodes began postpartum (40.1%), followed by during (33.4%) and prior to (26.5%) pregnancy (Wisner et al. 2013). Depression can occur in a single episode or in multiple episodes throughout life. Box 6–2 describes the symptoms of MDD, including use of the peripartum onset specifier. All mothers should be screened for depression during pregnancy and postpartum with a validated screening tool such as the Edinburgh Postnatal Depression Scale (American College of Obstetricians and Gynecologists 2018). The American Academy of Pediatrics recommends screening all mothers for PPD at infant well-child checks for the first year of the child's life (Earls et al. 2019). Screening, detection, referral, and treatment of perinatal depression can prevent adverse outcomes, including tragedies such as infanticide, filicide, and legal system involvement.

Multiple risk factors are associated with the development of PPD, the number one risk factor being depression or anxiety during pregnancy. Other factors include lack of social support, stressful life events, relationship problems including domestic violence, low socioeconomic status, and obstetric or medical complications (Robertson et al. 2004). Women with a family history of psychiatric disorders and subclinical symptoms of mood, anxiety, or psychotic disorders are at risk of developing psychiatric complications during the perinatal period (Ross et al. 2005). Available research shows no difference in incidence of PPD between different races and ethnicities. However, rates of treatment initiation, follow-up care, and continuation of care were higher in white women than in Hispanic or African American women (Kozhimannil et al. 2011).

The rate of maternal filicide in MDD with psychosis is 4.5%, which is higher than the rate of filicide in PPP without overt depression (Brockington 2017). Alice experienced subclinical anxiety symptoms during her pregnancy and also had obstetric complications resulting in a cesarean section, both of which are risk factors for the development of PPD. It should be noted that once a woman experiences a perinatal depression episode with psychotic features, the risk of recurrence with each subsequent pregnancy is between 30% and 50%, which is important for women and their families to know when planning future pregnancies (American Psychiatric Association 2013).

FORENSIC ASSESSMENT AND OUTCOME

During the legal proceedings, a forensic psychiatrist was hired to evaluate Alice for a plea of not guilty by reason of insanity (NGRI). Many countries in the world, including Canada, Australia, England, and the Netherlands, have specific laws that address infanticide and reduce the crime from murder to manslaughter. However, in the United States, the defense must rely on the state's NGRI laws or mitigation strategies to change the penalties for these cases. In Chapter 3, Feingold and Lewis discuss Illinois law PA 100-0574, which took effect June 1, 2019. This law recognizes postpartum psychiatric illnesses as mitigating factors in sentencing. Nevertheless, in most of the United States, forensic evaluation and testimony must follow that state's specified NGRI conditions.

Despite differences in state laws and requirements, the general principles for forensic evaluations for insanity are similar and should include a full history of the mother's childhood, young adulthood, and adulthood, including her education, family, occupation, and military experience (if any) and the medical, psychiatric, and behavioral aspects of her life. A clear and full timeline of events, starting from the birth of the infant to the critical incident, is helpful to track progression of the mother's symptoms and aid in establishing an accurate diagnosis.

In Alice's case, the presence of a psychotic thought process and behavior, including delusional beliefs about her child's development that were unwavering despite evidence of normal development; evidence that the thoughts were ego-syntonic; and her isolation and withdrawal from her family were key features to focus upon. These factors, in combination with her lack of sleep for 5 days, illustrated a sharp and profound decline and were major risk factors that would warrant immediate intervention. Unfortunately, this did not occur in Alice's case, and 2 days later she drowned her 5-month-old baby. The crescendo of symptoms that ultimately led to the child's death was an opportunity for intervention, treatment, and, potentially, prevention of the tragic outcome.

Alice was diagnosed with MDD with psychotic features based on her poor sleep, anhedonia, low mood, low energy, lack of care of herself and the baby, and presence of a delusional thought process. Her delusional thoughts remained fixed despite medical evidence to the contrary, which also dissuaded her from seeking further medical workup or assistance for herself or the baby. The ongoing progression and worsening of symptoms in the absence of medication intervention led to her delusions intensifying and ultimately the death of her infant. To answer the question of Alice's state of mind, gathering as much contemporaneous information as possible was helpful in establishing the thought process and possible motivations present at the time.

Despite having a timeline of Alice's deterioration since her child's birth, with an abrupt decline 5 days before the filicide, the court and opposing counsel were likely to highlight that the crime occurred 5 months postpartum. DSM-5 states that peripartum onset is limited to 4 weeks following the birth of the child; however, literature on PPP and PPD with psychosis often states a timeline of 6 months to 1 year (Yawn et al. 2012). This difference in timeline poses a challenge to expert witnesses who must present multiple pieces of literature that support their opinion rather than referring to DSM. They should be able to present the literature from which they drew to inform their opinion and acknowledge the differences present in the literature. Forensic experts should also be ready to discuss limitations within the evidence base. In summary, not only is PPP not directly classified in DSM-5, the peripartum onset timeline is limited to only 4 weeks after birth, and these barriers can produce catastrophic outcomes in the judicial system in terms of NGRI determination and sentencing of these mothers.

Postpartum Psychosis in a Case of Altruistic Filicide

CASE DESCRIPTION

Raphia was a 31-year-old woman who had had an uncomplicated delivery. When she was 10 days postpartum, she accused her husband of poisoning her food and believed that the baby was looking at her strangely. She also noted hearing the voice of God speaking to her, but she would not share with her husband the content of what the voice said. She experienced insomnia and was only sleeping 2 hours per night. Her hygiene declined, and she stopped tending to the baby's needs. The day before psychiatric evaluation, she told her husband that she figured out "how he is doing it" and again accused him of poisoning her and the baby. Raphia continued to report auditory hallucinations of the voice of God, which were becoming stronger and more intense. The following morning, her husband described her as happier and more affectionate toward the baby, but she would not speak to him.

DISCUSSION

The five classifications of motive as identified by Resnick (1969; see Chapter 9) are fatal abuse, unwanted child, altruistic, acute psychosis, and spousal revenge. When a parent decides to kill a child "out of love," believing that death is what is best for the child and serves the child's best interests, it is called *altruistic filicide*. Mothers experiencing psychosis may project their symptoms onto the child and then take the life of that child in an attempt to relieve their own psychotic symptoms (Resnick 1969). Filicide that occurs during an acute psychotic episode is attributed to the perceptual disturbances observed in psychosis, such as command auditory hallucinations or delusional beliefs (e.g., saving the baby by taking its life).

Of mothers who are filicide offenders, 16%–19% eventually go on to commit suicide (Hatters Friedman and Resnick 2007). Furthermore, a 4% risk of infanticide and 5% risk of suicide are estimated in patients with untreated PPP (Hatters Friedman and Sorrentino 2012). Chandra (2001) studied filicidal thoughts in mothers who were emerging from a perinatal psychiatric illness. Among 60 women with PPP, 30% experienced thoughts of infanticide. Of those, one had committed infanticide and one had fatally injured an older child, indicating a 3.33% ($n=2$) risk of infanticide in the population studied. Of the women who attempted to harm themselves deliberately, 50% had also tried to harm their child, representing a 20% filicidal risk ($n=12$) in PPP (Chandra 2001).

FORENSIC ASSESSMENT AND OUTCOME

In Alice's case, an expert witness evaluated the potential for an NGRI plea. Alice's diagnosis was consistent with PPP rather than a psychotic depression or other mental disorder. Raphia reported no prior psychiatric history and had not experienced symptoms of depression during her pregnancy or following the birth of her son. She was, however, experiencing auditory hallucinations and delusions that her husband was poisoning her and her infant. Although Raphia was clearly not able to function normally or care for herself adequately, her family did not seek professional care, and thus she did not get the medical and psychiatric help she needed. After her husband left for work, Raphia, in an acutely psychotic state, placed the 2-week-old infant in his crib and suffocated him. Her husband returned home unexpectedly after forgetting something and found her in their son's room with a plastic bag over the baby's head. She told him she was saving herself and their son from his poisoning. Raphia committed filicide while in a state of acute psychosis, and she did so for altruistic motives: she felt death was in the best interest of her child to save him from her delusional belief that they were being poisoned by her husband.

PPP is officially classified as a rare psychiatric disease in Orphanet, a worldwide online index of rare diseases, yet it is regretfully absent from DSM-5. It is, however, found in the *International Classification of Diseases*, 10th Edition (ICD-10) as code F53.1 (World Health Organization 1992). The absence of PPP in the current edition of DSM makes this diagnosis difficult to use in court. For this reason, a *Daubert* challenge or similar challenge to the validity of the diagnosis could come up in court (*Daubert v. Merrell Dow Pharmaceuticals, Inc.* 1993). This type of challenge functions as a way to only allow scientifically validated information into the courtroom and requires experts to describe the scientific, technical, or other specialized knowledge they possess that will help the court understand the issue. Experts must show that their opinion is based on sufficient facts or data and is the product of reliable principles and methods that they have reliably applied to the facts of the case (*Daubert v. Merrell Dow Pharmaceuticals, Inc.* 1993). These challenges often require presentation of large amounts of scientific data; in Raphia's case, textbooks and scientific literature describing the phenomenon of PPP, including its diagnostic features and how those applied in this situation, were presented. Use of textbooks and meta-analysis publications rather than individual research articles can be more persuasive in these challenges.

It is common, as part of these types of cases, for the court to ask about the risk of future violence. Because PPP is not a manualized diagnosis with clear diagnostic criteria, standardized assessment tools are typically not applicable in this setting. The existing violence risk assessment tools (e.g., Violence Risk Appraisal Guide; Historical, Clinical, and Risk Management–20) are not specifically tailored to the postpartum population and generally do not address factors unique to this period, such as the lack of previous psychiatric history, the challenges faced by mothers in the perinatal period, and the additional stresses inherent to being a new parent. Therefore, violence risk assessments should be used with caution because the results may not be reliable. What is known is that mothers who have perpetrated filicide are not a danger to society when properly treated with medications and psychotherapy. It is very rare for this subpopulation to commit further acts of violence in the future. Although research in the area is limited, one study found that no repeated cases of filicide demonstrated psychotic motivation for the killings (Klier et al. 2019).

Summary

Each of the cases described here focused on a different postpartum presentation that could lead to forensic consultation for either assessment of risk of violence or evaluation of the role of that diagnosis in the commission of infanticide or filicide. Although the level of risk of violence in OCD with peripartum onset is virtually nonexistent, the risk in PPP and MDD with psychotic features is elevated due to the presence of psychotic symptoms, including delusions and hallucinations. The key difference between these categories of risk is the egocentricity of the thoughts or hallucinations. In OCD, intrusive thoughts are ego-dystonic, whereas in psychosis the thoughts or voices are ego-syntonic. This distinction, combined with the mother's previous psychiatric history, history of violence, presence of current suicidal or homicidal thoughts, level of support, and severity of current psychiatric symptoms, can help determine level of risk, diagnosis, and recommendations for monitoring and intervention. The screening, detection, referral, diagnosis, and treatment of perinatal psychiatric disorders are essential to prevent tragic outcomes and legal system involvement. Increased publicity, awareness, research, education, training, and resources for the accurate identification and treatment of perinatal psychiatric complications are urgently needed to adequately address these underrecognized and often misunderstood disorders.

MAIN CLINICAL/LEGAL POINTS AND CULTURAL PERSPECTIVES

- Perinatal psychiatric complications are common. Depression and anxiety disorders are the most common (nearing 20%), with postpartum psychosis (PPP) being less common (0.1%–0.2%). Screening and guidelines for treatment in this population are available but not universally utilized.

- Available data show that rates of postpartum mental health issues are equal among different races and ethnicities but that access to and compliance with treatment is significantly higher among white women than among Hispanic or African American women. This disparity in access and adherence to care can have downstream effects on their mental health issues, including, at its most severe, an increased risk of filicide, neonaticide, and maternal suicide.

- Perinatal psychiatric complications, including mood disorders with psychotic features and PPP, have increased risks of aggression and violence, particularly when untreated. Mood disorders (e.g., major depressive disorder and bipolar disorder) with psychotic features have a higher risk for infanticide, filicide, and suicide when compared with psychotic disorders (e.g., schizophrenia).

- Differentiation of OCD from a psychotic disorder is important for both treatment and the assessment of risk of violence. No cases have been reported in the literature of a mother acting on violent intrusive thoughts associated with OCD.

- Because perinatal psychiatric complications are not well described in DSM-5, medicolegal experts must rely on data from textbooks and scientific literature that describe the phenomenon and its presentation. Although a new edition of DSM may identify PPP, the task force is still considering addition of the diagnosis, with current proposed criteria including psychotic symptoms, mood instability, and cognitive disorganization. The most current edition of DSM must be considered when discussing PPP in a courtroom, including acknowledging the absence of this diagnosis in previous editions of DSM and any other diagnoses listed in DSM that fit the clinical picture.

- In the perinatal population, forensic assessment should follow the same general guidelines as all other types of assessments, with special attention to the unique features and stressors of the perinatal period and the possibility of PPP.

Practice and Discussion Questions

1. Discuss the role of psychiatric testimony in the courtroom in cases of infanticide and altruistic filicide. Do the existing not guilty by reason of insanity (NGRI) laws adequately allow for psychiatric testimony in these cases? If not, why? Are these laws fair to the defendant mother? The public?

2. Discuss the presentation of a woman with major depressive disorder with psychosis versus that of one with postpartum psychosis. What

similarities exist? What differences exist? How do you explain these differences in the courtroom?

3. What are your personal beliefs about filicide and infanticide? How do these beliefs introduce bias into your work with these defendants? What other biases are present in the judicial system? How about in our culture?

4. In the three cases described in this chapter, what would you like to see as the sentence or treatment recommendation? What evidence would you use to support those recommendations?

5. What would you like to see change about NGRI or infanticide laws in these types of cases? What reasons or beliefs are your thoughts founded on?

6. Given the disparity in understanding how ethnic groups differ in access and response to treatment, how can we ensure that these women receive as much care and consideration as other nonminority groups?

References

American College of Obstetricians and Gynecologists: Screening for perinatal depression. ACOG Committee Opinion No 757. Obstet Gynecol 132:208–212, 2018

American Psychiatric Association: Diagnostic and Statistical Manual of Mental Disorders, 5th Edition. Arlington, VA, American Psychiatric Association, 2013

Bergink V, Burgerhout K, Koorengevel K, et al: Treatment of psychosis and mania in the postpartum period. Am J Psychiatry 172(2):115–123, 2015

Bergink V, Rasgon N, Wisner KL: Postpartum psychosis: madness, mania, and melancholia in motherhood. Am J Psychiatry 173(12), 1179–1188, 2016

Brockington I: Suicide and filicide in postpartum psychosis. Arch Womens Ment Health 20:63–69, 2017

Brandes M, Soares CN, Cohen LS: Postpartum onset obsessive-compulsive disorder: diagnosis and management. Arch Womens Ment Health 7:99–110, 2004

Chandra PS: The interface between psychiatry and women's reproductive and sexual health. Indian J Psychiatry 43(4):295–305, 2001

Cohen L, Altshuler L, Harlow B, et al: Relapse of major depression during pregnancy in women who maintain or discontinue antidepressant treatment. JAMA 295(5):499–507, 2006

Daubert v. Merrell Dow Pharmaceuticals, Inc., 509 U.S. 579 (1993)

Earls MF, Yogman MW, Mattson G, Rafferty J: Incorporating recognition and management of perinatal depression into pediatric practice. Pediatrics 143(1), 2019

Fairbrother N, Janssen P, Antony M, et al: Perinatal anxiety disorder prevalence and incidence. J Affect Disord 200:148–155, 2016

Forray A, Focseneanu M, Pittman B, et al: Onset and exacerbation of obsessive-compulsive disorder in pregnancy and the postpartum period. J Clin Psychiatry 71(8):1061–1068, 2010

Gaudiano BA, Dalrymple KL, Zimmerman M: Prevalence and clinical characteristics of psychotic versus nonpsychotic major depression in a general psychiatric outpatient clinic. Depress Anxiety 26(1):54–64, 2009

Gavin N, Gaynes B, Lohr K, et al: Perinatal depression: a systematic review of prevalence and incidence. Obstet Gynecol 106(5):1071–1083, 2005

Gaynes BN, Gavin N, Meltzer-Brody S, et al: Perinatal depression: prevalence, screening accuracy, and screening outcomes. Evid Rep Technol Assess (Summ) 119:1–8, 2005

Hatters Friedman S, Resnick PJ: Child murder by mothers: patterns and prevention. World Psychiatry 6(3):137–141, 2007

Hatters Friedman S, Sorrentino R: Commentary: postpartum psychosis, infanticide, and insanity—implications for forensic psychiatry. J Am Acad Psychiatry Law 40:326–332, 2012

Karakasi M, Markopoulou M, Tentes IK, et al: Prepartum psychosis and neonaticide: rare case study and forensic-psychiatric synthesis of literature. J Forensic Sci 62(4):1097–1105, 2017

Kessler RC, Petukhova M, Sampson NA, et al: Twelve-month and lifetime prevalence and lifetime morbid risk of anxiety and mood disorders in the US. Int J Methods Psychiatr Res 21(3):169–184, 2012

Klier C, Amon S, Putkonen H, et al: Repeated neonaticide: differences and similarities to single neonaticide events. Arch Womens Ment Health 22(1):159–164, 2019

Kozhimannil K, Trinacty C, Busch A, et al: Racial and ethnic disparities in postpartum depression care among low-income women. Psychiatr Serv 62(6):619–625, 2011

Lawrence PJ, Craske MG, Kempton C, et al: Intrusive thoughts and images of intentional harm to infants in the context of maternal postnatal depression, anxiety and OCD. Br J Gen Pract 67:376–377, 2017

Maina G, Albert U, Bogetto F, et al: Recent life events and obsessive-compulsive disorder (OCD): the role of pregnancy/delivery. Psychiatry Res 89:49–58, 1999

Masters GA, Brenkle L, Sankaran S, et al: Positive screening rates for bipolar disorder in pregnant and postpartum women and associated risk factors. Gen Hosp Psychiatry 61:53–59, 2019

Namouz-Hadad S, Nulman I: Safety of treatment of obsessive compulsive disorder in pregnancy and puerperium. Can Fam Physician 60(2):133–136, 2014

Resnick PJ: Child murder by parents: a psychiatric review of filicide. Am J Psychiatry 126(3):73–82, 1969

Robertson E, Grace S, Wallington T, et al: Antenatal risk factors for postpartum depression: a synthesis of recent literature. Gen Hosp Psychiatry 26(4):289–295, 2004

Ross LE, Murray BJ, Steiner M: Sleep and perinatal mood disorders: a critical review. J Psychiatry Neurosci 30(4):247–256, 2005

Russell E, Fawcett J, Mazmanian D: Risk of obsessive-compulsive disorder in pregnant and postpartum women: a meta-analysis. J Clin Psychiatry 74(4):377–385, 2013

Sharma V, Mazmanian D: The DSM-5 peripartum specifier: prospects and pitfalls. Arch Womens Ment Health 17(2):171–173, 2014

Spinelli MG: Maternal Infanticide Associated with Mental Illness: Prevention and the Promise of Saved Lives. Am J Psychiatry 161(9):1548–1557, 2004

Spinelli MG: Postpartum psychosis: detection and risk and management. Am J Psychiatry 166(4):405–408, 2009

Stewart DE, Vigod S: Postpartum depression. N Engl J Med 375(22):2177–2186, 2016

Suppes T, Dennehy EB, Hirschfeld RM, et al: The Texas implementation of medication algorithms: update to the algorithms for treatment of bipolar I disorder. J Clin Psychiatry 66(7):870–886, 2005

Torres A, Prince M, Bebbington P, et al: Obsessive compulsive disorder: prevalence, comorbidity, impact, and help-seeking in the British National Psychiatric morbidity study of 2000. Am J Psychiatry 163:1978–1985, 2006

VanderKruik R, Barreix M, Chou D, et al: The global prevalence of postpartum psychosis: a systematic review. BMC Psychiatry 17:272, 2017

Veale D, Freeston M, Krebs G, et al: Risk assessment and management in obsessive-compulsive disorder. Adv Psychiatr Treat 15:332–343, 2009

Wesseloo R, Kamperman AM, Munk-Olsen T, et al: Risk of postpartum relapse in bipolar disorder and postpartum psychosis: a systematic review and meta-analysis. Am J Psychiatry 173(2):117–127, 2016

Wisner KL, Sit DK, McShea MC, et al: Onset timing, thoughts of self-harm, and diagnoses in postpartum women with screen-positive depression findings. JAMA Psychiatry 70(5):490–498, 2013

World Health Organization: The ICD-10 Classification of Mental and Behavioural Disorders: Clinical Descriptions and Diagnostic Guidelines. Geneva, World Health Organization, 1992

Yawn B, Olson A, Bertram S, et al: Postpartum depression: screening, diagnosis, and management programs 2000 through 2010. Depress Res Treat 2012

CHAPTER 7

Altruistic Filicide

A TRAUMA-INFORMED PERSPECTIVE

Diana Barnes, Psy.D., LMFT, PMH-C

The societal conversation around motherhood idealizes mothers (Badinter 1981; Barnes and Balber 2008; Douglas and Michaels 2005; Thurer 1994). Even the word *mother* is imbued with qualities applicable to sainthood: limitless availability, unrelenting love and affection, omniscience and omnipotence. Although the instinct to nurture and protect exists (Dobson and Sales 2000; Gauthier et al. 2003), other stereotypical ideas about a mother's inherent capacity to instinctively know, spontaneously understand, and automatically anticipate her infant's needs pervade the maternal dialogue (Barnes 2014). However, the grand narratives of the good mother overlook the realities of human frailty that originate in a young woman's story of her relationship with her own mother and the ways in which her early psychosocial environment informs her thinking as she becomes a mother (Barnes 2014).

Because we revere mothers, we demonize them when their actions refute those constructs of the "good mother" embedded in the cultural perspectives and expectations we have shared throughout many generations. When a mother kills her child, it defies logical thought and violates a fundamental law of nature—that is, nurturing and protecting one's young to ensure their survival. When a mother harms or takes the life of her babies, we have no mental space to grasp the possibility that this mother might have been so mentally ill that she committed this incomprehensible act firmly out of altruistic motives, believing it was in the very best interests of that child. *Altruistic filicide* is murder committed out of a mother's love and her desire to relieve her child's real or imagined suffering because she is convinced that keeping the child alive is a fate worse than death. Women who commit infanticide are generally laboring under psychotic delusions that fuel their beliefs about their child's safety in the present. In the courtrooms of the United States, altruism has been identified as one of five motives for filicide (Resnick 1969). The other motives include the unwanted child, accidental filicide as a consequence of abuse, spousal revenge, and the acutely psychotic mother (Resnick 1969). The latter is discussed later in this chapter.

Having specialized in the field of women's reproductive mental health for 25 years, I have evaluated and talked with countless young women incarcerated for crimes against their children that occurred when they were in the throes of postpartum psychotic illness. In the course of our conversations, what has become clear is that the origins of their psychotic thinking run much deeper than genetics alone. Understanding a mother's state of mind in order to explain why she would commit the unthinkable goes beyond symptoms and is rooted within her own entrenched memories of real personal experiences of violence, neglect, and abandonment. This chapter looks at postpartum psychosis (PPP) and infanticide from a biopsychosocial perspective, addressing the significant connections between early experience, its impact on brain development, and the onset of serious mental illness (i.e., PPP). The following discussion challenges the idea that mothers with PPP are criminals who should be punished for life, instead presenting the science and fact that women with PPP are the psychiatric hostages of this illness, which distorts reality to such an extent that past and present become fused in a maelstrom of sensory distortions and false beliefs.

In the Beginning: Childhood Trauma and Disrupted Attachment

Our earliest attachment experiences create a psychological template for other relationships across the lifespan, setting up expectations and response patterns for future circumstances and situations that are reminders of original events (Bowlby 2008). From infancy, we rely on the care and goodwill of our primary caregivers to give meaning to our experiences. We are biologically programmed as we enter this world to seek out the comfort of an attachment figure in the service of our own survival (Bretherton 1992; see Chapter 13 for further discussion of trauma and attachment). Consequently, when a woman experiences childhood trauma and has no opportunity to make meaning of these earliest events with consistently responsive, caring and loving caregivers, it makes perfect sense that she would struggle to feel safe. She has never been able to establish a framework for trust and safety.

John Bowlby, the grandfather of attachment theory, enhanced our understanding that early relational experiences and events are a psychological launching pad for feelings of trust and safety across the lifespan. This sense of safety is predicated upon four basic tenets of attachment theory: 1) proximity; 2) separation; 3) safe haven, and 4) secure base (Bowlby 2008). Developmentally, even from infancy, the knowledge that one can maintain closeness or proximity to the primary caregiver is essential. Distress upon separation is expected for the young child; in essence, it indicates that an important interpersonal connection has been established. Primary attachments provide a safe haven for comfort when needed. The ultimate sense of trust and safety comes from knowing that the attachment figure provides a secure base and will be emotionally available when needed. Women with histories of childhood trauma, such as sexual or physical abuse, neglect, abandonment, and disrupted attachments, have no assurances that any of these fundamental attachment requirements exist. The absence of these attachment imperatives eventually has a negative impact on mood and overall mental health as the young woman matures and reaches childbearing years (Liotti 2004).

For women with traumatic histories, the onset of motherhood frequently revives and triggers those memories, often thought to have perished with the past. This revival creates confusion between then and now, not only for the new mother herself but also for the relationship she has with her children. Under extreme stress, past and present can become fused to the extent that they ultimately become indistinguishable from one another. In my many years of experience working with countless mothers, it has become clear to me that this psychological enmeshment between complex childhood trauma and current circumstances fuels the altruistic delusions of PPP. Just as instinctive impulses and spontaneous behaviors exist for nonpsychotic mothers and serve to safeguard their infants, a maternal instinct to protect exists within the confines of the delusional mind.

The Psychology of Trauma

A logic is woven through the disordered thought process of a psychotic mother in which she unwittingly relies on her own experience of past traumatic events to make decisions about the safety of her children in the present. A psychotic delusion is not simply an isolated symptom of an altered mind but a psychological marker that reflects a longstanding accumulation of unresolved loss, traumatic events, and disrupted attachments. Numerous researchers have found a causal relationship between childhood exposure to adverse experiences and later psychotic illness (Read et al. 2014) as well as a graded relationship between the number of childhood exposures to traumatic events and the degree of risk conferred (Anda et al. 2006; Shevlin et al. 2007). Some researchers found emotional abuse and neglect to be the most represented of traumatic childhood experiences, followed by physical neglect, physical abuse, and sexual abuse (Duhig et al. 2015; Larsson et al. 2013). Trauma disrupts attachment security that is so necessary for healthy psychological and social/emotional development, especially when the source of that trauma is the parents themselves. Such experiences induce a sense of terror, fear, and helplessness in the children victimized.

There is no doubt that fear changes the thoughts, emotions, and behaviors (Read et al. 2014) of people who experience complex childhood trauma. When they are threatened with abuse, children often dissociate; this reflexive defense strategy enables them to endure the untenable circumstances of the unfolding abuse while psychologically distancing themselves from it (Liotti and Gumley 2008). For victims of abuse, dissociation creates a psychological separation between the body and mind that alters conscious awareness of what is occurring in the present. The combination of the undue stress and circumstances of pregnancy and a history of trauma is frequently what sets the wheels of PPP in motion. The earliest relational experiences create a foundational road map for future experiences reminiscent of the original trauma. Thus, although to the nonpsychotic mind it may seem paradoxical to take the infant's life in order to save that infant, for a mother in the throes of psychotic illness, an altruistic filicide is actually a demonstration of maternal love and protection.

The Neurobiology of Trauma

The neurodevelopmental changes caused by trauma in the early years slowly chip away at rational thought. These alterations in brain function and chemistry are consistently found in individuals with psychotic disorders (Larsson et al. 2013; Read et al. 2014; Varese et al. 2012). Read et al. (2014) found that the brains of traumatized children looked strikingly similar those of people with schizophrenia. Their traumagenic neurodevelopmental model of psychosis explains the relationship between early trauma and later psychotic illness by attempting to integrate biological and psychological processes toward a further understanding of some of the origins of psychosis. Over time, repetitive trauma dysregulates the stress response system, which results in the heightened reactivity to stress seen in individuals with psychotic disorders as well as in those with PTSD. Continuous exposure to traumatic events also affects brain chemistry, structure, and functioning.

Changes in the chemistry and even in the architecture of the brain resulting from trauma can occur as early as the womb, ultimately altering the course of normal brain maturation. These injuries may lead to structural changes in the frontal lobe, the part of the brain implicated in executive functioning, as well as to shrinkage in the hippocampus, the part responsible for memory (Teicher et al. 2012). Elevation in cortisol levels is a normal physiological reaction to stress; however, when the body's fight-or-flight mechanism is continuously pummeled by traumatic and toxic stress, over time, it can have a deleterious effect.

Walker et al. (2010) identified that heightened cortisol levels often precede psychosis onset. Research has also shown a link between traumatic events in childhood and the persistence and severity of auditory hallucinations (Bartels-Velthius et al. 2012). One researcher noted that the time span between the onset of hearing voices and the traumatic or stress-inducing event was short (Escher et al. 2002). One mother I evaluated was charged with the murder of her three young children. She had been experiencing psychotic hallucinations and delusions at the time of the act. This mother reported hearing voices beginning at age 5, which was in close proximity to the death of her grandmother, with whom she had been exceptionally close.

Postpartum Psychosis

PPP is an insidious illness that reconfigures rational thought. Although rare, occurring in only 1 or 2 of every 1,000 births (Vanderkruik et al. 2017), it is considered a potentially life-threatening medical emergency that can threaten the life of both mother and child when left untreated (Sit et al. 2006; Spinelli 2009). For women with a diagnosis of bipolar disorder, the prevalence rate for PPP is 100 times that of the general population of pregnant women (Stewart et al. 1991). In a classic study, Kendall et al. (1987) found that among patients with PPP, 72%–80% had comorbid bipolar disorder or schizoaffective disorder, while 12% were comorbid with schizophrenia. Thus, any assessment of a mother's risk must consider her personal/family history of serious mood disorders as well as psychotic disorders. Studies also indicate that in the United

States, 5% of women with PPP commit suicide and 4% take the life of their child or children, with the birth of the baby as the catalyst for infanticide (Brockington 2017; Lindahl et al. 2005; Sit et al. 2006).

Psychosis in childbearing women looks quite different than in other psychotic disorders, particularly because of the strong mood component along with extreme cognitive disorganization (Bergink et al. 2015; Boyce and Barriball 2010; Wisner et al. 1994). Conceptualized as a variant of bipolar disorder, PPP has an atypical and complex presentation of symptoms that includes amnesia, extreme shifts in mood from euphoria to melancholia, cognitive confusion and disorganized thought, dissociation, agitation, disrupted sleep, neglected hygiene, and paranoia along with expected auditory hallucinations and delusions. In many ways, PPP presents like a delirium and has been termed by some as a "cognitive disorganization psychosis" (Wisner et al. 1994, p. 77).

The behavior of women with PPP is often disorganized. A woman may experience dissociative symptoms, such as depersonalization and derealization. Women often lack insight about the seriousness of their illness; as a result of her break with reality, she does not recognize that her delusions are just that—false beliefs without any foundation in fact. A woman with delusions of control may feel driven by a powerful force that overtakes her, leaving her devoid of any personal agency over her own behavior. Delusions of reference and persecutory/paranoid delusions are often a significant part of the clinical presentation of PPP. Their suspiciousness and subsequent mistrust may prompt some women to hide their delusional thinking from their families. Likewise, it is not uncommon for a diagnosis of PPP to be missed because symptoms often wax and wane, leaving a woman lucid one moment and floridly psychotic the next. In addition, women with PPP may present with depressed mood that is mistakenly diagnosed as major depressive disorder rather than a bipolar episode (Bergink et al. 2016). An undiagnosed bipolar episode can cause potentially serious mood complications when the woman is prescribed an antidepressant medication alone instead of a mood stabilizer to address her bipolarity (Sharma et al. 2008).

The Case of Ashley N

The story that follows reflects the experience of a young woman who was charged with murder for the death of her 7-month-old infant and facing life imprisonment because of untreated perinatal illness. Her history is strikingly similar to the stories of many women I have seen who find themselves in the criminal justice system under similar circumstances, a background filled with multiple examples of abuse, neglect, abandonment, and terror. Her narrative offers a glimpse into the unraveling of a mind, with complex childhood trauma as the catalyst. This mother, Ashley N, agreed and even encouraged me to share the details of her case in the hope that her experience will shed light and perspective on the fragility of pregnancy and motherhood, especially when this psychological and emotional milestone is preceded by a traumatic history.

> Ashley was no stranger to complex childhood trauma. Her father had alcoholism and became unpredictably enraged and even violent whenever he was drunk, which was frequently. Ashley had been repeatedly molested by a female cousin starting in early childhood until age 11 and was a victim of sexual abuse again at the hand of her father's close male friend when she was just 12 years old. By age 15, Ashley was experiencing anxiety and panic; she made her first suicide attempt at age 17, which resulted in a psychiatric hospitalization. Ashley made a second attempt at age 20, a third at age 21, and her fourth at age 23 on the same day as and just prior to her arrest for the murder of her 7-month-old baby. In my assessment, Ashley was in the throes of a delusional thought process in which she believed that taking her own life and the life of her baby would send them to heaven to start over and give them a better chance at fulfilling lives.
>
> In my role as an expert witness in the case, I discovered that Ashley's family psychiatric history spanned both the maternal and paternal sides. Both great-grandmothers had had major depression that resulted in hospitalization. In addition, Ashley's paternal aunt had attempted suicide after losing a child to a fatal infection, and her maternal grandmother had been diagnosed with schizophrenia before Ashley was born. Ashley's own mother had multiple depressive episodes as Ashley was growing up, and although her father had never been clinically diagnosed, he showed clear signs of major depression and suicidal behavior. On one occasion, he pointed a gun at his head while breaking down in tears in front of Ashley. Together, the mental illness of her family and the history of family chaos and trauma placed Ashley at a significantly elevated risk for a psychotic episode in the postpartum period.
>
> Although her pregnancy was unplanned, Ashley was excited at the prospect of becoming a mother. She stopped her mood stabilizer during her pregnancy because she was afraid the medication would result in birth defects. At about 4 months' gestation, the doctors discovered fluid on the fetal brain and expressed concerns about Down's syndrome. Ashley was given the option of terminating the pregnancy but chose not to because subsequent tests showed no fluid on the fetal brain. However, this uncertainty caused her considerable worry and uncertainty about the baby's health throughout the rest of her pregnancy. A difficult birth resulted in an unexpected cesarean delivery of a healthy baby boy.
>
> Ashley recalls the downward spiral into depression at 2 months postpartum and the dramatic shift between her initial joy and subsequent suspicion: "I was so mistrusting of everybody. I wouldn't let anyone hold

him. I felt like I was the only one who knew what he needed." It was clear that Ashley's fears were further aggravated by her boyfriend, who was preoccupied with conspiracy theories including government invasions, others altering textbooks to manipulate history, and people being kidnapped out of their homes.

When Ashley and I sat together and talked, she recognized that her extreme caution with regard to safety and trust had its origins in family messages and her childhood trauma, especially pertaining to the sexual abuse she endured. She revealed, "I've never trusted people, but it kept getting worse and worse. I was always paranoid about the world—everything going wrong." As a child, Ashley was not allowed to leave the house because her father did not trust anyone to be alone with her out of fear that something bad would happen to her. She was repeatedly told, "What's rule #1 in life, Ashley? Trust no one, just me and your mom. No one else is allowed in the circle of trust." It was only on one occasion that her father allowed, and even encouraged, her to go with one of his male friends, whom he trusted, so that Ashley could be outfitted for go-cart races. This friend molested her.

On the day Ashley took the life of her 7-month-old son, faulty early messages about trust and safety, along with unresolved experiences of betrayal and her maternal instinct to protect, sparked a delusional terror. Her capacity to differentiate her own childhood trauma from the current circumstances evaporated. Laboring under extreme paranoia, guardedness, and a psychotic belief that she and her baby were in grave danger and being followed by men who intended to kill them, she firmly believed she had to protect her son either from death or from the alternate possibility that he would grow up without her in the same "dangerous and disgusting world" in which she had been raised. Ashley reported to police officers at the scene that she believed she was being followed and was terrified that she herself would be dismembered, repeatedly insisting that her only intention was to protect her child and save him from suffering. She explained to the officer that she was so scared the people chasing her were going to hurt her baby that she believed taking her son's life was the better and only way out. In her own words, Ashley said, "I was scared that people are going to hurt him and someone's going to touch him in an inappropriate place." Such a statement of belief exemplifies an unconscious reference to the traumatic memories of her own history of sexual abuse.

Even in her delusional state, Ashley's behavior had been governed by a maternal instinct to protect her baby and to do what she believed would keep him safe. It is this steadfast belief that a mother is saving her baby from perceived harm that encompasses the term *altruistic*.

On that day, Ashley had driven her boyfriend to work, and her encounter with several of his male coworkers set in motion the paranoid delusion that she was being followed. Believing she was being followed by a band of unknown men, Ashley jumped into her car to escape and drove onto the freeway, eventually becoming lost and finally ending up in an unknown park. She grabbed a couple of jackets from her car so she could bundle her son up, because it was a chilly outside. When she was unable to run any deeper into the woods to hide from the perceived assailants, she believed that she and her son were trapped and that he would be taken from her. Ashley sat down and fed her son a bottle, then wrapped him in a blanket and rocked him to sleep with a prayer. In her haste to protect him, she decided to use a knife because she thought stabbing would be a quicker escape than smothering and that he would suffer less. Ashley then slit her own wrists so they could die together and he would not be alone. She was convinced at that moment that, "maybe if we die, we get to start over again and do a better job next time."

Ashley did not die from her self-inflicted wounds and was charged with premeditated murder. Fearful that a jury might not understand her mental illness and would hand down a verdict of life in prison, she agreed to a plea bargain that reduced her sentence to 10 years. No discussion of altruistic filicide, the impact of childhood traumas, past family mental illness, and so on were taken into consideration or part of the deconstruction of the events that led to her son's death. As of this writing, Ashley remains in state prison for the death of her child.

Identifying Risk

When preparing for trial any case that involves maternal mental illness, personal and family history becomes exceedingly important in establishing the circumstances that put this particular woman at grave risk for the onset of PPP and the eventual outcome that led to criminal charges. Numerous risks in Ashley's background could have been identified long before she gave birth, including her family history of alcoholism, major depression, and schizophrenia on both the maternal and paternal line; her preexisting history of anxiety and mania, along with her multiple suicide attempts; her history of sexual molestation and abuse; the cesarean birth of her son; and her boyfriend with paranoia.

In cases of infanticide, reproductive events are invariably intertwined with personal and family psychiatric histories in addition to any psychosocial stress pertaining to the current pregnancy. For Ashley, even though her motives were pure—believing she was protecting her unborn child by ceasing her medication during pregnancy—given her preexisting psychiatric history and her family's mental health background, the absence of medication to stabilize her mood during her pregnancy laid the initial groundwork for the critical incident that turned lethal (Gabriel and Sharma 2017).

Even though Ashley's concerns regarding the health of her unborn child were unfounded, they acted as a trigger for her escalating anxiety and worry. An unplanned cesarean birth can have a detrimental psychological impact on a new mother because it is unexpected, physically and mentally taxing, and presents a stark departure from the ideal vision that most women expect from the birth of their children. A birth itself can revive traumatic memories for women who have experienced childhood sexual abuse, with the delivery acting as a catalyst for prior experiences of helplessness and powerlessness. Had she received periodic screening during her pregnancy and early postpartum period along with appropriate attention to the obvious risks imposed by her extensive personal and family history of psychiatric illness, the epilogue of her story might have looked quite different.

Infanticide Is Not Altruistic

Dr. Phillip Resnick, in his early study on filicide in which he established categories of motive to explain possible reasons for infanticide (Resnick 1969), identified as one of his categories the acutely psychotic mother whose behavior and actions were solely governed by psychotic symptoms, including hallucinations and delusions.

> On A11ugust 5, 2011, Sarah J. called 911 for help because her 3-week-old daughter was not breathing and was cold to the touch. She was instructed by the emergency operators on how to perform CPR until medical personnel arrived. Physical examination of the infant showed no bruises, no injuries, and no signs of trauma. One of the detectives noted in his summary report that he saw no indications that Sarah was "not being a good mom." Her sister relayed to detectives that Sarah was quite depressed and had gone to the emergency department the night before because she was having suicidal thoughts. The medical examiner's office reported that the autopsy was inconclusive as to the manner of the child's death.

The established links between early trauma and psychotic illness exist independent of motive. Like Ashley, Sarah's psychotic illness originated in a backdrop of trauma and family chaos that included verbal and emotional abuse, alcoholism, drug abuse, and a personal and family history of eating disorders and depression. For Sarah, understanding her reproductive history is essential because it establishes a foundation for her downward spiral into depression and ultimately an acute psychotic episode. It also offers an explanation as to how a young woman with no criminal record and no involvement with child protective services who had served her country and been honorably discharged from the Coast Guard due to depressed mood would take the life of the baby she so desperately wanted.

> Sarah became pregnant twice at age 19, deciding with her husband to terminate those pregnancies because the couple was financially unstable and did not feel emotionally ready to start a family. At age 30, by mutual agreement, she became pregnant again. At 20 weeks' gestation, an ultrasound revealed a lethal anomaly called thanatophoric dysplasia, and they were presented with three untenable options: 1) let the baby decease in the womb; 2) let the infant pass from respiratory failure if she survived the birth, or 3) terminate the pregnancy. Sarah and her husband decided to terminate the pregnancy; however, she paid for the procedure with her own money and traveled out of state by herself, where she went through it alone. Grief stricken and severely depressed, Sarah became obsessed with the idea of becoming pregnant again and took multiple pregnancy tests—*hundreds of them*. Six months later, she was pregnant.
> Similar to Ashley's pregnancy, high alerts for problems with the unborn child turned out to be false alarms. Early in the pregnancy, doctors told her the fetal head size looked abnormal, then revised their opinion a couple of weeks later. At 36 weeks' gestation, Sarah was advised of a heart arrhythmia, then told again soon after that everything was normal. This only served to intensify her anxiety. She recalled that, "The whole pregnancy was like walking on eggshells." She went through the entire pregnancy "not expecting her to make it," referring to the unborn child.

Constructing the Narrative

MEDICATION

The use of medication to treat mood can be a critical piece in sustaining mental health during pregnancy and the postpartum period. The absence of appropriate medication management in high-risk women can set the stage for potentially lethal consequences, as seen with both Ashley and Sarah. Ashley stopped her mood stabilizer during pregnancy for fear of birth defects. Sarah had a history of using antidepressant medication, Prozac that she had gotten from her sister. She titrated the doses on her own, moving from one dosage to another as she felt was necessary. From 2006 to 2008, she took Prozac to treat an eating disorder and then stopped when she became pregnant in 2009. After she terminated that pregnancy due to the fetal anomaly, she resumed the Prozac, but stopped again when she became pregnant in 2010. She was only a few days postpartum when she began to feel debilitated by depression, so she started taking pills left over from a clinic where she had previously received care. She took the medication for 3 weeks and then stopped because she felt no improvement. Years of inconsistent medication management left her at serious risk for relapse.

SIGNIFICANCE OF BEHAVIOR
IN THE THIRD TRIMESTER

Pregnancy is not protective against mood disorders. In fact, it is an extremely vulnerable time for the onset of depression and anxiety (Shakeel et al. 2015). Even PPP often begins to rear its ugly head during the last trimester of pregnancy and is noticeable in the kinds of manic behaviors that some women demonstrate. To the nonclinical eye, doing research and preparing for baby can appear to be quite normal behavior for an expecting mother. The excessiveness of the behavior, coupled with other identifiable risk factors, such as family history of bipolar disorder, is the most telling. Sarah was on the computer more than 5 hours a day every day researching proper car seats, the merits of cloth versus paper diapers, and breastfeeding clothes that would not be itchy. She was driving aimlessly around the neighborhood in the middle of the night and remembered being exceptionally anxious.

ESCALATION OF SYMPTOMS

Sarah had a constant fear that her baby would die. Upon bringing her infant daughter home, she held her most of the time because she did not want her to cry or be sad, an unconscious reference to her own very unhappy childhood. Sarah slept on the floor so that if she inadvertently fell asleep, the baby would not fall out of her arms. Due to the relentless requirements of a newborn, and with no one to help her, she became exhausted, only getting 30 minutes of sleep each night. Eventually, the separation between day and night became a blur. She described feeling like she was "suffocating" and being so sleep deprived that she felt she was on "automatic pilot" and "emotionally numb."

By the day of the critical incident, Sarah was living in a "foggy haze, either staring out the window or bawling," feeling alone and "going through the motions." She described her state of mind as "drowning" and "mentally gone." Then she panicked about her daughter's future, not wanting the child to experience the same kinds of trauma that she had suffered. In the midst of the panic, "something just switched inside of me suddenly." It felt as though her daughter was "an extension of me." "I didn't see her as a person with her own needs and wants." She had lost agency over her own behavior, with the sense that she was "on the outside looking at myself," "watching myself do the acts." She used the word "hyper-focus." It felt to her as though she was suffocating and unable to distinguish herself from her daughter. In a state of tremendous confusion and cognitive disorganization, she smothered her daughter.

Brief Psychotic Disorder

Defense counsel's objective in retaining me was first to evaluate Sarah in order to offer an opinion about her mental state in the weeks preceding and following the birth of her daughter and then to testify as to that opinion. Alaska uses a modified version of the M'Naghten rule, referred to as the "right and wrong test," in determining insanity, with the burden of proof on the defendant. I opined that Sarah had experienced a brief psychotic disorder with postpartum onset and a temporary loss of contact with reality that would have made it impossible for her to distinguish between right and wrong at the time of the commission of the act. Because this case was tried in 2011, I used the terminology of DSM-IV (American Psychiatric Association 1994); if Sarah had gone to trial after May 2013, her diagnosis would have been brief psychotic disorder with peripartum onset (DSM-5; American Psychiatric Association 2013).

The essential feature of a brief psychotic disorder involves the sudden onset of symptoms that include either delusions, hallucinations, or grossly disorganized speech. Sarah came to believe that there was no personal boundary between herself and her infant, ultimately believing she was taking her own life and not that of her daughter. With postpartum onset, brief psychotic disorder typically occurs within 4 weeks of birth, and the onset is generally sudden. It lasts as short as 1 day and no longer than 1 month, after which individuals eventually return to their level of functioning before the onset of symptoms (American Psychiatric Association 2013). Although this postpartum psychotic episode may be brief, the cognitive and psychological impairment is so severe that individuals are in grave danger of hurting themselves or others, which was exactly the case with Sarah. Most often, a brief psychotic disorder occurs in reaction to trauma or prolonged, undue stress; women in the throes of this brief psychosis experience overwhelming confusion and cognitive disorganization. Sarah's symptom presentation fit the clinical picture of a brief psychotic disorder with postpartum onset for a number of reasons:

1. The psychotic episode occurred at 3 weeks postpartum, so it fit the time frame.
2. She experienced a sudden onset of symptoms, described by her as "feeling as though something switched inside of me suddenly."
3. She had the bizarre delusion that she and the infant were one and that "there was a defect inside of me that needed to be fixed."

4. Sleep deprivation was the proverbial "straw that broke the camel's back"; extreme sleep deprivation can be a contributory factor in the onset of psychotic symptoms (Sharma and Mazmanian 2003; Sharma et al. 2004).
5. Within a month following the critical incident, Sarah had resumed normal functioning.

Postpartum Psychosis in the Courtroom

A frequently used argument by the prosecution against insanity maintains that the accused mother became angry at the child because of the demands of infant care, such as persistent crying, or that she killed the child as revenge against an unsupportive or emotionally abusive partner. However, a number of factors distinguish the new mother who is gravely disabled by her illness from the woman who might be acting with intention (Resnick 1969; Twomey 2009). Women who commit infanticide are not generally violent mothers whose abuse gradually escalates to homicide; this is not a dominant characteristic of women with PPP. They may have already been seeking or receiving medical help but been misdiagnosed (Resnick 1969). In most cases, they make no attempt to conceal what has occurred. In fact, these women are the first to alert 911 and call for help. In addition, women with PPP often exhibit strange or bizarre behavior within hours or days prior to the tragic incident (Twomey 2009).

Sharing the story of a woman's life humanizes her. Emphasizing the extreme dichotomy between the loving mother everyone knew and her ultimate actions helps the jury understand that although symptom onset is sudden, women typically do not spontaneously transform from good mother to murderer unless a psychotic illness is driving their behavior. Symptoms may go unnoticed by professionals for weeks, months, and even years before the critical incident finally occurs because PPP waxes and wanes, remitting and reoccurring with a growing vengeance in subsequent pregnancies. Andrea Yates had already begun hearing voices after the birth of her first child, but it was not until shortly after the birth of her fifth child that she drowned her children in the bathtub.

PPP is a treatable illness. With appropriate psychiatric care, women do get well. Jurors need to understand that when a woman has PPP, the psychosis is the perpetrator of the criminal act, and the new mother is a victim of this insidious illness that strips her of the capacity to exercise rational and logical thought and to determine right from wrong. By its very nature, PPP renders a woman insane; delusions are fixed and cannot be willed away.

Relevance of Trauma in the Courtroom

The challenge for mental health experts is in helping juries understand that a woman's history of trauma is *not* just an isolated piece of background information with no relevance to her mental state in the present. Mental disease does not occur in a vacuum. The current scientific understanding of childhood trauma's negative influence on healthy psychological functioning also recognizes the impact these adverse experiences have on brain structure, functioning, and chemistry. These neurobiological consequences have a clinical impact in altering one's thought processes and behaviors to such a degree that it can ultimately result in criminal behavior. Although the American courts have yet to fully understand the nuanced relationship between childhood trauma and PPP, they have begun to acknowledge somewhat that psychosocial history, namely chronic childhood trauma (e.g., sexual abuse), has some significance as a mitigating factor in sentencing. From a defense perspective, telling a woman's "life story," backed by the scientific confirmation that early adverse experiences are a precursor to mental disease, paves the way for a deeper understanding of the role of trauma as a critical piece of evidence in the courtroom.

Conclusion

This chapter addresses the connections between PPP and infanticide, keeping in mind that PPP has both a scientific and a clinical trajectory that often begins as early as childhood. The current legal statutes regarding insanity create a roadblock because their definition of *criminally insane* bears no resemblance to the current scientific understanding of PPP. Although the law states that a person is only insane if she could not distinguish right from wrong at the time of the crime, psychology understands that psychosis creates a mental state that makes logical thought improbable, if not impossible. It is a clear challenge for jurors and courts to step out of their logical minds and into the extraordinary world of the mother with PPP, a world crafted by early experience and its neurobiological consequences. Successfully proving insanity is more likely when counsel can show that although the mother might have understood that her actions were wrong, within her delusional mind existed a logic independent from the thought processes operating in a rational mind.

MAIN CLINICAL/LEGAL POINTS AND CULTURAL PERSPECTIVES

- Always look for childhood trauma because of the links between early trauma and the potential for later psychotic illness.
- Listen to the language women use to describe their state of mind before, during, and after the critical incident, such as "autopilot," "detached," or "a force outside my control."
- Pay attention to a woman's reproductive history and any milestone events, such as a prior stillbirth or unusual or odd behavior around menses.
- Look for a personal and family history of prior mood or psychotic illnesses.
- Even within the context of delusional thinking and other psychotic symptoms, a woman may behave in a way that demonstrates maternal care and protection.

Practice and Discussion Questions

1. What are the legal statutes for insanity in your particular region? If your state uses the M'Naghten rule, how are the cognitive and volitional prongs of that rule interpreted? How do you anticipate that would affect your defense of a woman with postpartum psychosis?
2. What aspects of a woman's psychosocial history do you think would be most compelling to a jury?
3. Postpartum psychosis as a specific entity does not exist in DSM-5. Given that the court looks to DSM as the knowledgeable source of mental disease, how would you argue its existence as an actual mood disorder?
4. The next revised edition of DSM may include postpartum psychosis as a formal diagnostic category. How might this impact cases of altruistic maternal filicide?
5. When constructing a defense for a woman accused of what are described as "heinous crimes" when referring to infanticide, awareness

of one's own biases is essential. What are your initial reactions when you hear that a woman has taken the life of her infant/child?

References

American Psychiatric Association: Diagnostic and Statistical Manual of Mental Disorders, 4th Edition. Washington, DC, American Psychiatric Association, 1994

American Psychiatric Association: Diagnostic and Statistical Manual of Mental Disorders, 5th Edition. Arlington, VA, American Psychiatric Association, 2013

Anda RF, Felitti VJ, Bremner JD, et al: The enduring effects of abuse and related adverse experiences in childhood. Eur Arch Psychiatry Clin Neurosci 256(3):174–186, 2006

Badinter E: Mother Love: Myths and Reality: Motherhood in Modern History. New York, Macmillan, 1981

Barnes DL: The psychological gestation of motherhood, in Women's Reproductive Mental Health Across the Lifespan. Edited by Barnes DL. New York, Springer Publishing, 2014, pp 75–90

Barnes DL, Balber LG: The Journey to Parenthood: Myths, Reality and What Really Matters. Oxford, UK, Radcliffe Publishing, 2008

Bartels-Velthius AA, van de Willige G, Jenner JA, et al: Auditory hallucinations in childhood: associations with adversity and delusional ideation. Psychol Med 42:583–593, 2012

Bergink V, Boyce P, Munk-Olsen T: Postpartum psychosis: a valuable misnomer. Aust NZ J Psychiatry 49(2):102–103, 2015

Bergink V, Rasgon N, Wisner KL: Postpartum psychosis: madness, mania and motherhood. Am J Psychiatry 173(12):1179–1187, 2016

Bowlby J: A Secure Base: Parent-Child Attachment and Healthy Human Development. New York, Basic Books, 2008

Boyce P, Barriball E: Puerperal psychosis. Arch Womens Ment Health 13(1):45–47, 2010

Bretherton I: The origins of attachment theory: John Bowlby and Mary Ainsworth. Dev Psychol 28:759–775, 1992

Brockington I: Suicide and filicide in postpartum psychosis. Arch Womens Ment Health 20:63–69, 2017

Dobson V, Sales BD: The science of infanticide and mental illness. Psychology, Public Policy and Law 6(4):1098–1112, 2000

Douglas S, Michaels M: The Mommy Myth: The Idealization of Motherhood and How It Has Undermined All Women. New York, Simon and Schuster, 2005

Duhig M, Patterson S, Connell M, et al: The prevalence and correlates of childhood trauma in patients with early psychosis. Aust NZ J Psychiatry 49:651–659, 2015

Escher S, Romme M, Buiks A, et al: Independent course of childhood auditory hallucinations: a sequential 3-year-follow-up study. Br J Psychiatry Suppl 43:S10–S18, 2002

Gabriel M, Sharma V: Antidepressant discontinuation syndrome. CMAJ 189(21):E747, 2017

Gauthier DK, Chaudoir NK, Forsyth CJ: A sociological analysis of maternal infanticide in the United States, 1984–1996. Deviant Behav 24(4):393–404, 2003

Kendall RE, Chalmers JC, Platz C: Epidemiology of puerperal psychosis. Br J Psychiatry 150:662–673, 1987

Larsson S, Andreassen OA, Aas M, et al: High prevalence of childhood trauma in patients with schizophrenia spectrum and affective disorder. Compr Psychiatry 54:123–127, 2013

Lindahl V, Pearson JL, Colpe L: Prevalence of suicidality during pregnancy and the postpartum. Arch Womens Ment Health 8(2):77–87, 2005

Liotti G: Trauma, dissociation and disorganized attachment: three strands of a single braid. Psychotherapy: Theory, Research, Practice, Training 41:472–486, 2004

Liotti G, Gumley A: An attachment perspective on schizophrenia: the role of disorganized attachment, dissociation and mentalization, in Psychosis, Trauma and Dissociation: Emerging Perspectives on Severe Psychopthology. Edited by Moskowitz A, Schafer I, Dorahy M. Hoboken, NJ, Wiley-Blackwell, 2008, pp 117–133

Read J, Fosse R, Moskowitz A, Perry B: The traumagenic neurodevelopmental model of psychosis revisited. Neuropsychiatry 4(1):65–79, 2014

Resnick PJ: Child murder by parents: a psychiatric review of filicide. Am J Psychiatry 126(3):325–334, 1969

Shakeel N, Eberhard-Gran M, Sletner KS, et al: A prospective cohort study of depression in pregnancy, prevalence and risk factors in a multi-ethnic population. BMC Pregnancy Childbirth 15:5, 2015

Sharma V, Mazmanian D: Sleep loss and postpartum psychosis. Bipolar Disord 5(2):98–105, 2003

Sharma V, Smith A, Khan M: The relationship between duration of labour, time of delivery, and puerperal psychosis. J Affect Disord 83(2–3):215–220, 2004

Sharma V, Khan M, Corpse C, Sharma P: Missed bipolarity and psychiatric comorbidity in women with postpartum depression. Bipolar Disord 10(6):742–747, 2008

Shevlin M, Dorahy MJ, Adamson G: Trauma and psychosis: an analysis of the National Comorbidity Survey. Am J Psychiatry 164 (1):166–169, 2007

Sit D, Rothschild AJ, Wisner KL: A review of postpartum psychosis. J Womens Health 15(4):352–368, 2006

Spinelli MG: Postpartum psychosis: detection of risk and management. Am J Psychiatry 166(4):405–409, 2009

Stewart D, Klompenhouwer J, Kendall R, Huist A: Prophylactic lithium in puerperal psychosis: the experience of three centres. Br J Psychiatry 158:393–397, 1991

Teicher M, Anderson C, Polcari A: Childhood maltreatment is associated with reduced volume in the hippocampal subfields CA3, dentate gyrus, and subiculum. Proc Natl Acad Sci USA 109:E563–E572, 2012

Thurer S: The Myths of Motherhood: How Culture Reinvents the Good Mother. New York, Houghton Mifflin Harcourt, 1994

Twomey TM: Understanding Postpartum Psychosis: A Temporary Madness. Westport, CT, Praeger Publishing, 2009

Vanderkruik R, Barreix M, Chou D, et al: The global prevalence of postpartum psychosis: a systematic review. BMC Psychiatry 17(1):272, 2017

Varese F, Smeets F, Drukker M, et al: Childhood adversities increase the risk of psychosis: a meta-analysis of patient-control, prospective and cross-sectional cohort studies. Schizophr Bull 38(4):661–671, 2012

Walker E, Brennan P, Esterberg M, et al: Longitudinal changes in cortisol secretion and conversion to psychosis in at-risk youth. J Abnorm Psychol 119:401–408, 2010

Wisner KL, Peindl K, Hanusa BH: Symptomatology of affective and psychotic illnesses related to childbearing. J Affect Disord 30(2):77–87, 1994

CHAPTER 8

Understanding the Mysteries of Pregnancy Denial

Diana Barnes, Psy.D., LMFT, PMH-C

Anne Buist, M.D., FRANCP

Fear has the power to distort reality in any number of ways. As pertains to women's mental health, pregnancy is often the catalyst for reproductive aberrations that are rooted in fear and have psychological implications. Pregnancy denial and subsequent neonaticide are driven by fear and panic (Meyer and Oberman 2001). I (D.B.) had my first experience as an expert witness for a case of pregnancy denial and neonaticide in 2002, when I received a call from an attorney with the Los Angeles Office of the Public Defender. The attorney represented a 23-year-old client who had given birth to a baby in the bathroom of her home and, in a brief psychotic episode and governed by voices, had stabbed the baby. The client was completely unaware that she had even been pregnant or gone into labor. It is hard to imagine that a young woman would not know she is pregnant given that the physical manifestations of pregnancy are so clearly obvious to most of us, especially toward the end of gestation and during the process of birth, yet in 1 out of every 475 pregnancies (Beier et al. 2006; Wessel and Buscher 2002), a young woman's conscious knowledge of pregnancy does not emerge. In some cases, she may have an initial awareness of pregnancy that then disappears. In other cases, however, she has no recognition of pregnancy at all through the 9 months of gestation. What is clear, whether the woman is initially aware of her pregnancy or not, is that a strong connection between pregnancy denial and neonaticide exists (Amon et al. 2012; Hatters Friedman and Resnick 2009).

Having heard of my (D.B.) expertise as a psychotherapist who specializes in assessing and treating pregnancy and postpartum-related mood disorders, the attorney was hoping I could explain to the court the client's state of mind during the 9 months of pregnancy and at birth and how that led to the death of the newborn. Since that initial phone call in 2002, I have been retained by other defense counsel, often several times a year, on cases in which a denied pregnancy and subsequent neonaticide resulted in criminal charges of murder and premeditation with potentially lengthy prison sentences, often ranging between 25 years and life in prison. Depending on the particular state where the incident occurred, parole may or may not be a possibility.

In this chapter, Dr. Anne Buist and I examine the clinical presentation of neonaticide along with the psychological underpinnings that set the stage for pregnancy denial. This chapter differentiates between psychotic and nonpsychotic denial using an actual case from my files that highlights the impact of psychosocial history on psychological defenses and subsequent death of a newborn. The first section of the chapter captures my experiences as a veteran expert witness in neonaticide cases in the United States, followed by Anne's insights into neonaticide in Australia. Anne has more than 30 years of experience in this unique area, identifying the intersection between women's reproductive mental health and the law. We highlight the difference in legal perspectives between Australia and the United States when addressing the criminal implications of pregnancy denial that leads to neonatal death. We conclude our chapter with main clinical and legal points and discussion prompts. Some of the key terms raised in this chapter are defined in the glossary at the end of this book.

Concealment or Denial

In the specialized field of women's reproductive mental health, a dialogue is ongoing about the use of the word *concealment* versus *denial* because the confusion of terms creates difficulties for understanding this reproductive syndrome. *Concealment* and *denial* of pregnancy describe the same phenomenon but with differing degrees of recognizing the pregnancy. *Concealment* is frequently misunderstood in the courtroom as an intentional hiding of the pregnancy and tends to carry a more pejorative meaning, whereas *denial* indicates a refusal to accept the fact of the pregnancy accompanied by emotionally distancing oneself from the realities of that fact. Although a concealed pregnancy does involve a more conscious thought process, the symptoms and behavioral patterns are highly similar to the extensive lack of conscious awareness that exists in pervasive pregnancy denial (Meyer and Oberman 2001). Because of these parallels, concealment and denial are sometimes linked, particularly around labor, birth, and the eventual coping strategies that lead to the death of the newborn. For example, in cases of both concealment and denial, mothers do not experience the expected symptoms of pregnancy, such as morning sickness or feeling of fetal movement. Likewise, in denial as well as concealment, the woman has no recognition of the onset of labor. Consequently, the term *negation of pregnancy* has been used to encompass both concealment and denial given their close clinical association (Beier et al. 2006).

What Is Pregnancy Denial?

The mind has an uncanny ability to remove from conscious view things that are too unbearable to tolerate in the present. Psychological denial is a defense mechanism intended to protect a person from the anticipated negative consequences of a present or past reality. It is an emotion-focused, rather than a problem-focused, solution when one has a firm perception that a given situation cannot be changed (Miller 2003). Ironically, although denial serves a protective function intended to prevent the mother's mind from fragmenting or becoming so overloaded and overwhelmed that it leads to a mental breakdown, the act of giving birth in this state of denial is itself so traumatic that it results in the very psychological breakdown she has spent 9 months avoiding and envelops her in a dissociative process. It is pregnancy denial, also known as *pervasive denial of pregnancy* (Brezinka et al. 1994; Miller 2003) in the scholarly literature, that so often catches the attention of the media and the public because these babies are frequently discovered in dumpsters or trash cans.

Research on pregnancy denial indicates several ways in which pregnancies are "denied" (Miller 2003). In *affective denial*, a woman acknowledges the fact of her pregnancy but, without intention, creates emotional distance between herself and her unborn child. Instead of the heightened emotional sensitivity generally seen when a pregnant woman is in good mental health, a dampened or flat affect is more likely, which looks to the nonclinical eye like indifference. She rarely talks about the pregnancy or her baby and makes no plans for the upcoming birth. Any discussion about the pregnancy results in significantly heightened anxiety. To a nonclinical eye, this can look like difficulty adjusting to the surprise of an unplanned pregnancy, but it is as though the very fact of the pregnancy is a reminder of past or future circumstances that are too painful to tolerate in the present.

Consequently, affective denial acts as a traumatic response to the feeling of being trapped by the pregnancy. In *psychotic denial*, on the other hand, a woman experiences her pregnancy in a delusional way—as a blood clot, a foreign object lodged internally, or a tumor that needs to be removed. These cases are generally more easily identified because of the distinct break with reality and absence of rational thought. However, *pervasive pregnancy denial* is what finds its way to the headline story on the evening news and more often than not into the criminal courts.

Pervasive Pregnancy Denial

In pervasive pregnancy denial, the pregnancy has been obliterated from conscious awareness. As contrasted with affective or psychotic denial, in pervasive denial both the emotional significance and the actual existence of the pregnancy are absent from conscious awareness. The clinical presentation of symptoms is reflective of a dissociative disorder. Dissociation, an involuntary psychological reaction to stress often seen in women with histories of trauma, is a temporary disruption in conscious awareness that alters a woman's ability to respond to the situation before her and her current circumstances. Dissociation has been described in the literature as an atypical psychotic phenomenon (Spinelli 2010). Although a dissociative episode does not have the typical hallmark psychotic symptoms of hallucinations or delusions, it has a dramatic effect on one's ability to think logically; consequently, the immediate environment appears unreal.

Women who experience a pervasive denial of their pregnancy tend to have fewer and less obvious physical indications of pregnancy. In fact, the absence of those hallmark symptoms seen in normal gestation often confirms the diagnosis of pervasive denial. These women typically do not have any morning sickness, and pregnancy tests may be surprisingly negative. They have minimal weight gain, often accompanied by no awareness of fetal movement; more often than not, these women experience spotting or periods during the pregnancy that confirm their negation of the pregnancy because they believe they are menstruating.

It is not unusual in neonaticide cases for the woman's family or close friends to suspect a pregnancy but unintentionally participate in the denial by accepting her word that she is not pregnant and then subsequently dismissing it themselves. When labor occurs, it takes the woman by surprise, and contractions are attributed to other causes such as severe menstrual cramps, food poisoning, or an intestinal flu. The pushing that happens during labor is generally felt as the need to have a bowel movement, and labor most often occurs in the bathroom, with babies commonly being birthed into the toilet (Meyer and Oberman 2001; Neifert and Bourgeois 2000; Spinelli 2001).

Most women in the midst of this psychological disconnect describe an out-of-body sensation along with a feeling that the external environment appears unreal; this sense of being enveloped by a fog is known as *derealization*. Women who negate their pregnancies repeatedly describe watching themselves during the birth. As though in a dream, they become observers of their own actions, unable to intervene or redirect what they are witnessing before them. Their sensory input and perception are severely compromised, as is an accurate awareness of their surrounding environment and their capacity to control their behavior and respond appropriately. Women frequently talk about feeling robotic or on autopilot. These young women experience a separation between body and mind in which they become an observer, not a participant, in their own actions. This split is referred to as *depersonalization*.

UNASSISTED DELIVERIES

Women with pervasive pregnancy denial tend to give birth unassisted, often with others nearby having no sense of what is transpiring in the bathroom next door. Because dissociation distorts sensory input, vision is often blurred and hearing frequently muffled so that the women's perception of what is occurring in the present is grossly skewed. Several of the women I (D.B.) have evaluated described the interruption in consciousness as lights going off and coming on again. This dissociative experience of depersonalization and derealization accounts for the gaps in memory so many women report. In some cases, these women do not even recognize that they have given birth. After spending 9 months psychologically disconnected from the pregnancy, they have developed no emotional connection or loving attachment to the unborn child as expected in a normal pregnancy. This becomes a critical contributory factor to neonaticide because an attachment relationship protects the newborn against the threat of harm from the mother (Crittenden and Ainsworth 1989; Oshri et al. 2015). The disrupted or absent attachment that develops over 9 months of denying the reality of a pregnancy may explain why these women are not even certain they have birthed a child.

Even in situations in which the women do realize what has occurred, in their dissociative state they typically believe the baby is stillborn because they do not see movement or hear a heartbeat. These negated pregnancies are closely linked to the subsequent death of a living newborn within hours of birth because these women commonly wrap the baby in a towel or bag and place them in dumpsters. In addition to exposure to the outside elements, neonaticides in these cases typically occur through suffocation or drowning, in contrast with other filicide cases in which the child deaths are the result of battering or assault (Resnick 1970).

THE CASE OF SHAVAUGHN

In 2013, I (D.B.) received a call from the Virginia Office of the Public Defender regarding a 27-year-old client, Shavaughn, who had given birth in the bathroom of an office building where she was employed as a massage therapist. Similar to my first case in Los Angeles, this young woman also had no awareness of her pregnancy and thus had received no prenatal care. The baby was later found in a dumpster next to the office where the woman worked.

During her pregnancy, Shavaughn had believed that her weight gain was the result of overeating, because she knew she had a tendency to turn to food as a way to cope with stress. She had misinterpreted her morning sickness as food poisoning, and her menstrual periods, which she reported had always been irregular and ceased when under stress, had continued inconsistently throughout gestation. At some point, suspecting that she might be pregnant, she had taken two pregnancy tests, both of which were negative, which served to confirm the denial. Because she had no knowledge of her own pregnancy, Shavaughn continued her employment as a massage therapist, using massage oils daily, some of which were contraindicated for pregnant woman giving or receiving massage.

When Shavaughn went into labor, she identified her contractions as very severe menstrual cramps and recalled feeling as though she needed to have a bowel movement. She could not understand why the cramps were so severe. Hoping they would subside, she took four Percocet pills and went to work. By the afternoon, she remembered feeling hot and close to fainting. Worried that she might throw up, she went to the office bathroom. Shavaughn did not connect that she was birthing a baby, although she had been pregnant 4 years earlier with her son. She also had been unaware of that prior pregnancy until 7 months' gestation, but upon discovering it, she had sought regular prenatal care and follow-up appointments postpartum. This was additional evidence of her psychological propensity to become physically and emotionally numb.

Shavaughn described the events as "an out-of-body experience": "I did not feel like me. It was like being in two different places at once." What she saw in the toilet looked like a "purple Cabbage Patch doll." She recounted that she never saw the baby move or cry. She recalled blood everywhere but had no understanding of where the blood came from, so she started to clean up the bathroom with paper towels. She remembered, "I was scared and panicked, like on autopilot," like "being in a tunnel" and "spaced out." She had no memory of pulling the baby out of the toilet or of putting the baby in the dumpster. When later confronted by detectives, she explained to them that the baby looked dead to her upon its birth. She was charged with violating Section 18.2–323.02, "transport, secrete, conceal or alter a dead body," as defined in Section 32.1–249, "with malicious intent and to prevent detection of an unlawful act or to prevent the detection of the death or the manner or cause of death" (Code of Virginia 2007).

OTHER CASES OF PREGNANCY DENIAL AND CONCEALMENT

Shavaughn's descriptions of pregnancy and birth are repeatedly echoed by both women who deny and those who conceal pregnancies. One adolescent who had been raped and became pregnant shared, "I didn't know I was pregnant throughout the whole pregnancy." This young woman reported an absence of morning sickness and a continuation of menstrual bleeding. She reported never feeling any fetal movement and had actually lost weight, which surprised her because she had "never been that thin." Similar to Shavaughn, she never heard the baby cry or saw any movement after birthing. This young woman, at the time, did not identify that what she held in her arms was a baby. She sensed "it was something bad. I knew it was a mouth, but not what kind of mouth. I don't know what was going through my head exactly, that's the part I'm really trying to understand."

An example in which the mother knew that she was pregnant involves a young mother with three children who became pregnant with a fourth child as a result of rape. She reported feeling confused when giving birth because it did not feel like her prior experiences of labor. She described no labor pains, only intense heat. As labor progressed, she remembered a tremendous amount of bleeding and shared that it felt like "everything inside me just came out," but she added she had no realization that she had actually birthed a baby. She remembered wanting to talk but feeling unable to do so, similar to a nightmare in which you scream but no sound emerges. In her words, it felt as though "the light in the bathroom was on, then it went off by itself, then when it [the birth] was over, the light came back on again." In her mind, she believed she had passed a huge blood clot, so she wrapped it up and hid it in the bathroom, not wanting to leave a mess.

In another case, the mother reported the baby's birth as when "I stopped being me." She woman believed the baby was stillborn. She recalled observing herself stabbing the dead baby but that it felt as though "this other person was doing it." She revealed, "I felt stiff and frozen. Everything slowed down, and I couldn't stop it....I kept thinking the stabbing needed to stop, but I couldn't move." Afterward, she lay on the floor in her room with the baby for about 10–20 minutes and then went upstairs, where she passed the placenta. She remembered putting the baby in a large black plastic trash bag but did not remember first wrapping the baby in a brown paper bag. She had no memory of putting the baby in the trash can outside nor of cleaning up blood. "After everything happened, I went upstairs and took a handful of Tylenol. I was thinking, if this is a dream, let me wake up, and if it's not a dream, let me die." About an hour later, this young mother woke up and realized she had to get to work. She reported that she went back downstairs, grabbed her clothes out of the dryer, and left for her job as a cashier at a local market. Initially she did not understand why the police came to her workplace to bring her to the police station. There she reported having bits of memory return and explaining to the detectives that she had given birth to a stillborn baby. Only when she was taken to the hospital, where she thought she heard babies crying, did she start having flashbacks about the stabbing.

Demographic Profile

Regarding demographics, a number of psychosocial and personality characteristics are consistent among women who experience pregnancy denial. They are most often socially isolated young women, generally teenagers or adults younger than 25 who have grown up in chaotic families with poor boundaries (Friedman et al. 2007; Spinelli 2001, 2003). These are predominantly authoritarian homes where discipline is harsh and strict and conversation about important issues such as sex is taboo. As a result, the women's cognitive styles tend toward distancing themselves from unduly stressful circumstances and working hard not to think about emotionally intense situations, mostly because they have learned that no one is able to respond in an attuned way. With no internal nor external resources, these young women find it untenable for their mental state to integrate the reality of an unexpected pregnancy.

Neonaticide is most often committed by women who have never had interactions with law enforcement. In addition to rigid and authoritarian parents, conditions of alcohol and drug abuse, physical abuse, and emotional neglect are often the norm. Consistent with the emotional neglect reported, adolescents who deny pregnancies frequently describe their mothers as emotionally unavailable or hostile. Personal and family histories of sexual trauma are also commonly reported. Still, despite these challenges and dysfunctions, these women often depend on their families for economic survival. Additionally, women who experience pervasive pregnancy denial are frequently unemployed or may be students. Interestingly, although these women do not seek prenatal care because they lack awareness of their pregnancy, when they see a doctor for other reasons, the provider frequently does not identify the pregnancy either. This psychological phenomenon is referred to as *iatrogenic participation* and serves to reinforce the woman's denial (Amon et al. 2012; Wessel et al. 2003).

While women who deny their pregnancies and subsequently commit neonaticide do not generally have a history of serious mental illness (Meyer and Oberman 2001; Riley 2006), they are reported to have a child-like demeanor that affects their judgment and problem-solving capabilities. They are typically emotionally immature and present with *la belle indifférence* (Spinelli 2001, 2010). In *la belle indifférence*, the woman who has just gone through the stress of birthing a child alone remains remarkably calm; she may seem detached and emotionally distanced from the reality of what has just occurred, despite being confronted with what would appear to be an emotionally charged and intense circumstance. To the outside observer, and most often to the detectives who conduct interrogations, her seeming indifference is often misinterpreted as deviance and malevolence.

Motivation for Pregnancy Denial/Concealment

The driving emotion for most young women who deny a pregnancy is fear (Amon et al. 2012; Meyer and Oberman 2001). They may fear the reactions of an abusive romantic partner or a parent and, in either case, are terrified of being abandoned or emotionally or financially cut off from those closest to them. In addition to fear, feelings of shame and guilt about having engaged in sexual relations and consequently disappointing or humiliating their family frequently precede the concealment and subsequent denial of a pregnancy.

Regarding sexuality, the pregnancy itself may also be a reminder of previous sexual trauma, such as rape. The threat of abandonment and recrimination by her family is the foremost catalyst for a woman's suppression of a pregnancy (Amon et al. 2012; Meyer and Oberman 2001). In some cases, fear does not result in pervasive denial of the pregnancy but in concealment. The crux of the expert witness's work is in distinguishing the nuances through assessment and then explaining the continuum of the woman's consciousness about the pregnancy, because the denial/hiding is so readily admonished to these women by the general public. For example, one young girl who became pregnant with her second child had been told by her mother, in no uncertain terms, that the mother wanted absolutely nothing to do with her if she became pregnant again—to the extent that the mother did not even want her living in the same house. Another teenage girl shared her worry that if her mother found out she was pregnant, she "would disown me." She was afraid she would be "kicked out of the house and be all on my own." Although the level of conscious awareness differs between concealment and pervasive denial, the absence of pregnancy-related symptoms looks similar for both defenses.

Assessment and Evaluation

Pervasive denial of pregnancy is a traumatic response to a situation that feels life threatening. The fact of a pregnancy, along with the perceived consequences of revealing that pregnancy, is terrifying to these young women. Any assessment should pay particular attention to a woman's psychosocial history along with an in-depth understanding of her important relationships, given that pregnancy denial most often occurs as a reaction to undue fear and panic created by environmental and interpersonal factors. Listening to the story of a young woman's circumstances and the words she uses to describe the sequence of events is critical in determining whether she meets the clinical criteria for pervasive denial of pregnancy. Her presentation, if pregnancy denial, often looks and sounds like the profile described herein. Questions that help assessment include

- Was there an absence of normally expected pregnancy symptoms?
- How does she describe labor and birth?
- What is her demeanor when initially confronted by police?
- What are the family dynamics?
- Does she have any history of childhood trauma?

Women with histories of early trauma share an additional neurobiological impact because repeated trauma compromises and overstimulates the more primitive parts of the brain such as the limbic system, the emotional seat of the brain, which is highly reactive, especially as it relates to fear. Under extraordinary stress, the frontal lobe, that part of the brain responsible for organizing one's thoughts and problem solving, shuts down and becomes unavailable, while the brain stem, the primitive part of the brain that operates on instinct, impulse, and reflex, takes over in a fight-or-flight mechanism (Anda et al. 2006). In addition, before age 25, the frontal lobe is still developing and undergoing enormous neurobiological changes that have a significant impact on the way these young women ultimately make decisions (Luciana et al. 2005). Assessing the extent to which a history of trauma may have contributed to a woman's dissociative response may also act as mitigation in eventual sentencing.

Researchers have recently recognized a graded relationship between trauma history and psychological outcomes, including major depression, PTSD, dissociative disorders, and even psychosis (Althoff 2017; Felitti 2019; Raman 2016). The Adverse Childhood Experiences Scale (ACES) is highly recognized as a valid assessment instrument that is helpful in determining the kinds of trauma and number of different traumatic events a person has experienced (Anda et al. 2006; Chapman et al. 2004). The ACES questionnaire includes 10 questions organized into three categories: abuse, neglect, or household dysfunction. The questions inquire as to whether the person has experienced a particular adverse childhood experience; an affirmative answer to any question constitutes one point. With 10 being a maximum score, any score of 4 or above is considered clinically significant in terms of its implications for mental health. In my evaluations of women who are charged with murder as a result of a denied pregnancy, it is rare to find a woman with an ACES score below 4.

Shavaughn, described earlier, had an ACES score of 5. She had had a chaotic and traumatic childhood. By the time she was 6 years old, she had already lived in four different countries because her mother was in the military. Her father was mostly absent from her life, and she recalled feeling abandoned by him. She also had an extensive history of personal and familial sexual assault. At age 12, she was raped by three boys. An extended family member was sexually inappropriate with her, engaging in conversation in the bathroom, pulling back the curtain and watching her while she showered, and attempting to cuddle with her on the couch. Although this made her extremely uncomfortable, she never told anyone because she was afraid of getting someone in trouble.

Shavaughn's mother was physically and emotionally abusive, punching her in the chest and demeaning her with name calling. Shavaughn received confusing messages about sexuality and had a family history of multiple concealed pregnancies. The sexual and physical trauma left her feeling mistrustful, guarded, and frightened. At an early age, she began to sleep with a knife by her side because she had come to believe that she might have to defend herself at any moment. Eventually, whenever she felt anxious or scared, Shavaughn began to have visual hallucinations in the form of black and white clowns staring at her, peering through windows, vents, and even walls.

Because women who deny or conceal their pregnancies describe a dissociative experience particularly around labor and birth, the Dissociative Experiences Scale (DES) is especially useful (Miller 2003; Spinelli 2001, 2010). Designed as a screening instrument for dissociative disorders, the DES is a 28-question self-report validated measure that identifies the frequency of dissociative experiences that occur for individuals in their daily lives when they are not under the influence of alcohol or drugs (Bernstein and Putnam 1986). The percentage scores from this screen are not intended to produce a diagnosis but to act as an indicator of dissociative experiences that the individual is aware have occurred and with what frequency.

Dissociative experiences are quantified for each item on the DES as happening from 0% to 100% of the time. Among young women who have experienced repetitive complex trauma, dissociation often develops as a reflexive and adaptive coping mechanism during future times of extreme stress. Dissociation disrupts conscious awareness, making it possible for an individual to tolerate psychological pain and painful reality occurring in the present from which no perceived escape is apparent, such as an unplanned and unanticipated pregnancy. It also affects the quality and timing of a person's responsiveness because of the visual and aural distortions that occur. For example, Shavaughn not hearing the newborn's heartbeat or seeing the baby move is reflective of a dissociative process. Memory loss for situations and events that have occurred are not at all uncommon.

Because abandonment fears as well as shame around issues pertaining to sexuality are often the driving force behind a pervasive denial of pregnancy (Meyer and Oberman 2001), Shavaughn's history of abandonment and the mixed messages about sex from her mother—for example, calling Shavaughn a "bastard child" because she had been born out of wedlock, while at the same time preaching abstinence—created the underpinnings for the dissociative disorder that surfaced when Shavaughn became pregnant. The rampant negation of pregnancies among her other family members reinforced these sexual taboos and the terror of retribution should a pregnancy be revealed.

Shavaughn's responses on the DES confirmed the presence of dissociative symptoms. For example, she had very often had the experience of feeling as though she was standing next to herself or watching herself do something and seeing herself as though she were looking at another person. This reflects the dissociative symptom of depersonalization. Shavaughn also noted, with some frequency, the experience of feeling that other people, objects, and the world around her were not real, a dissociative symptom known as derealization. She indicated a high degree of frequency with respect to the dissociative experience of sometimes finding that she could not remember whether she had actually done something or just thought about doing it.

REVIEW OF MEDICAL RECORDS

Another critical part of assessment is a thorough review of all medical and mental health records, including any jail documentation. These records offer a window for understanding additional contributing factors to the denial as well as potentially laying the foundation for a woman's state of mind at the time she gave birth. Shavaughn's records were notable for postpartum depression in 2011 after the birth of her first child. Discovering this first pregnancy in the third trimester was significant because it indicated physical and emotional numbing, which are symptoms of PTSD or a dissociative disorder. Progress notes 3 years before the critical incident revealed the presence of visual hallucinations, which Shavaughn described as chronic. In addition, the counseling documentation as well as certain medical records indicated a diagnosis of bipolar disorder with consideration for chronic PTSD or a generalized anxiety disorder. Although these diagnoses, along with the presence of psychotic symptoms, are generally rare in pregnancy denial, they made this case all the more compelling in the courtroom. One study found that the "defense mechanisms of pregnancy negation seem to be more related to dissociative disorders or complex PTSD" (Amon et al. 2012, p. 172).

Establishing Mental Disease or Defect and the Law

The *Diagnostic and Statistical Manual of Mental Disorders* (DSM) is the official guidebook of the courtroom. Consequently, any diagnosis an expert establishes regarding pervasive pregnancy denial must conform to diagnostic criteria in DSM. Although the research and literature describing denied as well as concealed pregnancy—and their strong connection with neonaticide—is widely substantiated, DSM-5 (American Psychiatric Association 2013) does not recognize pregnancy denial as a valid psychological condition with specific diagnostic indicators. As a result, expert witnesses are tasked with finding a diagnosis of mental disease or defect that fits the profile of the woman who negates her pregnancy. The language women use to describe their experience, particularly during labor and immediately post birth, is highly descriptive of dissociative-like symptoms. Therefore, a diagnosis of a dissociative disorder or of PTSD, dissociative subtype would be apt. Because dissociation disrupts conscious awareness and strips the individual of agency over her own actions, dissociative disorder would explain why a woman in the throes of giving birth would be unable to control any aspect of the events as they unfold before her.

Shavaughn met the DSM diagnostic criteria for depersonalization/derealization disorder. DSM-5 notes the following: "Episodes of depersonalization are characterized by a feeling of unreality or detachment from, or unfamiliarity with one's whole self or aspects of self" (p. 302). The person may feel as though her thoughts are not her own and may experience sensory distortions and a "diminished sense of agency" that she describes as robotic or on autopilot. She may lose control of speech or movement. DSM-5's criteria for depersonalization details a split between body and mind, with one part observing and the other participating; the observing self is unable to intervene and stop what is happening. In its extreme form, depersonalization feels like an "out-of-body" experience.

According to DSM-5, derealization, the feeling of being enveloped by a fog or encased in a bubble, is often accompanied by visual distortions, such as blurriness or a narrowing visual field, along with auditory distortions, such as voices or sounds that are either muted or heightened. The overall goal of any diagnostic conclusion with respect to pregnancy denial is twofold: 1) to reduce the charge of murder by demonstrating that the death of the child was not premeditated, and 2) to reduce the potential sentence by demonstrating that the dissociative episode during labor and birth affected the mother's cognition to such an extent that it made it impossible for her to have any control over her actions, behavior, or impulses.

Neonaticide preceded by a concealed or denied pregnancy is not a premeditated killing. Instead, the panic that ensues following birth creates thought disorganization and dissociation that affects the mother's perceptions and resultant decision making, inadvertently leading to the neonaticide. Pervasive pregnancy denial rarely meets the legal criteria for insanity given that most young women who deny their pregnancies are driven by psychosocial stress and not often by the kind of mental illness seen in postpartum psychosis and subsequent infanticide as described in Chapter 7.

Among the many cases of pregnancy denial in the United States that have come to my attention since that first phone call in 2002, women are almost always charged with intentional or premeditated murder. A com-

mon argument by the prosecution is that this was an unwanted pregnancy and that these young women coped by hiding their condition and
then intentionally killing the infant at birth as a way of solving the problem. Sentencing guidelines vary from state to state and can range from
25 years to lifetime incarceration. Although there is generally no dispute
in the courtroom as to a young woman's involvement in the death of her
infant, questions remain as to her intentions as well as the extent of her
responsibility in causing her baby's death, which is usually addressed in
the guilt phase of trial.

In Shavaughn's case, the jury returned a lesser verdict of second-
degree murder. In Virginia, this means the murder did not meet the qualifications for either capital or first-degree murder. Sentencing guidelines
in Virginia for second-degree murder range between 5 and 40 years. The
jury returned a verdict of 7 years, and the presiding judge suspended
2 years of that sentence, citing three similar cases of infant deaths that
had resulted in prison terms of 3, 5, and 5 years, respectively. One of
those cases involved a conviction for manslaughter, one for first-degree
murder, and one for second-degree murder. While this was a positive
decision for Shavaughn, given that she was initially facing a life sentence, it may be considered an isolated verdict. Another judge in the same
state with a different jury, a different judge in a different state with a similar jury, or even a bench trial in a different state might have ruled differently because there is no continuity of law in these cases across the
United States.

Sentencing guidelines are broad and vary dramatically from state to
state depending on the nature of the criminal act. A young woman in a
Midwestern state who concealed her pregnancy was given a life sentence without parole. Another woman in California with circumstances
similar to Shavaughn's case faced a sentencing range from 25 years to
life and was eventually sentenced to 15 years in state prison as part of a
plea agreement on charges of voluntary manslaughter and felony child
abuse, along with allegations of using a deadly weapon and inflicting
great bodily injury on a child under the age of 5 years. Although she had
originally pled not guilty by reason of insanity (NGRI), an uncommon
plea in pregnancy denial cases, she withdrew that plea and pled no con-
test 1 week before her jury trial was set to begin. As part of the plea agreement, she waived all credits for time already served in custody.

In each of these cases, the women fit the profile. They were younger
than 30 years of age and had been raised in chaotic families in which
they experienced physical, emotional, or sexual abuse. Their childhood
histories of trauma, in concert with threats of abandonment, isolation,
and confusing messages about sexuality, laid the groundwork for their

absence of coping skills, inability to manage the undue stress of an unplanned pregnancy, and maladaptive defenses such as dissociation that are predictive in these cases. Regardless of circumstances, their descriptions of their pregnancies, absence of pregnancy-related symptoms, what they felt at the beginnings of labor, and recall of the birth itself and the language they use to describe the onset of the dissociative episode and the altered sensorium during and in the immediate aftermath are identical across each of their narratives.

Neonaticide and the Law in Other Countries

In the United States, mental health and the law are in direct conflict with each other as pertains to cases involving women's reproductive mental health. Other countries, such as Australia, have a greater sensitivity to the changes in mental health that surface during the childbearing years and in some cases have a more compassionate approach to events that have criminal implications, such as maternal filicide, although state differences also reveal significant discrepancies in sentencing (Bartels and Eastel 2013). Australia (population 25 million) consists of six states and two territories, each with variations in how they legally and, to a large extent, morally approach and deal with complex cases like Shavaughn's. Historically, the country has adopted the Westminster legal system and maintains ties to the United Kingdom and the Queen through her delegate, the Governor General.

Pertaining to the Infanticide Law, however, only three states currently have this law as in the Westminster system: Tasmania, Victoria, and New South Wales (NSW). Western Australia removed the law in 2008. The Infanticide Law in Victoria relates to infants up to 24 months, whereas in Tasmania and NSW it is up to 12 months. Its origin can be traced to legal empathy for complex psychosocial circumstances in order to avoid an otherwise mandatory death sentence (Brennan 2013). Conversely, in New Zealand (also a constitutional monarchy), Infanticide Law holds compassion for mothers who take the lives of their children and can include children up to 10 years old (New Zealand Government 1961). It is important to note that in Australia and New Zealand, no legal differentiation is made between cases of neonaticide and infanticide, and scholarly reviews and researchers also tend not to separate them (De Bortoli et al. 2013). As such, the term *filicide* relates to a broader range of child homicides perpetrated by both men and women and includes those without mental illness as a key factor.

Australian Cultural Context

State laws aside, cultural context must also be considered in examining the incidence of infanticide in Australia (much lower, at 2–3 per 100,000 compared with 8 per 100,000 in the United States) and the attitudes and responses to these crimes. Although based upon Anglo-Saxon Christian values, Australia is considered multicultural, with 29% of the more than 25 million residents being born overseas (Australian Bureau of Statistics 2019). Christianity remains the predominant religion (52%), but this has declined from 88% in 1966, and 30% of the population now has no religion (Australian Bureau of Statistics 2017).

Abortion is readily available everywhere in Australia except in NSW, where risk to the mother of carrying a baby to full term must be shown. Conversely, Australia does not have safe-haven capacity for anonymous births, and adoption is possible but not without stigma and hurdles. The barriers to adoption are evident; from 1994–1995 to 2018–2019, overall adoptions declined 64% (Australian Institute of Health and Welfare 2018–2019). Contributing to this drop is the reduced births of unwanted children due to the availability of abortion and of single-mother benefits that enable women to raise their infants without a partner.

Unlike Canada and the United States, sex education is widespread in most schools in all Australian states (despite some resistance to sex education in religious schools) and contraception is readily accessible and inexpensive for adolescents (including oral contraception and intrauterine devices, providing the adolescent is 14 years of age or older and the doctor believes she is competent to consent) (McMicking and Lloyd 2017). Such practices have resulted in a decreasing rate of teenage pregnancies from 17.6 per 1,000 to 9.2 per 1,000 in 2017 for 15- to 19-year-olds (Australian Institute of Health and Welfare 2020). Teenage pregnancy rates in the United States, although higher, are also dropping: 18.8 per 1,000 in 2017 (7% lower than in 2016) (Centers for Disease Control and Prevention 2019).

The openness that Australia has achieved regarding sexuality is most likely due to multiple factors. Between 2001 and 2005, a nationwide campaign was launched to reduce stigma for postnatal depression through screening, educational booklets, and materials as well as television advertisements. Such maternal mental health awareness strategies resulted in general acceptance of routine screening for all mothers during pregnancy and postpartum. Widespread acknowledgment of women's vulnerability to mental health issues (Buist et al. 2006) may have had a positive influence on the judiciary's attitudes toward maternal infanticide becoming more compassionate. In Victoria, leniency in sentencing was evident prior to this, possibly dating back to the first mother–baby unit implemented in this state in 1983 in a psychiatric hospital. More mother–baby units were added in the early 1990s in other obstetric and private hospitals (Buist et al. 2004).

This judicial attitude of compassion seen in sentencing (the maximum under the Infanticide Law being 5 years) has tended to be noncustodial, meaning that community orders are given, and good behavior and adherence to treatment where appropriate are the only restrictions. In NSW, where the Infanticide Law is less often invoked (and "child homicide" is used), and in Queensland, where it is not available, sentencing sometimes involves more than 20 years in prison when a woman is convicted of murder. Nevertheless, throughout Australia, leniency is more likely to be applied regardless of whether murder or infanticide is determined. De Bortoli et al. (2013) noted eight Australian cases of a mother killing a child younger than 1 year in Australia in which mental illness was considered. Half of the women were charged with infanticide and half with manslaughter. Only one woman actually served jail time, with a sentence of 15 months; her original charge had included attempted murder. The remainder of the women were given bonds, released on parole, or given a community order. In neonaticide cases, sentencing has also appeared to take into account the range of psychological and social factors that contributed to the crime.

CASE ILLUSTRATIONS IN AUSTRALIA

Mitigating factors help reduce sentencing—including survival of the infant. The following is a case from my (A.B.) practice:

> When I saw a 28-year-old woman I will call Jasmine, she was in Silverwater jail in NSW awaiting trial. Several months earlier, she had delivered her baby in the hospital and been discharged the following day. She had then abandoned the infant in a dumpster on her way home. The infant's cries had been heard, and the baby was recovered. Later, the baby was identified by the hospital, leading to Jasmine's arrest.
>
> Jasmine had been brought up in a strict Christian family in Fiji and sent to Australia at the age of 25 to stay with extended family, in the hope that she would find a husband. She had struggled at school and dropped out when she was 15 years old. A Wechsler Adult Intelligence Scale administered while she was in prison showed her IQ to be 69, which is in the range of intellectual disability. In Australia, Jasmine had difficulties adjusting to the increased freedom and lack of support available to her. She was unable to find work and spent most of her time at shopping malls. Jasmine came across as sweet and naive and more like a teenager than her 28 years. At the mall, she met a Fijian-Australian man, and they

began a casual sexual relationship. She was well into her third trimester when she suspected she was pregnant.

Jasmine told no one and sought no obstetric care. She went to the hospital when she was in pain, guessing it was labor. There was clear evidence of concealment, and Jasmine spoke of her fear about her family rejecting her as the primary underlying reason. Although Jasmine was shocked by the delivery, the support of obstetric staff in some ways mitigated against a full dissociation. When she described what happened the next day, after she and her baby were released from the hospital, she had still clearly been in shock; she described her thoughts at the time as being frozen and, after discharge, feeling like a robot, watching her actions rather than thinking about them, which is consistent with depersonalization. Although Jasmine did not provide nor recount a history of abuse, her childhood was similar to Shavaughn's in that she was given mixed messages about sexuality and was driven by fear of abandonment and shame. Jasmine left the baby in the dumpster because her fear, coupled with a complete inability to visualize or problem solve about what would happen if she took the baby home, drove her panic and her psychological response of depersonalization.

Jasmine was initially charged with attempted murder. The sentence was lessened to abandonment of a child under 7 years old and causing the child to be in danger of death and recklessly causing grievous bodily harm. The judge had compassion for Jasmine and took into account her intellectual disability, poor problem-solving capacity, and isolation—as well as the unlikelihood that she would be a repeat offender. As a result, she served less than 2 years of a 3-year sentence.

Further examples of compassion by judges, in which they have taken into account the complex psychosocial factors involved in neonaticide, include two cases in which, like Jasmine's case, the babies survived. In these two cases, neither woman did jail time; one was not charged but was repatriated to her own country. The other was charged with abandonment (the child was found quickly and with no negative effects). Both of these women had had childhoods in which shame around sexuality and fear of abandonment were deeply rooted.

For completed maternal neonaticides, I (A.B.) have seen two cases and testified in one of them. I was involved in one case through my work as a consultant in the gynecology ward at the Preston and Northcote Community hospital (now relocated and renamed), after retained placental products were discovered in a young woman who presented with bleeding to the emergency department. She was reported to the police by the treating doctor, and the infant was found partially buried in the back garden of the family home. Given that the autopsy of the infant was inconclusive, and with consideration of the psychiatric report, the 15-year-old mother was not charged. This young woman described having no idea she was pregnant as well as experiencing dissociation throughout the delivery. She displayed *la belle indifférence* as she spoke and, like the other cases discussed, had had a poor emotional connection with her parents and had received admonishing messages about her sexuality that drove her shame and fear.

The other case involved a young woman, Karen, who was charged with and convicted of infanticide. Despite a confession that she "struck the baby several times in the head, intending to kill him, for she did not want him," she was sentenced to a community order that specified she comply with treatment and not reoffend within 5 years. In this case, the judge accepted my testimony of a brief dissociative episode as her state of mind. This fits in DSM-5 under other dissociative disorders, in which there are mixed features of dissociation, often brief and in relation to stress. Karen's background was similar to the other cases described. Although her mother was open to the idea of this young woman being on contraception, her father was perceived as rigid and judgmental. The judge concluded: "you know that jails are nasty, violent places. All the purposes of punishment can be achieved without putting you [Karen] in jail" (Garner 2017, p. 124).

Psychosocial History in the Courtroom

An awareness of the psychological complexities shown in these cases is in contrast to the majority of infanticide cases I (A.B.) have been involved with in NSW and those reported in the United States, in which the woman's psychosocial history has less or no acknowledgment or weight in the courtroom. In 2005, Victoria amended its Infanticide Law in consultation with psychiatrists and acknowledged the complexity of psychological aspects related to these cases. They expanded the Infanticide Law to include children up to 24 months of age rather than making it harsher or choosing not to use it. In more recent cases of infanticide in 2018, the (new) Victorian prosecution was less willing to consider the complex psychological factors, which highlights the need for forensic mental health specialists to be constantly looking for opportunities to educate both the public and those in the legal profession.

Lack of education leads to a tendency to simplify these cases as "bad" rather than what is in most cases tragic and driven by multiple psychological and social factors. Punishment is unlikely to act as a deterrent for others. The vastly different outcomes in sentencing that occur in these cases, even within Australia, and certainly between Australia and the

United States, suggest that the state of mind of the prosecutor, jury, and judge has a significant outcome on both verdict and sentencing.

MAIN CLINICAL/LEGAL POINTS AND CULTURAL PERSPECTIVES

- Pregnancy denial cases are complex and involve multiple factors such as attachment and trauma, which affect neurobiological development and alter personality development and stress responses in adulthood.

- Concurrent poverty, intrapersonal violence, and lack of support further disadvantage women and undermine any ability to cope with the physical and psychological aspects of pregnancy and the acute, potentially life-threatening event of childbirth.

- The absence of pregnancy-related symptoms in most of these cases contributes to the ongoing denial and the inadvertent collusion by family and medical staff in preventing early detection.

- The complexities often do not fit neatly into a DSM-5 category, and trying to make them do so risks minimizing the factors that contribute to this tragedy.

- There is a constant tension between psychiatry and the law in these cases. As forensic experts in perinatal illnesses, our role is to help the court make sense of these complexities in order for justice to be served, with mercy when indicated.

- Societal attitudes play a significant part in the prosecution of these cases. The defendants are up against the stigma not only of mental illness but also of being "bad" mothers.

- Although not officially recognized by DSM-5, a common diagnostic pattern to symptoms and a demographic profile can be found among women who deny or conceal their pregnancies.

- Lack of uniformity in the law across the United States results in substantially different rulings in similar cases.

- Australia has states with and without the Infanticide Law, and even in states where it exists, it is not always used, also resulting in different rulings.

- Compared with the United States, Australia is more likely to consider the complex psychosocial factors that contribute to infanticide and to offer lenient, often noncustodial sentences.

Practice and Discussion Questions

1. Debate the merits of the Australian Infanticide Law. How well does research support the balance of mind being affected by childbirth and lactation? Is this law sexist?
2. The Australian Infanticide Law was primarily brought into legal practice for psychosocial reasons. Without it, are there other ways to ensure that complex psychosocial and mental health issues are considered and that there is more uniformity in sentencing?
3. In your professional role, how might you be involved in neonaticide cases? What are your beliefs regarding the role of trauma, psychosocial history, and dissociation in the culpability or nonculpability of women who kill their newborns? Where do these beliefs come from?
4. In your country, what has been the trend over the past 5–10 years regarding the conviction and sentencing of women in pregnancy denial or neonaticide cases? Can you connect that trend to cultural factors, such as religiosity, abortion laws, sex education in schools, maternal mental health education and attention, and so on?
5. Considering the case of Shavaughn, do you think she was malicious (as per the charges)? What can you learn from her background and the way it shaped her personality and response to trauma that could inform a better understanding of others you see with trauma histories?
6. Considering the case of Karen, reflect on how this might have been handled in other countries. Would a custodial sentence have achieved anything more than her community order?
7. How does the media contribute to societal attitudes toward women who conceal/deny their pregnancy and kill their children? What language is used, and what are their views about mental illness and trauma?

References

Althoff R: Adverse childhood experience (child psychiatry consult). Pediatric News 51(3):14, 2017
American Psychiatric Association: Diagnostic and Statistical Manual of Mental Disorders, 5th Edition. Arlington, VA, American Psychiatric Association, 2013

Amon S, Putkonen H, Weizmann-Henelius G, et al: Potential predictors in neonaticide: the impact of the circumstances of pregnancy. Arch Womens Mental Health 15(3):167–174, 2012

Anda RF, Felitti VJ, Bremner JD, et al: The enduring effects of abuse and related adverse experiences in childhood. Eur Arch Psychiatry Clin Neurosci 256(3):174–186, 2006

Australian Bureau of Statistics: 2016 census data reveals "no religion" is rising fast (press release), June 2017. Available at: http://www.abs.gov.au/ausstats/abs@.nsf/mediareleasesbyReleaseDate/7E65A144540551D7-CA258148000E2B85. Accessed August 16, 2020.

Australian Bureau of Statistics: Migration, Australia, 2017–18 (Publ No 3412.0), ABS.gov.au, April 3, 2019. Available at: https://www.abs.gov.au/ausstats/abs@.nsf/mf/3412.0. Accessed December 12, 2019.

Australian Institute of Health and Welfare: Adoption Australia. Child Welfare Series No 71, Cat No CWS71. Canberra, Australia, AIHW, 2018–2019. Available at: https://www.aihw.gov.au/reports-data/health-welfare-services/adoptions/overview. Accessed September 2, 2020.

Australian Institute of Health and Welfare: Australia's children. Cat No CWS69. Canberra, Australia, AIHW, 2020. Available at: https://www.aihw.gov.au/reports/children-youth/australias-children/contents/health/teenage-mothers. Accessed September 2, 2020.

Bartels L, Eastel P: The forensic use and judicial reception of evidence of postnatal depression and other psychiatric disorders in Australian filicide cases. Melbourne University Law Review 37(2), 2013

Beier KM, Wille R, Wessel J: Denial of pregnancy as a reproductive dysfunction: a proposal for international classification systems. J Psychosom Res 61(5):723–730, 2006

Bernstein EM, Putnam FW: Development, reliability, and validity of a dissociation scale. J Nerv Ment Dis 174(12):727–735, 1986

Brennan K: Traditions of English thought: a history of the enactment of an infanticide law in Ireland. Irish Jurist 50:100–137, 2013

Brezinka C, Brezinka C, Biebl W, et al: Denial of pregnancy: obstetrical aspects. J Psychosom Obstet Gynecol 15(1):1–8, 1994

Buist A, Minto B, Szego K, et al: Mother-baby psychiatric units in Australia: the Victorian experience. Arch Womens Ment Health 7(1):81–87, 2004

Buist A, Bilszta J, Milgrom J, et al: Health professionals' knowledge and awareness of perinatal depression: results of a national survey. Women Birth 19(1):11–16, 2006

Centers for Disease Control and Prevention: Reproductive Health: Teen Pregnancy, 2019. Available at: https://www.cdc.gov/teenpregnancy/about/index.htm. Accessed December 12, 2019.

Chapman DP, Whitfield CL, Felitti VJ, et al: Adverse childhood experiences and the risk of depressive disorders in adulthood. J Affect Disord 82(2):217–225, 2004

Code of Virginia § 18.2–323.02. Prohibition against concealment of dead body; penalty. 2007

Crittenden PM, Ainsworth MD: Child maltreatment and attachment theory, in Handbook of Child Maltreatment. Edited by Cicchetti C, Carlson V. Cambridge, UK, Cambridge University Press, 1989, pp 432–463

De Bortoli L, Coles J, Dolan M: Maternal infanticide in Australia: mental disturbance in the postpartum period. Psychiatry, Psychology and Law 20(2):301–311, 2013

Felitti V: Origins of the ACE study. Am J Prev Med 56(6):787–789, 2019

Friedman SH, Heneghan A, Rosenthal M: Characteristics of women who deny or conceal pregnancy. Psychosomatics 48(2):117–122, 2007

Garner H: Punishing Karen, in Everywhere I Look. Melbourne, Australia, Text Publishing, 2017, pp 121–125

Hatters Friedman S, Resnick P: Neonaticide: phenomenology and considerations for prevention. Int J Law Psychiatry 32:43–47, 2009

Luciana M, Conklin H, Hooper C, Yarger R: The development of nonverbal working memory and executive control processes in adolescents. Child Dev 76(3):697–712, 2005

McMicking J, Lloyd J: Contraception in adolescents. O&G Magazine 19(3), 2017

Meyer CL, Oberman M: Mothers Who Kill Their Children: Understanding the Acts of Moms From Susan Smith to the "Prom Mom." New York, NYU Press, 2001

Miller LJ: Denial of pregnancy, in Infanticide: Psychosocial and Legal Perspectives on Mothers Who Kill. Edited by Spinelli MG. Washington, DC, American Psychiatric Publishing, 2003, pp 81–104

New Zealand Government: Infanticide (Crimes Act 178). Wellington, New Zealand Parliamentary Counsel Office, 1961. Available at: http://www.legislation.govt.nz/act/public/1961/0043/latest/DLM329332.html. Accessed December 19, 2019.

Neifert PL, Bourgeois JA: Denial of pregnancy: a case study and literature review. Mil Med 165(7):566–568, 2000

Oshri A, Sutton TE, Clay-Warner J, Miller JD: Child maltreatment types and risk behaviors: associations with attachment style and emotion regulation dimensions. Pers Individ Diff 73:127–133, 2015

Raman S: Adverse childhood experiences and theory of mind. Br J Psychiatry 208(1):94–95, 2016

Resnick PJ: Murder of the newborn: a psychiatric review of neonaticide. Am J Psychiatry 126(10):1414–1420, 1970

Riley L: Neonaticide. J Hum Behav Soc Environ 12(4):1–42, 2006

Spinelli MG: A systematic investigation of 16 cases of neonaticide. Am J Psychiatry 158:811– 813, 2001

Spinelli MG (ed): Infanticide: Psychosocial and Legal Perspectives on Mothers Who Kill. Washington, DC, American Psychiatric Publishing, 2003

Spinelli MG: Denial of pregnancy: a psychodynamic paradigm. J Am Acad Psychoanal Dyn Psychiatry 38(1):117–131, 2010

Wessel J, Buscher U: Denial of pregnancy: population-based study. BMJ 324(7335):458, 2002

Wessel J, Endrikat J, Kästner R: Projective identification and denial of pregnancy: considerations of the reasons and background of unrecognized pregnancy also undiagnosed by a physician (in German). Z Geburtshilfe Neonatol 207(2):48–53, 2003

FOUNDATION III

The Role of the Expert Witness in Maternal Infanticide and Filicide Cases

CHAPTER 9

Reflections of an Expert Witness in the Andrea Yates Case

Phillip Resnick, M.D.

On June 20, 2001, Andrea Yates drowned her five children. She then called 911 and requested that a police officer be sent to her home. When the police arrived, Ms. Yates told them she had killed her children and led them to the bedroom with the four dead children. The oldest, 7-year-old Noah, had been left in the bathtub. The Yates case received extraordinary publicity because of the number of children killed and the fact that Andrea's husband, Rusty Yates, was so open with the press.

When a mother kills her children, very strong emotions are evoked. When Ms. Yates's defense attorney George Parnham first heard about the killings, he changed the radio station due to his own emotional upset. Many think a mother must be severely mentally ill to take the lives of her own children. After all, she birthed and cared for them, and children provide a form of immortality for parents. Others respond with intense anger and disgust. They see *filicide* (child murder by a parent) as the ultimate betrayal, because children look to their mother for protection and nurturance. Most parents have had some angry thoughts toward their children. Some have even said in a rage, "I'm going to break your neck" or "I'm going to kill you if you do that one more time." When a mother actually does kill her children, some parents want to impose severe punishment on the murderers to reinforce their own controls to not harm their own children.

My Role in the Yates Case

Within the first 2 days of the Yates filicides, the TV show *Nightline* and various publications called me to ask why a mother might kill her own children. I am uniquely qualified as a forensic psychiatrist to respond to this because of my long-standing research interest in child murder. Very early in my career, I treated two women who had murdered their children. I became quite interested in the topic and wrote a seminal article that reviewed the world literature on filicide and proposed a classification for child murder (Resnick 1969). I taught courses about filicide to mental health professionals, lawyers, and law enforcement officers including the U.S. Federal Bureau of Investigation. By the time of the Yates filicides, I had personally examined more mothers who had killed their children than any other psychiatrist in the country, so I was not surprised when, a few days after the *Nightline* episode, George Parnham contacted me. He had by then been retained as Ms. Yates's attorney, and he told me that when he inquired about who would be the best psychiatric expert for the trial, "all the paths" led to me.

When Mr. Parnham told me that he anticipated raising an insanity defense for Ms. Yates, I made two requests. First, I wanted to see her as soon as possible to reduce the chance that her state of mind at the time of the filicide would be altered by psychiatric treatment she received in jail. Second, I wanted to video record my interview with her to preserve her thinking about the crime. That recording was shown to the jury to convey how Ms. Yates looked and how she explained her actions while she was still in a psychotic state. When juries see criminal defendants free of psychosis at their trial, they often find it hard to think of them as out of touch with reality at the time of their crime.

It is ideal if the forensic examiner can review all of the collateral information before interviewing a mother who has killed her children so that the examiner can confront the mother with any discrepancies. Prenatal records and birth records may contain statements made to hospital staff indicating whether a pregnancy was "wanted." Evidence of child neglect may be found in pediatric records. Records from child protective agencies may also be helpful. In Ms. Yates's case, medical records revealed that each of her pregnancies had been desired. She had had some contact with a child protective agency because of her filicidal thoughts after her earlier pregnancies. However, taking the time to gather complete collateral data must be weighed against the desirability of seeing a mother as soon as possible after her filicide. I determined that seeing Ms. Yates quickly was my first priority.

When assessing a criminal defendant for an insanity defense, I always keep in mind the possibility that the defendant may be malingering psychiatric symptoms for the purpose of avoiding prison or the death penalty. Clinical assessment and psychological tests are available to assess malingering (Resnick and Knoll 2018). In the case of Ms. Yates, substantial evidence of the genuineness of her serious psychiatric illness had accumulated long before her homicides. There were records from four prior psychiatric hospitalizations that included evidence of postpartum psychosis and thoughts of harming her children years before the crime. In fact, she was under the care of a treating psychiatrist at the time of her filicides. None of the experts who testified at the trial suggested that Ms. Yates was not genuinely mentally ill when she killed her children.

My Evaluation of Andrea Yates

When I arrived at the Harris County jail, I had my first opportunity to see the medical records of Ms. Yates by the jail's treating psychiatrist, Dr. Melissa Ferguson. Dr. Ferguson wrote on June 21, 2001, one day after the homicides, that Ms. Yates had been hearing human voices telling her to "grab them" and "she would struggle to resist the command." Ms. Yates told Dr. Ferguson, "My children were not righteous…I let them stumble," and they were "doomed to perish in the fires of hell." Later progress notes stated that Ms. Yates had heard the voice of Satan on a radio station and believed that Satan resided within her body.

When I met Ms. Yates on July 14, 2001, she was dressed in orange prison garb and her hair appeared unwashed and stringy. She was sad and very slow in her speech and movements. I learned that she had been a devoted mother and a highly regarded registered nurse at MD Anderson Cancer Center before she began having children. Her love for her children was evident. I found her to be a sympathetic woman ensnared in the tragic consequences of her psychosis. She had no insight into the nature of her psychotic delusions.

Ms. Yates told me that her children were "not righteous." She thought that they would never be right "before God" and would be punished and "burn in hell." Upon inquiry, she told me that at the time she drowned her children, she believed that taking their lives was in their best interest. If she took their lives while they were still "innocent," she thought that they would go to heaven. She believed she would be executed for killing her children and that Satan (the one and only Satan) who was "within her" would also be executed. She explained that she took her children's lives out of love for them. She did not feel any anger toward them. Later interviews with psychiatrists revealed that Ms. Yates had specific delusional ideas about each of her children before her filicides. She believed that her son John would become a serial killer, her son Luke would become a mute homosexual prostitute, and her other two sons would have early tragic deaths.

Ms. Yates told me that after drowning each child, she placed four of the children on the double bed in the master bedroom. Her son John had been a particularly good big brother to his 6-month-old sister, Mary, so she placed Mary in the crook of John's arm so he could protect her in the afterlife. Noah, age 7, was the most difficult child to drown because he was the strongest. He managed to get his head above the bathtub water and say, "I'm sorry, Mommy." This detail would prove to be one of the most disturbing for jurors to hear—evoking strong sympathy for the child and rage at Ms. Yates.

When I am asked to evaluate a defendant for a not guilty by reason of insanity (NGRI) defense after she has committed filicide, I keep my own classification of filicide in mind (see "Glossary" at the end of this book). After I evaluated Ms. Yates, it was clear to me that her filicides fit into the altruistic category because she believed that if she did not take her children's lives, they would burn in hell for eternity. She saw that outcome as worse than death for her children. I ruled out spouse revenge filicide because she viewed Rusty as a good father and supportive husband. I ruled out child maltreatment filicide because she had never been physically abusive toward her children. I ruled out unwanted child filicide because Ms. Yates wanted a large family and was a devoted mother. Even though she was psychotic, I ruled out acutely psychotic filicide because she had had the comprehensible motive (even though psychotic) of protecting her children from "going to hell."

After my initial interview of Ms. Yates, I learned that Dr. Park Dietz, a distinguished forensic psychiatrist, had been employed by the prosecution to evaluate her. Dr. Dietz and I had been friends for more than two decades before we testified on opposite sides of the Yates case. We had worked together for the prosecution in the case of Theodore Kaczynski, the Unabomber. We also had worked on the opposite sides of other high-profile cases, such as that of Susan Smith, who drowned her children, and John DuPont, who killed gold medal Olympic wrestler David Schultz. We had both been active in the American Academy of Psychiatry and the Law and had each served as president. I knew that Dr. Dietz was meticulous and complete in his assessments. When I know an opposing expert is going to do a high-quality job, it causes me to be even more thorough in my own preparation.

The Insanity Defense

No crime in the United States is more likely to succeed with an NGRI defense than a mother killing her own children. Nonetheless, due to skepticism about insanity, most women who plead NGRI for filicide are not successful. The perception that mothers have unconditional love for their children means mothers are much more likely to be found legally insane than are fathers who kill their children under similar circumstances (see Chapter 5).

Every insanity trial can be viewed as a morality play in which a jury decides whether a defendant with mental illness is blameworthy. The public follows these dramatic trials with considerable interest. Contested insanity trials give people the false idea that mental health professionals never seem to agree. Actually, 80% of successful insanity cases are uncontested (Rogers et al. 1984)—that is, the expert psychiatrists and psychologists on both sides agree that a defendant was insane. Only a brief walk-through trial is held in these cases. The public estimates that an insanity defense is raised in 20% of criminal trials, but in reality, an insanity defense is raised only in 1 out of 100 felony indictments (1%) (Callahan et al. 1991).

The American public is highly skeptical about insanity defenses; they are especially concerned about the possibility of defendants faking insanity (Resnick 2016). Most believe that defendants who are found legally insane "beat the rap" (Hans and Slater 1983). In reality, insanity acquittees sometimes spend more time locked up than do those found guilty of the same crime (Perlin 1998). The public and media often respond with anger when a high-profile defendant is found NGRI. There was public outrage when John Hinckley Jr. was found insane for his attempted assassination of President Ronald Reagan in 1981 (Hans and Slater 1983). Many editorials and columnists attacked the verdict and the insanity defense. For example, columnist Carl Rowan (1982) said, "It's about time we face the truth that the insanity defense is mostly last gasp legal maneuvering, often hoaxes, in cases where a person has obviously done something terrible" (p. B4). In response to the Hinckley verdict, the U.S. Congress passed the Insanity Defense Reform Act (1984), which narrowed the federal insanity test and eliminated the irresistible-impulse portion of the test.

In 1994, Susan Smith drowned her two children by driving them into a lake. The prosecutor attempted to portray this as an unwanted-child filicide based on a letter from Ms. Smith's lover saying that he was reluctant to continue their relationship because she had two children. However, in an 8-hour evaluation of Susan Smith, I learned that she had planned to kill herself due to a categorical rejection by her lover earlier on the day of the crime and had intended to take her children to heaven with her. This placed her in the category of an altruistic filicide. She had lost her nerve to kill herself at the last moment and jumped from her car, allowing her two children to drown in the lake still strapped in their car seats. She then falsely claimed that her car, along with her children, had been "hijacked by a black man." She cried on live television and begged the alleged hijacker to return her children. When she later confessed to killing them, people were outraged and the majority of the public wanted her to receive the death penalty. Perlin (2003) observed that, "Smith told us the 'big lie' and betrayed the greater community—not by killing her children, but by appealing to our sympathy and empathy and then kicking us in our unconscious and leaving us with a 'sense of betrayal'" (p. 20). Smith was found guilty and sentenced to life in prison. Perlin suggested that by the time of the Yates filicide trial, jurors' disgust at such a vile act trumped feelings of empathy (Perlin 2003).

Although juries are given instructions about the specific test to apply in insanity cases, research suggests that about 79% of jurors do not actually apply the insanity instructions given by the judge (Skeem and Golding 2001). Instead, they use their own common sense in deciding whether a defendant is insane. One of the key factors that affects jury decisions is whether the jurors can emotionally forgive the defendant. Defense attorneys often portray defendants pleading insanity as victims of their own mental illness. Prosecutors seek to make these crimes unforgivable. In the Yates case, the prosecution employed a pediatric forensic pathologist to testify that a bruise on the tip of Noah's tongue suggested that he was "silently screaming" while being drowned. The real purpose of this testimony was to make the crime less forgivable by the jury. One juror said in a television interview that after hearing the detail about Noah telling his mother that he was sorry, he stopped listening to the rest of the trial. That juror found the evidence too upsetting to hear because he had a 6-year-old son at home.

After my first interview, I concluded that Ms. Yates knew that killing her children was against the law, but she had believed she was doing what was in their best interest. I asked Mr. Parnham whether any case law in the Texas insanity test indicated whether the word *wrong* meant *legally* wrong or *morally* wrong. The Texas Supreme Court had touched on the issue in one case but had given no definitive meaning to the word "wrong." Thus, it would be up to Ms. Yates's jury to decide how to interpret that in the insanity test. Furthermore, Texas had a narrow definition of insanity: To be found NGRI, the defendant must prove that at the time of the conduct charged, he or she, as a result of severe mental disease or defect, did not know that the conduct was wrong (Texas Penal Code 1973). Everyone in Texas is presumed to be sane.

Jurors tend to be disposition oriented. Some states require judges to inform juries that if a defendant is found NGRI, he or she will be committed to a psychiatric hospital and retained there until shown to no longer be a danger to society (Piel 2012). Other states, including Texas, do not permit judges to reveal the consequences of an NGRI verdict to juries. This lack of information means some jurors are more likely to reject an NGRI verdict out of fear that the defendant will be immediately released and commit further violence (Daftary-Kapur et al. 2011). If the Yates jury had been aware that Ms. Yates would not be immediately released upon an NGRI finding, some jurors may have considered insanity more favorably.

My Court Testimony in the First Yates Trial (2002)

DIRECT EXAMINATION

Mr. Parnham called 10 mental health professionals, mostly treating clinicians of Ms. Yates, to show the severity of her psychosis. I was the primary forensic psychiatrist to testify regarding her insanity because of my background in filicide insanity cases. The prosecution psychiatrist, Dr. Dietz, and I agreed on three critical issues: 1) Ms. Yates had had a severe mental disease on June 20, 2001, when she drowned her children; 2) Ms. Yates knew that drowning her children was against the law; and 3) Ms. Yates believed that killing her children was in their best interest. We disagreed, however, on the issue of knowledge of wrongfulness. Dr. Dietz testified that Ms. Yates knew her homicidal conduct was wrong in the eyes of the law and of God. I testified that Ms. Yates did not know the wrongfulness of her conduct due to her severe mental disease for the following reasons:

1. She believed it was right to drown her children because she held a delusional belief that her children were not righteous and would burn in hell if she did not take their lives before the age of accountability. She believed the age of accountability was 10. She psychotically believed that it was right to arrange for her children to go to heaven and be with God for all eternity while they were still "innocent."
2. She was not deterred from "saving her children's souls" by the fact that she expected to be executed by the State of Texas. In fact, she believed that she was doing the world a favor because Satan, who ex-

isted within her, would be executed along with her. This would bring about Armageddon.

3. She had not killed her children when she heard command hallucinations to do so in 1999 because she had then believed it was not in her children's best interest to die. Instead, she had twice attempted suicide rather than risk harm to her children. It was only when her psychosis recurred in 2001 that she came to believe it was in her children's best interest to die.

4. She made no effort to hide her crime or to avoid responsibility. She called the police, remained at the crime scene, confessed, and expected to be punished.

5. She had no alternative motive to take the lives of her children other than her psychotic beliefs. All the witnesses who testified in the trial agreed that Ms. Yates was a devoted mother who loved her children.

CROSS EXAMINATION

I was cross examined by assistant prosecutor Joe Oymby. He began by bringing up some quotations I had given to the press within 2 days of Ms. Yates's homicides. He asked if I had told a reporter that juries view mothers who kill their children as mentally sick. After I asked to see my quotation in full, I pointed out that he had taken my comment out of context. My remark about mothers being perceived as mentally ill was only in comparison to fathers who killed their children.

Mr. Oymby also brought up a statement I had made in 1995 that I would be comfortable allowing Susan Smith to babysit for my grandchildren. I responded that I had meant to convey that a mother's killing of her own children did not mean she would necessarily endanger other children in the community. Mr. Oymby then went through several different insanity tests that are not used in Texas in an effort to show that Texas had a narrow insanity standard. I responded that I had used the precise Texas standard in forming my opinion regarding Ms. Yates's sanity.

Mr. Oymby raised the issue of Ms. Yates knowing that killing her children was a sin. I conceded that this was true but added that she viewed the homicides as a "lesser sin" than having her children burn in hell forever. He challenged my opinion that Ms. Yates had no rational motive for her crime, asking, "Isn't it a rational motive to remove yourself from feeling tired and overwhelmed?" I replied that it is not rational to kill your children in response to feeling overwhelmed if you believe that doing so will result in your own execution. He also raised the possibility that Ms. Yates might have killed her children as a way to get back at a "controlling, dominating husband." I responded that Ms. Yates viewed her husband as a good father to the children and a good husband. She had no feelings of resentment toward Rusty.

Ms. Yates had been indicted with death penalty specifications and thus was tried by a death qualified jury in 2002. About two-thirds of the American public favored the death penalty in 2002; by 2018, only 53% of Americans favored the death penalty (Death Penalty Information Center 2019). In a capital case, each potential juror must agree before the trial to impose the death penalty if the facts call for it. Death qualified juries are more conservative and are less likely to find a defendant NGRI (Ellsworth et al. 1984). The jury in Ms. Yates's first trial deliberated for 3.5 hours before finding her guilty. They rejected the death penalty in less than 30 minutes.

Reaction to the First Yates Verdict

The trial evidence showed that Ms. Yates was deeply religious and had homeschooled her children. One question I was often asked by reporters after the first Yates trial was whether devoutly religious parents were more likely to kill their children. I responded that although religious people are more likely to have delusions of a religious nature, no evidence indicates that religious people are more likely to become psychotic or to kill their children. I explained that religion was like a trellis along which Ms. Yates's delusions grew.

The world press followed the Andrea Yates trial with great interest. When I lectured in Australia several months after the first trial, Australian psychiatrists were knowledgeable about the facts and extremely interested in the details of her case. When I presented her case in Norway a few months later to a group of forensic psychiatrists, they expressed outrage that Ms. Yates had been found guilty rather than NGRI. European countries had abolished the death penalty many years earlier. One psychiatrist stood up and asked, "How can you live in a country that would even consider executing such an obviously mentally ill woman?"

When Dr. Dietz, the psychiatric expert employed by the prosecution, was interviewed by *The New York Times* after the first Yates trial, he said that if Texas did not have such a narrow insanity test, he might have reached a different outcome: "For instance, I think I would have found her insane in a jurisdiction where the test is whether she emotionally appreciated the wrongfulness of her actions" (Toufexis 2002). He added, "It was obvious where public opinion lay. It was obvious she was mentally ill. It was obvious where the professional organizations would like the case to go. But it would be wrong to distort the law, to stretch the truth, and try to engineer the outcome" (Toufexis 2002).

Mr. Parnham appealed the verdict on several points of law. The Texas Court of Appeals overturned the Yates trial verdict due to an error by Dr. Dietz (*Yates v. Texas* 2005). A script consultant for the television show *Law and Order*, Dr. Dietz had incorrectly testified that shortly before Ms. Yates's homicides, an episode of the show had aired depicting a woman who was found insane after drowning her children in a bathtub. This erroneous statement had also been used by the prosecutor in closing arguments.

The Second Yates Trial (2006)

The second Yates trial occurred in the summer of 2006. The prosecution did not seek the death penalty in the second trial. Dr. Dietz's testimony for the prosecution and my own testimony for the defense changed little from the first trial. It is my opinion that the primary reason the second Yates jury was more receptive to an insanity defense was because the jurors were not "death qualified" and thus were likely to be less conservative. In addition, two other Texas mothers had been found NGRI for killing their children between Ms. Yates's first and second trials (Associated Press 2004). After 12 hours of deliberation, the second jury found Ms. Yates NGRI. The jury foreman, Todd Frank, said to a television interviewer, "We understand that she knew it was legally wrong. But in her delusional mind…we believed that she thought what she did was right" (Casey 2006). I found this comment particularly gratifying because it was the essence of what I had tried to get across to the jury.

Providing testimony in the Yates trials was a high point in my career. The extensive media coverage assured that all of my testimony would undergo intense scrutiny in addition to being tested by vigorous cross-examination. A number of subsequent filicide cases were referred to me because of my work on the Yates case. It was a privilege to work with George Parnham and to observe his humanity toward Ms. Yates. He has remained committed to supporting Ms. Yates for almost two decades.

Aftermath for Mothers Who Kill their Children

There is no greater tragedy than having a child pre-decease a parent. Children who lose their parents are called orphans. Women who lose their husbands are called widows. There is no word for parents who lose their children, perhaps because it is unspeakable. If a child dies by suicide, the parents' grief and guilt may last a lifetime and often results in divorce. If children die by their mother's own hand, the guilt and grief may be too much to bear. When I lecture about filicide, I sometimes ask the audience this question: "If you killed your children in a psychotic state, would you prefer to leave your psychosis untreated or would you rather be treated and face the reality of what you had done?" About 80% of people respond they would prefer to remain psychotic.

In addition to their grief, mothers who have killed their children experience real losses. They have lost their children. Most of the time their spouse leaves them. Finally, they lose their freedom, either in a forensic hospital or a prison. Mothers who are found NGRI for killing their children are doubly stigmatized as both "mad and bad." In prison they are often harassed and called "baby killer." When insanity acquittees are released after a filicide, the stigma is so great that they may change their name and move to a different city. Wherever she goes, Ms. Yates not only will have to deal with the ordinary stigma but also, because of the extreme publicity in her case, will be likely to be recognized by others wherever she goes.

Mothers who have killed their children while psychotic often find it difficult to forgive themselves even after society has forgiven them by finding them legally insane (Stanton and Simpson 2006). Some of these women realize that they were out of their minds when they killed their children but still blame themselves because they had recognized that they were becoming mentally ill and had failed to seek help. In my experience, some of these mothers feel that they deserve punishment for the rest of their lives, or at least that nothing good should ever happen to them. Some women I have seen who committed filicide based on religious delusions have pulled away from religion. Andrea Yates, however, never gave up her faith in God as an important source of support. She struggled with her faith for 11 years, believing she was "worthless and did not deserve God's love." Once she believed that God had forgiven her and still loved her, she was finally able to forgive herself.

Although Ms. Yates received some supportive mail, she received more hate mail, some from as far away as Australia. Some letters even threatened her with physical harm. She became so concerned about her safety that it affected her decision about when to seek release from the forensic psychiatric hospital where she resides. I have had the opportunity to visit Ms. Yates several times since her insanity acquittal. She is no longer psychotic and is well liked by the nursing staff. She enjoys watching videos that she had made of her children.

Each filicide is a tragedy, not only for the dead children but also for the mentally ill mother and her family. The thoughts of Medea when she took the lives of her two sons convey the ongoing anguish of these mothers (Euripides, in Hamilton 1942):

> To die by other hands more merciless than mine.
> No; I who gave them life will give them death.
> Oh, now no cowardice, no thought how young they are,
> How dear they are, how when they first were born—
> Not that—I will forget they are my sons.
> One moment, one short moment—then forever sorrow.

MAIN CLINICAL/LEGAL POINTS AND CULTURAL PERSPECTIVES

- Filicide cases evoke strong emotions in people.
- Mothers who kill their children are more likely to be found insane than are fathers who kill their children.
- Video recording psychiatric interviews of defendants close in time to the crime allows juries to see the mental state of potentially not guilty by reason of insanity (NGRI) defendants while they are still mentally ill.
- It is desirable to obtain collateral information before a forensic expert sees a defendant in a potential insanity case, but this may be less important than seeing the defendant as soon as possible after the crime.
- Malingering should be considered in all insanity cases.
- Categories of filicide include 1) altruistic, 2) acutely psychotic, 3) unwanted child, 4) child maltreatment, and 5) spousal revenge.
- Juries are skeptical about insanity defenses.
- Forensic examiners should learn the exact legal definition of *insanity* in the relevant jurisdiction, including whether the word *wrongfulness* is limited to legally wrong or allows for a defendant's belief that an act is morally right.
- Prosecutors try to portray crimes as unforgivable in insanity trials.
- Women who kill their children find it hard to forgive themselves, even if they were found NGRI.

Practice and Discussion Questions

1. Debate whether the insanity defense should be abolished. Four states have abolished the insanity defense.
2. What are the advantages and disadvantages of juries being allowed, or not, to know what happens to defendants after they are found NGRI?
3. Do you believe that the United States should adopt infanticide laws that reduce the penalty for women who kill their children younger than 1 year of age? Why or why not? Such laws exist in 26 countries, including Canada.
4. Discuss the pros and cons of requiring all psychiatric insanity evaluations to be video recorded.

References

Associated Press: Religiosity common among mothers who kill children. Tyler Morning Telegraph, December 14, 2004, p B-1

Callahan LA, Steadman HJ, McGreevy MA, Robbins PC: The volume and characteristics of insanity defense pleas: an eight-state study. Bull Am Acad Psychiatry Law 19(4):331–338, 1991

Casey R: Yates jury wiser than hired guns. Houston Chronicle, July 28, 2006. Available at: http://www.chron.com/news/casey/article/Yates-jury-wiser-than-hired-guns-1867381.php. Accessed August 16, 2020.

Daftary-Kapur T, Groscup JL, O'Connor M, et al: Measuring knowledge of the insanity defense: scale construction and validation. Behav Sci Law 9:40–63, 2011

Death Penalty Information Center: Facts About the Death Penalty. Washington, DC, Death Penalty Information Center website, 2019. Available at: http://files.deathpenaltyinfo.org/documents/pdf/FaceSheet.f1597410707. Accessed August 16, 2020.

Ellsworth PC, Bukaty RM, Cowan CL, Thompson WC: The death-qualified jury and the defense of insanity. Law Hum Behav 8(1–2):81–93, 1984

Hamilton E: The quest of the golden fleece, in Mythology. Boston, MA, Little Brown and Company, 1942

Hans VP, Slater D: John Hinckley, Jr. and the insanity defense: the public's verdict. Public Opinion Quarterly 47(2):202–212, 1983

Insanity Defense Reform Act of 1984 (codified as amended at 18 U.S.C. § 17)

Perlin M: Mental Disability Law: Civil and Criminal, 2nd Edition. New York, LexisNexis, 1998

Perlin M: She breaks just like a little girl: neonaticide, the insanity defense, and the irrelevance of "ordinary common sense." William and Mary Journal of Women and the Law 10(1), 2003

Piel J: In the aftermath of State v. Becker: a review of state and federal jury in-
    structions on insanity acquittal disposition. J Am Acad Psychiatry Law
    40:537–546, 2012
Resnick PJ: Child murder by parents: a psychiatric review of filicide. Am J Psy-
    chiatry 126(3):325–334, 1969
Resnick PJ: Filicide in the United States. Indian J Psychiatry 58:S203–S209, 2016
Resnick PJ, Knoll JL: Malingered psychosis, in Clinical Assessment of Malinger-
    ing and Deception, 4th Edition. Edited by Rogers R. New York, Guilford,
    2018, pp 98–121
Rogers JL, Bloom JD, Manson SM: Insanity defenses: contested or conceded?
    Am J Psychiatry 141(7):885–888, 1984
Rowan C: Justice system is crazy to allow insanity pleas. Plain Dealer (Cleve-
    land, Ohio), June 14, 1982, p B4
Skeem JL, Golding SL: Describing jurors' personal conceptions of insanity and
    their relationship to case judgments. Psychology, Public Policy, and Law
    7(3):561–621, 2001
Stanton J, Simpson AI: The aftermath: aspects of recovery described by perpe-
    trators of maternal filicide committed in the context of severe mental ill-
    ness. Behav Sci Law 24(1):103–112, 2006
Texas Penal Code § 8.01 Acts 1973, 63rd Leg, p 883, ch 399, Sec 1 (amended by Acts
    1993, 73rd Leg, ch 900, Sec 1.01; Acts 1983, 68th Leg, p 2640, ch 454, Sec 1)
Toufexis A: A psychiatrist's-eye view of murder and insanity. The New York
    Times, April 23, 2002. Available at: https://www.nytimes.com/2002/04/23/
    health/a-psychiatristseye-view-of-murder-and-insanity.html. Accessed
    August 16, 2020.
Yates v. Texas, 171 S.W.3d 215, 222 (Tex. App 2005).

CHAPTER 10

Becoming an Expert Witness in Maternal Filicide Cases

Gina Wong, Ph.D.

Kathryn Bell, M.C.

Stories in the media of mothers who kill their children make dramatic headlines, given our culture's fascination with morbidity and the well-known adage "if it bleeds, it leads." Despite this public fixation, scholarly emphasis directly elucidating the experience of becoming an expert witness in maternal filicide cases is scant. This role is not unlike the work of any expert witness involved in criminal investigations; however, maternal filicide cases are particularly charged, given the perniciousness and social misunderstanding of this crime. Expert witnesses serve a fundamental role because the outcome of legal proceedings rests heavily on their shoulders (Williger 1995).

The available literature regarding the expert witness role, while informative, was specific to other topics, such as employment discrimination litigation involving industrial organizational psychologists (Thornton et al. 2009), family court proceedings involving systemic psychotherapists (Hickman 2017), and autism spectrum disorder litigation involving counseling psychologists (Berryessa 2017). More general advice was focused on consulting experts, factual experts, or testifying experts who provide either consultation, testimony without opinion, or both opinions and expert testimony in court (Forkner 1987; Walton 2013). Bodiat (2019) provided guidance to medical professionals serving as expert witnesses in medical malpractice cases, outlining briefly what to expect in the process, what a report contains, and the ethical and legal duties involved.

Other scholars, such as Brodsky and Robey (1972), have provided practical but general advice to effectively orient expert psychologists in the courtroom. More recently, Brodsky et al. (2017) offered insights for psychiatrists, psychologists, and social workers to avoid problematic temptations in the courtroom by encouraging expert witnesses to be "a picture of a calm and confident teacher, whose job is to explain honestly to the triers of fact the evidence and logic that support each opinion" (p. 463). Gutheil (2009) also wrote survival tips for the psychiatrist in the courtroom and described the *Daubert* challenge, which is initiated by opposing counsel and requires the judge to assess the validity and methodology of expert testimony. Furthermore, best practices in forensic mental health assessments are offered in a 21-volume series published by Oxford University Press on a range of topics including criminal responsibility, evaluating sexually violent predators, and jury selection (Grisso et al. 2009–2021).

In light of the fact that many cases do not go to trial and the psychiatric report is often the culmination of the psychiatrist's work, Resnick and Soliman (2009) proposed practical steps to plan, write, and edit forensic psychiatric reports that effectively "translate information from the language of medicine into comprehensible language that elucidates the relevant psycho-legal issues" (p. 412) while avoiding common pitfalls in report writing. Dvoskin and Guy (2008) conveyed empirically supported strategies to manage expectations and advised witnesses to "think of themselves simply as evidence" (p. 203). Likewise, Ainsworth (2009) remarked on the ethical, technical, and practical considerations of hiring a linguistic expert witness.

General research findings can be found in the literature, such as jurors confirming the significant impact of expert testimony, particularly when the expert appears unbiased (Edens et al. 2012), is concise and confident, makes genuine eye contact, and has good academic qualifications (Blackwell and Seymour 2015). Other suggestions for the success of expert witnesses include their ability to be courtroom oriented rather than courtroom unfamiliar (Brodsky and Robey 1972), to be likable, to use lay language, to be confident without being arrogant, and to fully demonstrate their expertise and credentials (Valez et al. 2016). Although these guidelines are applicable to expert witnesses serving in maternal filicide cases, they fail to capture the nuanced and detailed practices of veteran expert witnesses.

Indeed, a dearth of research exists regarding the experiences of expert witnesses in maternal filicide cases. Several scholarly books are available:

- *Unwilling Mothers, Unwanted Babies: Infanticide in Canada* by Kirsten Kramar (2005) focuses on infanticide laws in Canada (and is further discussed in Chapter 4).
- *When Mothers Kill*, by Oberman and Meyer (2008), is a scholarly publication that proposes five reasons why mothers kill their children.
- *Women's Reproductive Mental Health Across the Lifespan*, edited by Barnes (2014), has a broad-based focus on girls' and women's mental health. In this work, contributors Nau and Peterson describe perinatal and postpartum mental health issues and touch upon infanticide and neonaticide.
- *Infanticide: Psychosocial and Legal Perspectives on Mothers Who Kill*, edited by Spinelli (2003), is considered a benchmark volume examining the legal, medical, neurohormonal, and psychosocial aspects of mothers who kill their infants.
- *Advocating for Women With Postpartum Mental Illness: A Guide to Changing Laws and the National Climate* by Feingold and Lewis (2020) (see Chapter 3 for details) discusses the process in moving the Illinois postpartum law PA 100-0574 through legislation in 2018.

Although these books are exceptional contributions and provide authoritative accounts addressing maternal infanticide and filicide, they do not directly investigate the experience of the expert witness.

Current Research Investigation

The purpose of our qualitative investigation was to capture the lived experiences of expert witnesses in the field of perinatal mental health who had been involved in filicide cases in Canada and the United States. Specifically, the focus was to capture their general experiences as well as identify best practices in becoming an expert witness in maternal filicide cases. Elucidating in-depth understanding of the role of expert witnesses in this area required qualitative data generation from novices and veterans. Our emphasis was on becoming an expert witness in maternal filicide. The research question was: What are the lived experiences of perinatal and maternal mental health expert witnesses involved in infanticide and filicide court cases in Canada and the United States from the perspective of novice and veteran expert witnesses? Gina Wong, a psychologist in Canada specializing in perinatal mood and anxiety disorders and a novice perinatal expert witness in maternal filicide cases, was the principal investigator. Kathryn Bell completed a

Master of Counselling in Alberta, Canada, and has a background in maternal mental health and publishing in this field.

RESEARCH PROCESS

Following university research ethics approval, key informants were asked to identify expert witnesses across Canada and the United States who met eligibility criteria. Depending on the number of maternal filicide cases with which participants had been involved, they were classified as either *novice* (one to three maternal filicide cases) or *veteran* (five or more cases) expert witnesses. This classification was distinctive in this research, given that expert witnesses with a variety of backgrounds engaged in the study. Some had been expert witnesses in hundreds of cases during their career but were classified as novices based on the number of maternal filicide cases in which they had participated. At the other end of the spectrum, some participants were classified as veteran expert witnesses given their involvement in a handful of maternal filicide cases although they generally did not work in the field of forensics or criminal justice. Participants were English speaking and primarily educated in Canada or the United States. Although perinatal expert witnesses from other countries expressed interest in participating, this initial phase of the study involved a local demographic. Expert witnesses without practice in maternal filicide cases were excluded from the study.

RESEARCH METHOD

Interpretive phenomenological analysis (IPA) was used to collect rich, descriptive qualitative data regarding the lived experiences of expert witnesses. IPA is dedicated to understanding and identifying meaning surrounding personal and social experiences (Larkin and Thompson 2012; Smith and Osborn 2007). This method is appropriate for investigating the lived experiences of expert witnesses and identifying, describing, and understanding how they comprehend and experience the world around them (Smith et al. 2009).

Research Interviews

The use of semistructured interviews allowed similarities between interviews, along with follow-up questions to query individual salient experiences. All of the interviews (each 2–4 hours in length) were conducted either in person or remotely using ZOOM Inc., a video teleconferencing platform, which is an established method for qualitative interview data generation (Grey et al. 2020). ZOOM interviews as well as in-person interviews were recorded, stored securely, and transcribed to facilitate analysis. Before the interview, participants were given the interview protocol and were prepared to share rich, descriptive accounts, responding to questions pertaining to their lived experiences in this role.

Data Analysis and Interpretation

Each participant's cognitive, linguistic, affective, and physical presentations of the phenomenon (Pringle et al. 2011) were taken into account. Inductive reasoning and interpretation helped with interview transcript analysis. Dr. Wong's own experience as an expert witness intimately connected her to the subject matter, which was an advantage with IPA research. Smith et al.'s (2009) guidelines for content coding and thematic analysis using NVivo 11 software were employed to organize the large data set.

PARTICIPANTS

Ten participants (five Canadian and five American; see Table 10–1 for countries of origin) were involved in this study. Four identified as male and six as female. Eight of the expert witnesses were white and two were of Chinese descent. Participants held a variety of professional designations (see Table 10–1), and a criminal defense lawyer was included who had expertise with hiring and working alongside perinatal expert witnesses in maternal filicide cases. In total, six participants were novice expert witnesses and four were veteran experts. Three novices and one veteran expert witness had not exclusively worked with the defense teams in these cases; they were employed in forensic psychiatry units or hospitals and performed evaluations as required of their work.

The six novices in our sample had been involved in one case each, whereas the four veterans had been involved in a range of 12–60 cases each. In terms of age, participants represented a five-decade age span— that is, two novices were in their thirties, three were in their forties, and one was in their fifties. Among veteran experts, two were in their sixties and two were in their seventies. The age demographic of study participants was evidence that veteran experts are among an aging population (Figure 10–1). The need to learn and excavate the wisdom of these masters is essential to foster the next generation of expert witnesses.

Results and Interpretations

Participants were asked general questions in the interview, such as how they had obtained their first case, what was most influential to them in fulfilling and conducting this role, and their experiences in becoming

TABLE 10–1. Participants' levels of competency and distinctions

Perinatal expert witness level	Nationality	Highest level of education	Level of competency		
			Maternal mental health	Criminal justice	Psychiatry
Novice	Canadian	M.D., Forensic Psychiatry	Little	Extensive	Extensive
Novice	American	Post-Master's Certificate M.F.T.	Extensive	Little	Moderate
Novice	American	Master of Social Work	Extensive	Little	Moderate
Novice	Canadian	Ph.D., Counselling Psychology	Extensive	Little	Moderate
Novice	Canadian	Ph.D., Clinical Psychology	Little	Extensive	Extensive
Novice	Canadian	Ph.D., Counselling Psychology	Little	Extensive	Extensive
Veteran	American	Ph.D., Clinical Psychology	Extensive	Extersive	Extensive
Veteran	American	M.D., Psychiatry	Extensive	Extensive	Extensive
Veteran	Canadian	Ph.D., Clinical Psychology	Moderate	Extensive	Extensive
Veteran	American	Doctor of Jurisprudence	Extensive	Extensive	Extensive

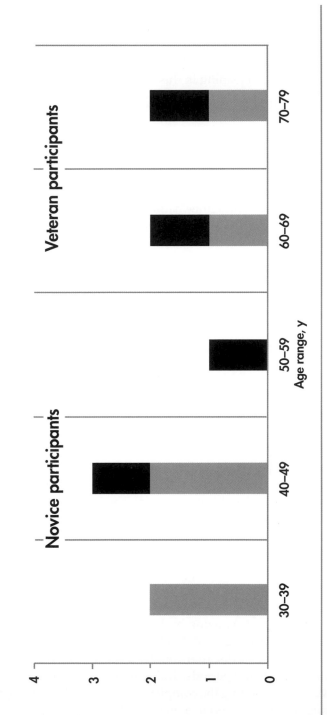

FIGURE 10–1. Participant demographics.

expert witnesses in these cases. As part of the larger study in becoming an expert in this field, findings were organized into five categories: 1) three domains of competencies, 2) how experts gained competencies, 3) initiation to their first maternal filicide cases, 4) necessary supports to this role, and 5) meaning in this work.

THREE DOMAINS OF COMPETENCIES

As we reviewed, re-reviewed, and coded the research interviews, areas of competency emerged as experts described the bodies of knowledge that facilitated their ability to perform this role. Some participants spoke of the domain areas as notable gaps in knowledge that they had when they started out and either had to learn in order to execute the role or did not learn and, in hindsight, wished they had. The three domains of competency identified in this research were 1) maternal mental health, 2) psychiatry, and 3) criminal justice. Each expert witness was identified according to his or her level of expertise in the domains (little, moderate, or extensive; see Table 10–1) and, upon participant verification, was depicted on the schematic diagram in Figure 10–2. It is important to note that these domains, although discussed herein as separate competency areas, are not entirely discrete bodies of knowledge.

Maternal Mental Health Domain

Maternal mental health is focused on the well-being of mothers during pregnancy or up to 1 year postpartum, when they are at significant risk for developing a mental disorder, such as depression (Gavin et al. 2005; World Health Organization, n.d.) or anxiety (Fairbrother et al. 2015), especially in low- or middle-income countries (Woody et al. 2017) and situations of "poverty, migration, extreme stress, exposure to violence (domestic, sexual and gender-based), emergency and conflict situations, natural disasters, and low social support" (World Health Organization, n.d., para 5). The World Health Organization emphasizes mental health disorders such as postpartum depression as a global major public health risk and has advocacy, support, and prevention as major objectives regarding maternal mental health.

Competency in maternal mental health involves knowledge and specialty training recognizing and treating symptoms of perinatal mood and anxiety disorders (PMADs), which include depression, anxiety, OCD, PTSD, panic disorder, bipolar disorder, and psychosis in the antenatal and postnatal periods. Training in perinatal mental health also involves understanding the complex biological and psychological sequelae during this time period in a woman's life.

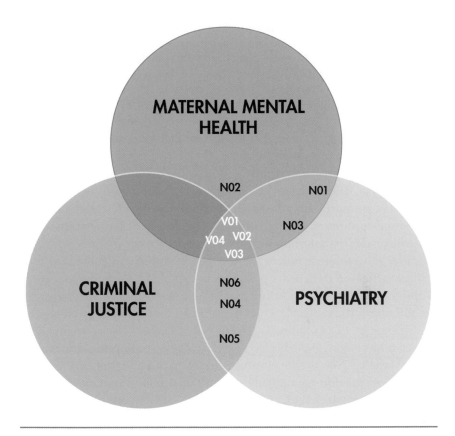

FIGURE 10–2. Schematic of participants' core competencies.
N=novice; V=veteran.

Related to maternal filicide, competency in this area denotes knowledge to identify characteristic signs and pattern of symptoms of PMADs in the woman's mental health before and at the time of filicide perpetration: in other words, determining the mother's psychological state and its impact, if any, on her ability to know right from wrong. Although the mental health of the accused is important to consider in criminal charges in general, an awareness of specialized knowledge in maternal mental health involving PMADs is distinct and imperative to know as an expert witness in maternal filicide cases.

Specialization in maternal mental health was the competency that led some participants into this area of work. For example, one novice indicated she was introduced to her first maternal filicide case through her work as a psychologist in the area of PMADs over the past 15 years:

> [T]here are forensic psychiatrists who typically do this kind of work. But forensic psychiatrists don't have perinatal expertise. So, that's what happened in my case. There was a forensic psychiatrist brought in, and she assessed [the mother]…but she had no expertise about postpartum mental health, so that's why [the lawyer] phoned me.

Novice expert witnesses also spoke of the need for "adequate training in perinatal mental health" as "one of the foundational pieces" to effectively do this work. Indeed, competence in maternal mental health disturbances was described as paramount.

Another novice emphatically stated that it would be seen "as malpractice if you didn't" have this background. Additionally, novices with experience primarily in criminal justice and psychiatry stated that they would seek out more understanding in the area in order to be involved in further cases of maternal filicide. One novice expert witness, who was employed in a forensic unit at a psychiatric hospital, indicated that "it'd be nice to find out if there are postpartum experts in the world to consult with them. It'd be nice to know that there are resources there." During the interview, the novice learned that indeed there are maternal mental health experts and exclaimed, "[A]nd now I know!"

All four veteran experts also vocalized the essential role of maternal mental health. One veteran emphasized, "You can't do this.…Any work with infanticide and neonaticide without understanding that field (maternal mental health), [be]cause it is unique." Other veterans stated that "an expert witness needs, first of all, to have some background in this whole area of mother and child." Veterans also identified the centrality of understanding nuances of perinatal mood disorders, as one perinatal psychologist underscored the importance of knowing "the basics of the different kinds of perinatal mood and anxiety disorders and very specifically how they look and how they present."

Psychiatry Domain

The field of psychiatry is a medical specialty devoted to the assessment, diagnosis, treatment, and prevention of mental, emotional, perceptual, and behavioral disorders. Maternal mental health is neither distinctly nor exclusively focused upon in the *Diagnostic and Statistical Manual of Mental Disorders*, Fifth Edition (DSM-5; American Psychiatric Association 2013), whereas psychiatry is informed by DSM-5 and other clinical manuals such as the *International Statistical Classification of Diseases*, Eleventh Revision (ICD-11; World Health Organization 2019). Clinical diagnosis draws credibility in the courts, and thus, the language, bases, and diagnostic criteria for mental disorders are set within the standards of these manuals.

The most recent version of DSM and evidence-based research are considered the major currencies against which mothers' diagnosis are held in criminal justice proceedings. In the role of the expert witness, an understanding of the acute psychosis, delusions, and related disorders that preclude mothers from being in touch with reality (e.g., schizophrenia, bipolar disorders) is essential in assessment and diagnosis. As these clinical manuals are revised and updated, the legal outcome is affected because of the weight given to psychiatric diagnosis. Spinelli referred to upcoming changes to DSM, in which she lobbied to have postpartum psychosis added to the formal diagnostic nomenclature (personal communication, November 24, 2019), which would "save lives" (personal communication, August 14, 2020) and increase the defense credibility in the eyes of the courts where it applies.

Trained psychiatrists also assess fitness to stand trial, including insanity defense evaluations. In the role of an expert witness in maternal filicide cases, competence in psychiatry is paramount, as was identified by participants: four of six novices and all of the veterans spoke of psychiatric assessment and diagnosis as a core competency in the expert witness role. One novice participant stated "You should really have some experience treating and diagnosing [postpartum psychosis], I think, to do a solid job." Another participant spoke about awareness of specific subtleties to diagnosis: "even postpartum psychosis doesn't present the way....It's not a very clear clinical presentation. It has a lot of nuance to it." They also underscored the credibility that psychiatric expertise brings to the courts: "I think, too, that psychiatry brings with it a certain jury acknowledgment about the expertise of the witness." Some novice experts had sought this domain of competence and acquired what they needed to know as they worked on cases, whereas others brought this specialty training into the role as their starting point and still others identified this as an area in which they were lacking competency.

Criminal Justice Domain

Criminal justice is an overarching term focused upon the processes, procedures, and delivery of justice. Schmalleger (2018) defined the American criminal justice system as involving "the criminal (penal) law, the law of criminal procedure, and the array of procedures and activities having to do with the enforcement of this body of law" (p. 10). Goals of criminal justice involve assessing innocence or guilt, fair treatment, rehabilitation, prevention, and safety of the public from perpetrators as well as respect for victims. It is the "system of law enforcement that is directly involved in apprehending, prosecuting, defending, sentencing, and punishing those who are suspected or convicted of criminal offenses" (Lexico.com 2020, para 1).

In relation to maternal filicide, competency in this area means the expert witness is familiar with court processes, local and national legislation pertaining to infanticide laws, and the criminal justice system in general. Several participants indicated that they did not feel pressure to be or to become legal experts but that some familiarity was important. They spoke about forensic sciences and understanding the importance of compiling history and direct and collateral evidence, as well as providing assessment and evaluations when involved in filicide cases.

All novice participants mentioned either their own competency (as forensic practitioners), "so to really know the law, to understand its application," or the need for competency in this area (as nonforensic practitioners): "That's what the attorneys are for, are to coach me on the forensics part." One veteran expert witness said, "There's a lot in forensics [that] would be helpful to know." This area was spoken about in-depth by three novice experts who had extensive forensic training and experience—"Yeah, I've had lots of experience in court"—and spoke of their experiences in criminal justice as informing their approach to the maternal filicide case with which they were involved: "[O]h, the question at hand was criminal responsibility. And I've done many, many, many criminal responsibility assessments, and the courts had no problem admitting me as an expert witness." All four veteran experts had extensive training or experience in criminal justice. They told stories and used case examples to explain intricacies of the law; sometimes, rather than outright state their knowledge base, they demonstrated it through their responses to interview questions.

HOW EXPERTS GAINED COMPETENCIES

According to participant accounts, to begin the work, they had expertise in at least one of the three domains of competency. In areas of weakness, they improved their knowledge by consulting with a mentor or taught themselves in order to fill knowledge gaps. Three veteran experts who had been involved in this work for decades spoke of a dearth of formal training in perinatal mental health and other relevant areas when they had first started. One veteran voiced, "There [were] no training programs in forensic psychology. None existed. None in the United States, none in Canada, so it wasn't like, 'No, you didn't have any training.' Well, no one else did either."

It was also clear that veterans and novices started out with roughly the same expertise, but over time and by working on multiple cases they had gained competency in all three areas. We recognized that any novice could become a veteran with continued practice in more and more cases.

Additionally, experts shared that a mentor was fundamental to their learning; as one veteran said, "I self-taught, but also I sought out those people who could help me get that knowledge that I didn't have." Mentors are further discussed in the section "Necessary Supports to This Role" later in this chapter.

With respect to self-teaching, participants reviewed research, read books, or googled information: "I looked for the templates and examples and that sort of thing," said one novice. Another novice expert researched the infanticide law because "I had to do a bit of research on that…about the frailty of the infanticide provisions and law." Another said, "I read about Andrea Yates and all these other things. I looked into the case law of different high-profile cases like this to kind of learn what has happened over the years, how has this been approached, to help inform my practice."

All veteran expert witnesses spoke of doing their own research, and most recommended that novices do the same or buy books to educate themselves, because "there are books like that; like becoming an expert witness or something like that." Novices and veterans acknowledged winging it or having a "fake it until you make it" attitude to learn what they needed to know in order to fulfill the role of expert witness in maternal filicide cases. One novice confessed, "It's been a lot of learning in the moment and on the spot." Another disclosed: "Oh, gosh, yeah. No. I just winged it, especially when writing reports."

Veteran experts also talked about the need to continue gaining competencies, to keep learning. It was obvious that the fields of maternal mental health, psychiatry, and criminal justice as they pertain to maternal filicide are not static competencies that one gains and then has complete mastery over; staying abreast of the research, legal changes, and so on was deemed essential as well. As one veteran put it, "All professionals, particularly in our work, have to approach it with 'our learning is never, ever done.' If you plateau, you should leave the profession. So, it's continual learning, and so when I do a case, if I don't know something about it, I go and research it." The attitude of continual learning and taking the initiative to self-teach was present in veteran participants still, and they spoke of starting their first case with the same attitude that carries them today.

INITIATION TO THE FIRST MATERNAL FILICIDE CASE

Regarding how expert witnesses became involved in their first case of maternal filicide, we identified no divide between how novice and veterans were introduced to the role. In our small sample, both novice and veteran experts may have come to their first case through forensic work, such as one novice who had been involved in many assessments: "Oh, it was just a regular assessment that was put on my desk" and another novice who had been working in a hospital setting: "[the mother] was remanded to our facility, and I was the only psychologist working there at the time. So, it fell into my lap." One veteran spoke of doing every case in their region because of the work: "It would come to you, so...." Others had been asked to serve in the role because of their reputation or experience in the area of criminal justice or maternal mental health, such as this novice: "A lawyer phoned me up one day and asked me if I would be interested in being an expert witness for her. I said okay." One veteran stated, "I think what qualified me at that time to be an expert was my understanding of the pertinent issues regarding women's mental health around the childbearing years." In effect, there were two main entry points to doing this work: 1) because it was part of the regular work conducted (three of six novices and one of four veterans) or 2) due to experience and reputation (three of six novices and three of four veterans) in at least one of the three competency domains (maternal mental health, psychiatry, or criminal justice).

NECESSARY SUPPORTS TO THIS ROLE

Two types of resources were identified as most helpful or most desired among novices and veterans. Having a network of supportive professionals and having a mentor were underscored throughout the research interviews as necessary, both practically and emotionally, to fulfill the role of expert witness in maternal filicide cases, not only for the first case but also for continuing to engage in this work. Having a network of supportive professionals was underscored by all participants as foundational to this work. Said one novice expert, "I have people I can turn for advice and for support and just like, 'Hey, I know if I don't know something, I know who does.'" About having a mentor, another novice stated, "I don't think I would have continued in the case if I didn't have somebody like her." This participant conveyed how much of a fledgling expert witness they had felt themself to be and that consultation with the mentor had been a saving grace. All but one novice expert witness and all veterans expressed the need for a mentor. We noted that the areas of practical, hands-on support that experts sought from other professionals and from their mentors were within the three domains of competency (maternal mental health, psychiatry, or criminal justice).

A Network of Supportive Professionals

Participants identified supportive professionals to be among those involved in the case itself and those in their place of employment. Some networks included colleagues, lawyers, social workers (often gathering collateral data for forensic reports), and clinical teams in hospitals. "Then we also had the multidisciplinary case conference, that includes a psychiatrist, social workers, nurses, mental health therapists. I think that's everybody, where we kind of talk about the case," explained one novice participant. Veteran experts also reflected back to when they were fledglings and the need for supportive professionals: "Well, I was fortunate because I had an attorney that was very.... She gave me a template.... I just kind of asked her, 'What would you like the report to look like?' And so, she gave me a template and then I worked with the template."

Novice expert witnesses described how it was extremely helpful to consult with professionals for practical advice and support: "We have a great base of people here in my facility where I can talk with, have very frank conversations with, and it's very liberating." Experts sought support from their network for practical purposes relating directly to performing the role and for emotional support and connection. Although some novices spoke of this in a professional capacity—"Talking to people who have been involved in those cases and getting a sense of what they considered or what do they wish they would have considered or how they approach the cases, those types of things"—others mentioned the value of having emotional support and validation. One novice stated,

> there were a few of them that I had confided in, that I was working with on this case. And it was really helpful to have them because I knew they understood. I didn't ever have to worry about talking about something that they were going to question like, "How can you even talk to someone like that [mother who killed her baby]?" They got it. So that, that is really what helped the most.

Veteran participants also spoke of the importance of receiving emotional support and validation from other professionals. For example, "The support, and the camaraderie, and the..'We all get it.' And when you're out there in the world doing this kind of work, [you need that]."

A Guiding Mentor in
Maternal Mental Health Forensics

Almost all novices spoke of having or wanting an experienced mentor to call upon: "I would have to say that my mentor...he was an excellent resource, [I am] very grateful for having him." One veteran expert "sought out those people who could help me and get that knowledge that I didn't have." Paralleling the type of support garnered from a network of supportive professionals, participants had mentors for practical purposes, such as sharing templates and looking over drafts of reports, and for emotional support and validation, a feeling of connection to another who understood the nuances of the expert role in maternal filicide cases. The difference was that their mentors were identified professionals to whom they felt they could, and did, consistently go for advice and support related to this work.

In general, veterans emphasized the importance of novices seeking out mentors: "I think they should be able to learn from more senior members." One novice relayed that when asked to write a letter to the judge and provide initial recommendations, they consulted with their mentor, who "read my draft of my letter and gave feedback." Another novice participant described the hands-on help they received:

> And really what I found most helpful was how he kinda talked about the step-by-step kind of things you should be familiar with, how to prepare, the types of questions they might ask you, how to qualify…the wording to suggest, to have you qualified as an expert witness, where to look, who to…look at when you're answering questions in court; all those types of things that aren't in any chapter or article that I have come across.

Likewise, the emotional support and validation was underscored by a novice who had contacted a veteran mentor: "I think the most important thing that I got from her, other than advice, was even just that the emotional part of reminding that you can't define how you did based on the outcome." Another novice said that it was also "just getting that reassurance that I was on the right track, doing what I should be doing."

MEANING IN THIS WORK

Sharing their experiences as experts, participants spoke about the tremendous meaning and reward in fulfilling this role. All 10 participants stated they wished to take on more cases in maternal filicide or were already involved in others at the time of the interview. Almost all participants conveyed the difficulty of doing this work, which one veteran described as filled with "such heartbreak and tragedy." In reference to the *meaning* that this role brought, one novice, who was in the midst of their first case and expressed a desire to continue this work, said, "[I]t's hard, it's difficult, but it's at the same time very meaningful." A veteran who had been involved in more than 45 maternal filicide cases spoke of the desire to continue doing this work despite sometimes being exhausted by it, highlighting the experience as being deeply rewarding, a privilege, and much more than just work: "It's just such meaningful work. And giving voice to women's experiences who otherwise would not be heard is very deeply touching to me.... In many ways, I feel very privileged and very honored to have these women share their stories with me."

Experts articulated the poignancy of working in maternal filicide cases, and their unwavering commitment was for reasons of justice and to save a mother's life. Relative to justice, they spoke about why the work mattered; said one veteran, "I felt this was such an injustice here that it didn't make sense....I felt very strongly about the way we were treating women here in the United States and felt I had to do something." Veteran experts overall discussed the difficult but worthwhile endeavor having to do with that sense of justice: "The greatest reward is knowing that they needed you, they needed your information and you gave it to them. And fair and just decisions were made." Likewise, one novice shared, "I think really feeling like I was part of the process that allowed this young, vulnerable mom to not stay in prison for years and years and years. Just really feeling like I was able to bring some information to the table that was helpful in shortening her sentence." One veteran thought about the significance in even changing one mind: "I really hadn't thought about this, but maybe the hope that even on a jury, even if you change one mind, you've changed a mind."

Another meaningful experience conveyed in working as an expert witness in maternal filicide cases was making a difference and saving a mother's life. Many participants spoke of this, such as this novice: "I'm still thankful for the opportunity just to have been a part of that, because that made a difference for her." A veteran poignantly expressed, "I think a verdict that is returned...that will basically save the life of your client, I think that's the greatest reward for me." Yet another novice participant said,

> I radically changed the direction of this woman's life, yes. So yeah, that's intrinsic. Indeed, it's in certain cases where my testimony can genuinely in the fullest sense of the term, change the course of someone's life. In this court, in this case, I would be one of two persons that did that for this person. Had I not done the job that I did or [if] these questions didn't come up, her life would be completely different right now... radically different.

Participants also indicated that success was difficult to define apart from reducing a woman's time in jail, but that it was important to do this. Experts described viewing success even in changing one mind or in educating the public and those in the courtroom about postpartum mental health and issues surrounding maternal filicide regardless of the verdict.

Discussion and Summary

This qualitative research utilized IPA to draw out experiences of becoming an expert witness in maternal filicide cases in Canada and the United States. Through interviews with six novice and four veteran experts in maternal filicide cases, we identified three domains of competency including 1) maternal mental health, 2) psychiatry, and 3) criminal justice. Participants were plotted on a schematic diagram (see Figure 10–2) illustrating that veteran experts, who had been involved in at least 12–60 cases each, had extensive knowledge in each of the three domains. Veterans started out in the field just as novices did, with little to no experience in at least one of the domains. Also, the way veterans and novices had obtained their first case in maternal filicide did not differ: either as part of their regular employment or via invitation due to their reputation in maternal mental health or criminal justice.

These findings are evidence that those interested in becoming perinatal expert witnesses have different professional entry points and qualify for this role with expertise in at least one of the domains. Growing into the role has been the trajectory for all experts in this study, who utilized similar types of supports and learning resources. In effect, most novices and veterans honed their competencies in the three domains via formal training in at least one domain and gained competence in the other domains through connection to professional networks, working with a mentor, and using their own self-learning strategies. Many spoke to said that they "winged it" and learned by performing the expert witness role. Veterans also acknowledged that they became increasingly knowledgeable as they took on more cases. Expert witnesses in maternal filicide cases expressed that having a network of supportive professionals either in their workplace or involved with the same case who were available for practical consultation (e.g., how to write a report, how to prepare for the role) and for emotional support and validation helped them the most. Likewise, a mentor was significant to participants' growth in the field, again in practical ways as well as for emotional support and validation.

Finally, immense meaning and reward through this work was emphasized by all participants. It was very hard and difficult, but it was more than *just* work; they found meaning in contributing to justice and having, almost single-handedly, the ability to save a mother's life by altering the course of her verdict or sentencing through their report or testimony. They also acknowledged that success and meaning could be found even when a guilty verdict was returned. Although difficult to achieve, success was also described as changing even one mind or educating others about the devastating tragedy of maternal filicide.

Limitations of the study included the fact that most participants were those who primarily worked with the criminal defense team in maternal filicide cases. Future studies involving expert witnesses and legal experts hired by the prosecution would be valuable to add more diversity to the perspectives offered, as would expert witnesses from other countries who would contribute their lived experiences. Given the relative homogeneity of participants (eight white and two Asian), involving expert witnesses of different ethnicities would also add to understanding diversity of perspectives. Continued investigation into the experiences of experts involved in maternal filicide cases and the dos and don'ts will add to the increasing knowledge base and assist in the training of other professionals. Further details into *what* aspects of knowledge and *how much* one needs to grasp to declare oneself an expert in the three domains are prudent to identify.

As maternal mental health forensics evolves further as a distinct subspecialty field, "winging it" is not a sustainable practice to train beginning expert witnesses. Historically, a mixed assortment of gained expertise was born of necessity, given the absence of integrated training. Veterans who blazed the trail have done so very successfully; however, it is not an enduring model. In this study, veterans were in their sixties, seventies, and eighties, which highlights the need for succession planning; ad-hoc mentoring is neither sustainable nor practical in the long term. Esteemed veterans, along with perinatal forensic psychiatrists, are our leaders.

Next steps involve creating a competency-based curriculum by establishing benchmarks and best-practice guidelines in the three domain areas, as well as exploring strategies to assess competency and initiate an enduring mentorship/supervision model. Future directions also include researching and publishing best practices for perinatal mental health forensic assessments and identifying the need for certification in the area. A maternal mental health forensics curriculum, once formalized, will offer state-of-the-art, up-to-date information to capture developments in the field and new discoveries informed by evidence-based research and practice, including any changing laws and updated DSM diagnostic classifications. Evaluating the need for board certification will be essential to consider in standardizing and maintaining rigor of practice.

From this research, no advantages were apparent, because the participants did not report any great detriment or negative outcome in a mother's case if the expert witness had limited or no experience starting out in one or two of the three domains.

RECOMMENDATIONS

This qualitative investigation confirms the richness and necessity of having a supportive community and a mentor for those starting out in this work. Ensuring ease of networking those who are new to a case with others who are more experienced would be invaluable. Building community and a network of supportive professionals, along with mentorship/ supervision for guidance, is not formalized at this point in time. Having a list of qualified and available mentors, perhaps adding suggestions for negotiating consulting fees at the outset, and rotating mentors so veteran expert witnesses are not overtaxed with mentees, would go a long way in cultivating new experts and fostering the longevity of others. Further community building and mentorship programs among expert witnesses, while currently existing on an ad-hoc basis with Postpartum Support International (see Chapter 15) and the International Marcé Society for Perinatal Mental Health, who are the most prolific in advocacy and treatment of perinatal mental health globally, will enhance the excellent strides these organizations are already making in this area.

The Forensic Expert Witness Association (FEWA) is a national non-profit organization that has been in operation since 1994 and includes nine geographically based chapters across the United States. Members have testified as an expert witness at least three times and practice within the association's code of ethics (see https://forensic.org/about/code-of-ethics). FEWA offers education and credentialing experiences to individuals at all levels of knowledge; publishes an online directory of expert witnesses in various areas of specialty; offers events such as a national annual conference, webinars, and online networking; and offers training and certification opportunities. Although the directory listed no expert witnesses specifically for filicide or perinatal mental health evaluation that we could find, and is only based in the United States, we see the potential value of set standards for those involved in maternal filicide cases in order to provide the most qualified experts in these difficult cases.

The need for increased rigor, facilitating networking, ensuring that supports are available, providing training opportunities, and having an accessible, like-minded community are recommendations that emerged from this research. More events, conferences, and continuing education courses and consideration of the need for board certification are essential to enhance the visibility and underscore the significance of the field of maternal mental health forensics.

Veteran expert witnesses in maternal filicide are among an aging population. They are in their sixties and seventies and should be honored for their extensive work. Their wisdom must be excavated and documented, which was an impetus for this study. Neophyte expert witnesses also have much to add, especially in understanding how one starts out in the role, how one navigates their first case, and the types of supports sought. This study elucidated the lived experiences of maternal mental health expert witnesses in Canada and the United States and will inform and shape the next generation of expert witnesses.

MAIN CLINICAL/LEGAL POINTS AND CULTURAL PERSPECTIVES

- Three domains of competency for the role of expert witness in maternal filicide cases confirmed in this study were 1) maternal mental health, 2) psychiatry, and 3) criminal justice. Each novice expert witness had extensive knowledge in at least one domain, whereas veteran experts had extensive knowledge in all three.

- Expert witnesses were brought into cases because of expertise in one or more of the areas or because it was part of their regular employment. Those who lacked competency in one or two of the other domains sought out supportive professionals, a mentor, or were self-taught, using and reviewing research, books on the topic, and the internet, as well as learning on the spot.

- Expert witnesses were interested in continuing to perform this role and found great meaning, such as enhancing justice for these mothers as well as saving a mother's life via possible reduced sentencing.

- The need for increasing professional networks and mentoring programs was identified as a recommendation emerging from the study.

- The need for advanced formal and integrative training concentrating on the three domains identified in this research—along with key competencies derived—was recommended in canonizing the subspecialty field of maternal mental health forensics.

• Indeed, next steps involve curriculum development, the assessment of competencies, and integrating an enduring mentorship/supervision program.

Practice and Discussion Questions

1. Does your experience in this field echo the findings of this research? In what ways are your experiences consistent and in what ways are your experiences discordant?
2. How might cultural differences such as societal norms, sociocultural factors, federal and provincial governments, and economic welfare impact the role and access to perinatal expert witnesses?
3. Discuss your level of competency in maternal mental health, psychiatry, and criminal justice and how your training and experience contribute to that level. Which domains are your forte, and which are your areas for growth? How can you build your competence in those areas, and how would you go about seeking training and experience?
4. In your areas of competence, what essential knowledge and experience do you have that you believe most greatly informs your knowledge base for the role of an expert witness?
5. What qualifies someone to be a mentor for a maternal mental health expert witness?
6. What resources and things can be put into place now to support the new generation of expert witnesses in maternal filicide cases?
7. In a group, discuss where you would place yourself on the schematic diagram of competencies (see Figure 10–2). Discuss and reflect on what informs you about where you would fit on this schematic representation.
8. If you are a veteran expert, what ways have you or would you mentor others and make yourself available to novices?

References

Ainsworth J: A lawyer's perspective: ethical, technical and practical considerations in the use of linguistic expert witnesses. International Journal of Speech, Language and the Law 16(2):279–291, 2009

American Psychiatric Association: Diagnostic and Statistical Manual of Mental Disorders, 5th Edition. Arlington, VA, American Psychiatric Association, 2013

Barnes D (ed): Women's Reproductive Mental Health Across the Lifespan. New York, Springer International Publishing, 2014

Berryessa CM: Educator of the court: the role of the expert witness in cases involving autism spectrum disorder. Psychology, Crime and Law 23(6):575–600, 2017

Blackwell S, Seymour F: Expert evidence and jurors' views on expert witnesses. Psychiatry, Psychology and Law 22(5):673–681, 2015

Bodiat A: Being an expert witness in a medical malpractice case. Professional Nursing Today 23(2):34–36, 2019

Brodsky SL, Robey A: On becoming an expert witness: issues of orientation and effectiveness. Prof Psychol 3(2):173–176, 1972

Brodsky SL, Dvoskin JA, Neal TMS: Temptations for the expert witness. J Am Acad Psychiatry Law 45(4):460–463, 2017

Dvoskin JA, Guy LS: On being an expert witness: it's not about you. Psychiatry, Psychology and Law 15(2):202–203, 2008

Edens JF, Smith ST, Magyar MS, et al: 'Hired guns,' 'charlatans,' and their 'voodoo psychobabble': case law references to various forms of perceived bias among mental health expert witnesses. Psychol Serv 9(3):259–271, 2012

Fairbrother N, Young AH, Janssen P, et al: Depression and anxiety during the perinatal period. BMC Psychiatry 15(1):1–9, 2015

Feingold S, Lewis B: Advocating for Women With Postpartum Mental Illness: A Guide to Changing the Law and the National Climate. Lanham, MD, Rowman and Littlefield, 2020

Forkner D: Expert advice on becoming an expert witness. Nursing 17(6):69–71, 1987

Gavin NI, Gaynes BN, Lohr KN, et al: Perinatal depression: a systematic review of prevalence and incidence. Obstet Gynecol 106(5):1071–1083, 2005

Grey L, Wong G, Cook K, et al: Expanding qualitative research interviewing strategies: Zoom video communications. The Qualitative Report 25(5):1292–1301, 2020

Grisso T, Goldstein AM, Heilbrun K (series eds): Best Practices in Forensic Mental Health Assessment. New York, Oxford University Press, 2009–2021

Gutheil TG: The Psychiatrist As Expert Witness. Washington, DC, American Psychiatric Publishing, 2009

Hickman S: Systemic psychotherapists as expert witnesses in the family court: 'visitors to another world'? J Family Ther 39(3):437–453, 2017

Kramar KJ: Unwilling Mothers, Unwanted Babies: Infanticide in Canada. Vancouver, BC, UBC Press, 2005

Larkin M, Thompson A: Interpretative phenomenological analysis, in Qualitative Research Methods in Mental Health and Psychotherapy: A Guide for Students and Practitioners. Edited by Thompson A, Harper D. Hoboken, NJ, John Wiley and Sons, 2012, pp 99–116

Lexico.com: Criminal justice system (Dictionary). Lexico.com, 2020. Available at: https://www.lexico.com/en/definition/criminal_justice_system. Accessed January 6, 2020.

Oberman M, Meyer CL: When Mothers Kill: Interviews From Prison. New York, NYU Press, 2008

Pringle J, Hendry C, McLafferty E: Phenomenological approaches: challenges and choices. Nurse Researcher 18(2):7–18, 2011

Resnick PJ, Soliman S: Planning, writing, and editing forensic psychiatric reports. Int J Law Psychiatry 35(5–6):412–417, 2009

Schmalleger F: Criminal Justice Today: An Introductory Text for the 21st Century, 15th Edition. London, Pearson, 2018

Smith JA, Osborn M: Interpretative phenomenological analysis, in Qualitative Psychology: A Practical Guide to Research Methods, 2nd Edition. Edited by Smith JA. Thousand Oaks, CA, Sage, 2007, pp 53–80

Smith JA, Flowers P, Larkin M: Interpretative Phenomenological Analysis: Theory, Method and Research. Thousand Oaks, CA, Sage, 2009

Spinelli MG (ed): Infanticide: Psychosocial and Legal Perspectives on Mothers Who Kill. Washington, DC, American Psychiatric Publishing, 2003

Thornton GI, Eurich TL, Johnson R: Industrial/organizational psychologists as expert witnesses in employment discrimination litigation: descriptions and prescriptions. The Psychologist-Manager Journal 12(3):187–203, 2009

Valez RE, Neal TMS, Kovera MB: Juries, witnesses, and persuasion: a brief overview of the science of persuasion and its applications for expert witness testimony. Jury Expert 28(2):1–5, 2016

Walton B: Being an expert witness. ISNA Bulletin 39(3):9–13, 2013

Williger SD: A trial lawyer's perspective on mental health professionals as expert witnesses. Consulting Psychology Journal: Practice and Research 47(3):141–149, 1995

Woody CA, Ferrari AJ, Siskind DJ, et al: A systematic review and meta-regression of the prevalence and incidence of perinatal depression. J Affect Disord 219:86–92, 2017

World Health Organization: Maternal mental health. WHO.int, n.d. Available at: https://www.who.int/mental_health/maternal-child/maternal_mental_health/en. Accessed January 6, 2020.

World Health Organization: International Statistical Classification of Diseases and Related Health Problems, 11th Edition. Geneva, World Health Organization, 2019

CHAPTER 11

Writing the Maternal Filicide Report

PEARLS OF WISDOM FOR EXPERT WITNESSES

Susan Hatters Friedman, M.D., DFAPA

Daniel Riordan, MBBS, M.A., M.Sc., MRCPsych, FRANZCP, MInstGA

Jacqueline A. Short, M.B.Ch.B., B.A., FRCPsych, Affiliate RANZCP, Dip.For.Psychotherapy, Dip.Soc.Pol&Criminology

Acts of neonaticide and filicide can be difficult for jurors and attorneys to fathom. Expert witnesses in these cases must therefore help the court understand the phenomenology of postpartum mental illness and child homicide. This chapter is crucial for the forensic mental health professional who is inexperienced in neonaticide and filicide cases, as well as the maternal mental health professional who is thinking of venturing into the forensic arena. We first focus on the general principles of report writing for the expert witness and then turn to discussing greater detail about being an expert witness in cases of neonaticide and filicide. The various types of reports that may be requested by attorneys and courts in child homicide cases are each discussed in turn. Important areas to cover in the interview and the framing of questions posed to the evaluee (the mother) are also described. Finally, we highlight common errors seen in neonaticide and filicide reports. The authors of this chapter are experts in forensic psychiatry as well as maternal mental health. We have each practiced in these fields for more than a dozen years. Among the three of us, we have each practiced in at least two nations, including the United States, United Kingdom, Australia, and New Zealand. We have each evaluated and treated multiple mothers who have allegedly harmed or have taken the lives of their children.

Distinctions Between the Therapeutic Role and the Expert Witness Role

Common concerns about expert witnesses in court include 1) that they act as hired guns with opinions for sale, 2) that they can be activists for a cause rather than unbiased evaluators, and 3) that they are professorial, speaking in jargon rather than lay language (Friedman et al. 2011). Fact or professional witnesses differ from expert witnesses. They may testify as to direct observations that they have made, but they do not offer expert opinions or draw conclusions from others' reports (Strasburger et al. 1997). Fact witnesses can be laypersons who have knowledge of facts in a particular case or treating psychiatrists or therapists. Treaters acting as fact witnesses may testify about observations they made about their patient during therapy or clinical treatment and their diagnosis and prognosis based on these observations. This would not be offered as an opinion but as a report of the treaters' thinking and actions during the therapy.

Expert witnesses, on the other hand, also known as forensic consultants, become involved in the case to provide evaluation and testimony that may help in the legal process, and they may offer opinions regarding legal questions. They do not see the mother for treatment as a patient but, rather, serve as forensic experts (Strasburger et al. 1997). Treating psychiatrists or psychologists should, in general, attempt to avoid acting as expert witnesses because these roles have different responsibilities (West and Friedman 2007). Whereas the goal of treatment is healing, the goal of the legal process is resolution of a criminal or civil matter. Forensic and clinical work are directed at "different (although overlapping)" realities. (Strasburger et al. 1997, p. 450). Therapy searches for meaning rather than facts, whereas the forensic evaluation seeks historical truth. Although the therapeutic evaluation may seek a narrative truth about the patient's inner reality, the therapist may not appropriately consider whether, for example, the patient is exaggerating or malingering. Forensic experts must consider malingering (reporting false or grossly exaggerated symptoms in the legal context) and must evaluate a case with objectivity.

The forensic evaluation does not involve a doctor–patient relationship, and an expert witness must usually gain informed consent regarding the purpose of the evaluation. A forensic interview is significantly different from a clinical interview, and a forensic report is different from a clinical report. Whereas the goal of a treater is healing and recovery of the patient, the goal of a forensic evaluator or expert witness is the social cause of justice in the individual case. A therapeutic evaluation is also less likely to seek the extensive collateral information on which a forensic evaluation relies heavily. Treating mental health professionals must "first do no harm," but in the courtroom, the evaluee may indeed experience harm from the report or testimony.

Additionally, Young (2016) described the "four Ds" of forensic work: dignity, distance, data, and determination. He noted that expert witnesses should behave with *dignity*, keep *distance* from the adversarial situation, and obtain valid *data* to judiciously arrive at their *determination*. Dual agency is a potential concern if the patient's treating mental health professional enters into the forensic arena, and this should be avoided whenever possible. However, the need for impartiality must also be balanced against the need to have the right professionals (those who have knowledge of the specific subject matter) commenting on care (Rix et al. 2015). In some cases, taking on both the role of the treating mental health professional and the expert is unavoidable; for example, rural locations may have significant human resource issues in which the dual role cannot be avoided.

The Forensic Report

COMPILING AND WRITING THE FORENSIC REPORT

Forensic reports should include information regarding

- the requester of the evaluation,
- the questions the report seeks to answer,
- the sources of information available,
- the nonconfidentiality warning provided to the evaluee,
- the relevant information gathered,
- the mental status examination,
- the diagnostic impression,
- the opinion of the evaluator regarding the question posed, and
- the reasoning behind that opinion (Berger 2008).

The expert witness should remember that "the success or failure of forensic psychiatric reports ultimately turns on how effectively they communicate information to courts" (Resnick and Soliman 2012, p. 412). Experts should carefully describe their reasoning in their opinions and marshal the supporting evidence (Resnick and Soliman 2012). This necessitates that even information that does not support their opinion be included in the report (Resnick and Soliman 2012). The ethical guidelines published by the American Academy of Psychiatry and the Law (AAPL; 2005) discuss the ethical principles for expert witnesses regarding confidentiality, consent, honesty and striving for objectivity, and having appropriate qualifications.

Necessary data should be gathered prior to writing the report, which may include interviews, medical records, police reports, depositions, and relevant literature (see tables later in the chapter for potential sources of information). If information that may be important to the case (e.g., medical records or interviews with important others) cannot be obtained, this should be noted in the report (Resnick and Soliman 2012). Expert witnesses should be familiar with the state of the literature regarding neonaticide or filicide. Resnick and Soliman (2012) further noted that if professional literature is cited in the report, it should be included as a source of information among the documents referred to while writing the report, and may appear at the beginning, as footnotes in the body, or at the end of the report.

For general recommendations about how a forensic evaluation is completed, interested readers are referred to the practice resource from the AAPL (Glancy et al. 2015). While it is beyond the scope of this chapter to comprehensively discuss writing a report, some important principles include considering the legal rather than clinical audience and thus not using mental health jargon and using headings in the report such that information can be easily found. Reports should have clarity, simplicity, brevity, and humanity (Resnick and Soliman 2012). Quotations used in a forensic report may help demonstrate or remind of the accused's humanity. The report itself should be self-sufficient, meaning that other documents should not need to be referred to for full understanding. Although clinicians might write in their medical records or notes that they wish to "rule out" a condition, this is not appropriate in court reports. Rather, expert witnesses provide a diagnosis when full evidence for that diagnosis has been found and clearly provided.

The psychiatrist or psychologist must be clear about the relevant legal standard that the report should address. Resnick and Soliman (2012) noted "the opinion is the most important part of the report. Thus it may require 50% of the writing time even if it makes up only 20% of the total report" (p. 416). Following the written opinion, each piece of supporting evidence should be explained to demonstrate the reasoning. The opinion section should be organized thusly: "My opinion is X. The following evidence supports this opinion: Y, Z." When writing the report, the specific source from which each datum was obtained should be described. When the evaluee has powerful motives to malinger, various data points may differ. If there are multiple versions of events, expert witnesses should acknowledge these inconsistencies in the report. Experts should limit their opinion to the psycholegal issue at hand rather than the ultimate issue of culpability in the filicide (Resnick and Soliman 2012).

Grisso (2010) analyzed reviewer evaluations of a national sample of forensic reports submitted by candidates for board certification in forensic psychology. More than half of the reports submitted offered opinions but did not sufficiently explain the evidence for those opinions, regardless of whether the written data supported them. Likewise, the forensic purpose was unclear in more than half of the reports. In other words, the legal standard or question was not stated, was inaccurate, or was unclear. Grisso examined reviewers' critiques of introductory material, organization and style, data reporting, psychological test reporting, and interpretations and opinions. Additional faults included

- Problems with organization (disorganized, without reasonable logic or lacking sequence of organization)
- Irrelevant data or opinions
- Lack of consideration of alternative hypotheses
- Inadequate data, either not obtained or not reported
- Data and interpretations mixed in the same section of the report
- Overreliance on a single source of data, such as the evaluee's self-report, rather than collateral information
- Problems with language such as jargon, pejorative terms, or gratuitous comments
- Improper uses of psychological testing

Another caution concerning expert witnesses is various potential biases. Experts must not advocate for the retaining party merely because they are the retaining party. Experts must also use caution to avoid gender bias in their analysis (Friedman 2015). Significant gender bias can occur in cases of filicide; the idea exists that for a mother to have killed her children, "she must have been mad." An alternative idea also exists for some that such mothers are monsters who deserve to pay for breaking a cardinal rule of mothering. The expert witness must also guard against confirmation bias, specifically, that only evidence supporting one's own preconceived notions is believed and used in the report. A circuitous notion exists that "the crime is punishment enough," meaning the death of a mother's children is enough punishment for the act itself, so she should be spared any sentencing. Expert witnesses must not succumb to personal bias for or against a mother's culpability or sentencing.

Finally, the expert witness must understand and address the limitations of assessment measures. For instance, no existing psychological test ascertains a mother's motive or culpability in these cases. A variety of tests may be used to help the expert; however, psychological testing is not compulsory in cases of neonaticide or filicide. One small American study (Spinelli 2001) used the Dissociative Experiences Scale and found high rates of depersonalization, intermittent amnesia, and dissociative hallucinations on the self-reports of mothers who committed neonaticide. However, self-report scales are of limited utility in a legal context, where there are strong reasons to exaggerate symptoms. Another study (McKee et al. 2001) considered the Minnesota Multiphasic Personality Inventory-2 (MMPI-2), finding a mean profile of 6–8 in a group of pretrial mothers charged with the murder of their child who were ordered by the court to be evaluated for competency to stand trial. This profile is commonly associated with psychotic symptoms, such as delusions, hallucinations, and disorganized thought. Psychological testing such as the MMPI-2 may be useful to understand the personality traits of these women.

TYPES OF FORENSIC REPORTS RELATED TO MATERNAL FILICIDE AND NEONATICIDE

The types of reports that perinatal forensic experts may be asked to write include

- Competency to stand trial reports (also known as fitness to stand trial reports)
- Infanticide Act reports
- Sanity reports
- Mitigation of penalty/diminished responsibility reports
- Disposition reports
- Conditional release reports

This chapter discusses general principles, and practitioners should be aware of the specific laws in their own jurisdiction. One or several different experts may provide reports at different stages of the legal process. Experts may be instructed by the defense or prosecution lawyers, which invites an adversarial approach, but a fundamental principle is that experts provide their opinions to help the court, regardless of which side is providing instruction and paying for the report. Experts may also be court appointed or may be asked to engage in a "hot-tubbing" exercise. Hot-tubbing, also known as *concurrent evidence*, is a procedure in which both parties sit down together to reach a consensus opinion. In some instances, more than one expert witness is involved in a case, and in others, there is only one. These reports are described in further detail in the following sections.

Competency/Fitness Reports

In a fitness or competency to stand trial report, the issue is the individual's capacity to stand trial at the time of the trial. This means that the person's mental state at the time of the act is not the issue at hand but, rather, the person's present mental state at the time of the trial. (Conversely, in a not guilty by reason of insanity [NGRI] report, the mental state at the time of the filicide is what is considered.) The principle that a person should possess a certain capacity in order to be taken to trial centers on fairness. Expert witnesses may be asked to provide an opinion on fitness to stand trial based on their clinical assessment, sometimes assisted by structured assessment tools depending on statute and case law interpretation and customary practices in the particular region (Brown et al. 2018; Rogers et al. 2008).

Intellectual disability (formerly known as mental retardation), as well as mental illness, may affect the offending mother's competency to stand trial. This may be remediable by teaching and treatment. For a full discussion of general principles in the evaluation of competency or fitness to stand trial, readers are referred to the AAPL practice guidelines for competence to stand trial (Mossman et al. 2007). In the opinion section of their report, experts should state at the outset their opinion as to whether the mother is fit to stand trial and then provide evidence for this opinion.

Infanticide Act Reports

Culpable homicide, in which the mother is considered liable for the death of the child, includes murder, manslaughter, and, depending on jurisdiction, infanticide. Expert witnesses must understand the elements of the charges laid in order to make an informed analysis of the case. As more evidence becomes available, the charges may change; a case initially charged as murder—that she intentionally caused the death of the child—may be revised to manslaughter, in which the death was not intended but was caused, for example, by failure to provide the necessaries of life for that child without lawful excuse when under a legal duty to do so as the mother. Less commonly, the charge may be revised to infanticide in some countries.

Infanticide is not a new practice but has occurred throughout history and, as such, must be contextualized within history and culture (Oberman 2003). In England at the turn of the twentieth century, attempts were made to find an appropriate legal means to compassionately dispose of mothers who killed their babies. This resulted in development of the Infanticide Act in 1938 in the United Kingdom. This Act amended the original 1922 Infanticide Act, adding two changes: extending the victim's age from a newborn child to a child younger than 12 months and including "lactation" as grounds for mental disturbance. In brief, in the United Kingdom, a mother may be convicted of infanticide instead of murder if she kills her baby who is 12 months of age or younger while she is experiencing a mental disturbance that results from giving birth or lactation. Twenty-four nations have adopted some version of the Infanticide Act, including Canada (Friedman and Resnick 2007). However, specific infanticide legislation does not exist in some parts of the world, and even in those countries and states that do have this legislation, interpretations, amendments, and important aspects differ, for example, the age limit of the child in New Zealand and parts of Australia (Bartels and Easteal 2013). Infanticide can be interpreted as both an offense in its own right or as a partial defense to murder. It is a partial and not a full defense because, if successful, it does not result in complete acquittal but instead reduces liability from murder to manslaughter. Depending on the legal jurisdiction, this distinction allows for discretionary sentencing.

The use of the infanticide defense remains controversial, especially when alternative legal routes are available to allow for insanity, diminished responsibility, or the equivalent, and several jurisdictions have questioned its use on ideological and medical grounds (New South Wales Law Reform Commission 1997). Critics of infanticide legislation have argued that infanticide is based on unsound and outmoded notions of mental disturbance, shores up outdated views on women and pregnancy, is gender biased and undervalues the life of the child, and conflates neonaticide and infanticide and that the social, medical (particularly the notion of "lactational insanity"), and legal bases of the Act are not supported by empirical evidence and are no longer relevant (Friedman et al. 2013; New South Wales Law Reform Commission 1997). However, the view of the U.K. Law Commission in 2006 was that empirical evidence at the time did not definitively refute the lactation theory and that, although inconclusive, some research suggested a possible link between lactation and the vulnerability of some women to develop puerperal bipolar disorder (Wieck et al. 2003). The reference has been retained in both the United Kingdom and New Zealand legislation (U.K. Law Commission 2006).

Infanticide laws in Canada, Australia, New Zealand, and the United Kingdom (among others) mean that infanticide reports may be requested by attorneys in these jurisdictions. Modern thinking has evolved since "lactational insanity." However, modern-day expert witnesses are faced with statutes that may include the terms *lactational insanity*, *imbecility*, or *defect of the mind*, concepts not presently used clinically. Use of outdated and inappropriate terms in statutes occurs not only in perinatal forensic reports but also in other types of forensic reports. Experts should consider how to comport this language with modern medical knowledge.

Not Guilty by Reason of Insanity Evaluations

Specifically, when expert witnesses evaluate a mother who has committed filicide, they should obtain the precise standard for NGRI in the relevant jurisdiction from the court or the retaining attorney. For example, many American jurisdictions consider whether the mother's mental illness caused her not to know the act was wrong (a "M'Naghten test"). In such evaluations, the expert queries the mother's mental state at the time of the filicide event and obtains records and other data indicative of her functioning around the time of the event. Specific jurisdictions that require analysis under Model Penal Code (MPC) or moral wrongfulness legislation are further described in Chapter 2.

Jurisdictions that use the MPC may consider whether the mother had the ability to refrain from the act despite knowing it was wrong, due to mental illness. In such jurisdictions, in addition to the M'Naghten-like criteria, a mother may be found insane if mental illness caused her not to be able to conform her behavior to the legal behavior (e.g., cases of mania in which the mother may have known that the killing was wrong but was unable to refrain from it). This necessitates a different analysis.

Experts should also be aware that "wrongfulness" in the insanity statute may include moral wrongfulness or legal wrongfulness depending on the jurisdiction (Friedman et al. 2012). In general, in jurisdictions that use the M'Naghten standard for insanity, evaluators must determine whether mental illness caused the mother not to know the wrongfulness of the act. In New Zealand, for example, moral wrongfulness is spelled out in the statute. Someone may know that the act of killing her children is illegal yet, for example, believe it is morally right because she killed after "hearing" the voice of God.

In forensic reports regarding insanity, discussion of motive for the crime is critical. Motive for filicide is relevant because of its relationship to culpability. One American study reviewed the motives of mothers found insane in filicide cases; most were altruistic or acutely psychotic (Friedman et al. 2005). Other motives for filicide (e.g., fatal maltreatment, partner revenge, unwanted child) are usually not directly related to serious mental illness. Mothers who have killed their children also may have a mental illness and still not qualify for the insanity defense; for example, a mother with depression, schizophrenia, or a personality disorder may kill related to one of the other motives. As such, it is critical that expert witnesses determine whether the mental illness was causally related to the filicide or if the mental illness was coincidental to the filicide (Friedman et al. 2012).

Thus, in the forensic interview, the motive for the filicide should be explored in significant detail. Each of the motives described in the literature (Friedman and Resnick 2007) should be considered when listening to the self-report of the forensic evaluee. Collateral information may be obtained from interviews of family members, friends, and neighbors. The relationship of the mother with the child victim should be explored and whether previous maltreatment of the child had been reported. Relationship problems with the other parent and partner revenge filicide should be explored. Friedman et al. (2012) noted "in assessing whether a parent believed their killing was morally wrong, the evaluator could ask perpetrators whether they believe they will meet their Maker with a pure heart" (p. 791). Not every filicide has only one motive; for example, the primary motive could be altruistic and a secondary motive could be partner revenge. If the mother attempted suicide at the time of the filicide or subsequent to the filicide, this should be explored in detail as well. Did the mother plan to kill herself first and then decide to kill the child, or vice versa? This can help elucidate her thinking. It is noted that "the evaluator should inquire about planning, and the offender's thinking, feelings, and behaviors around the time of their offense" (Friedman et al. 2012, p. 791).

A deific decree defense may be used in some jurisdictions in cases when mothers who were acutely psychotic killed because they believed they were responding to the command of God (Friedman et al. 2012). It is noted that, in Genesis 22, God commanded Abraham to kill his son Isaac. In some locations that otherwise limit NGRI to legal wrongfulness, mothers acting in response to a deific decree may qualify for an NGRI finding.

For mothers who kill in a fatal maltreatment case, the death may have been a one-off act of maltreatment or may be indicative of a longer pattern of child harm. These mothers do not believe that what they did was right. Similarly, mothers who kill a child because the child is unwanted usually are not experiencing mental illness. Mothers who kill in cases of partner revenge are usually acting out of feelings of anger and revenge rather than due to a mental illness (Friedman et al. 2012).

To formulate an opinion about sanity, expert witnesses first must determine whether mental illness was present at the time of the offense. Experts must be cognizant of the risk of malingering and compare the mother's report to collateral information. In addition, if she was taken to an emergency department for evaluation just after the filicide, that information will be quite useful. Expert witnesses should be aware that postpartum psychosis (PPP) may wax and wane quickly, and thus, different reports at different times of the day may vary (Friedman et al. 2019). Also, although PPP has been a diagnosis used since the time of Hippocrates (Friedman and Sorrentino 2012), it does not appear as a specific diagnosis in DSM-5 (American Psychiatric Association 2013). After describing the diagnosis, experts should describe the mother's motive for the homicide, which then leads logically to consideration of sanity versus insanity. For example, a mother who kills altruistically may believe she is doing what is right because she is sending her child to heaven.

Additional data that may help examiners to determine knowledge of wrongfulness may include the mother reporting that strangers kidnapped the child, attempting to hide the death of the child, or attempting to hide details about the death. Friedman et al. (2012) noted "societies often try to explain away various forms of female aggression. The evaluator may need to explain to the court that not all female aggression is related to mental illness and that there are some rational motives for maternal filicide" (p. 792).

When it comes to reporting a PPP diagnosis, a great deal of discussion has concerned perinatal mental illnesses and how they are diagnosed and codified in diagnostic manuals (Cox 2004; Monzon et al. 2014; Parameshwaran and Chandra 2018). This is important for experts to know when diagnosing mental illness in pregnancy and the postpartum period. The DSM and *International Classification of Diseases* (ICD) criteria are notably different for postpartum disorders. In DSM-5, peripartum is considered to include only pregnancy and the first 4 weeks postpartum. However, as research shows and perinatal psychiatrists know, the first postpartum year is a time of increased risk. Expert witnesses may need to explain this discrepancy to the court despite using proper DSM or ICD terminology and may need to explain current knowledge about postpartum depression (PPD) and PPP as well as the rather normative baby blues.

DSM-5 does not recognize PPP as a distinct clinical entity but as a specifier "with peripartum onset" for depressive disorders (pp. 186–187) or bipolar disorders (pp. 152–153) if the onset of mood symptoms occurs during pregnancy or within 4 weeks following delivery. Likewise, if the mother with PPP best satisfies the criteria for a brief psychotic disorder, then that diagnosis should be made, again with the specifier "with peripartum onset" if onset occurs during pregnancy or within 4 weeks postpartum (p. 94). ICD-11 has similar qualifiers with a 6-week postdelivery time frame (Parameshwaran and Chandra 2018; World Health Organization 2019). However, expert witnesses should be prepared to explain diagnosis and criteria issues to the court (e.g., that DSM-5 does not fully recognize the cognitive changes in PPP because PPP is not recognized as its own entity, and that PPP presents differently than a general psychosis, often with rapid onset of delusions) (Friedman and Sorrentino 2012).

Mitigation Reports

Some who fall short of meeting criteria for an insanity plea may still have mitigating evidence available to them. Forensic experts may be asked to write a mitigation of penalty report. In such a report, the expert describes the motive and diagnosis but then marshals evidence that the mother needs special consideration in sentencing. Mitigating factors might include significant stressors and mental illness for which she did not meet the NGRI criteria.

Disposition Reports

After a finding of NGRI, expert witnesses may be asked to author a report regarding the appropriate disposition for the mother. When contemplating criminal commitment to the forensic psychiatric hospital, experts must consider her treatment needs as well as her safety and that of the community. In the vast majority of cases, after a finding of NGRI, mothers are remanded to a psychiatric forensic hospital for treatment. Very rarely is a community disposal option appropriate at this phase.

Conditional Release Eligibility Reports

At a later point subsequent to an NGRI finding and criminal commitment, the patient/mother may seek release into the community, such as a community treatment order or a conditional release program, depending on the jurisdiction. To assess this readiness, expert witnesses evaluate her progress in treatment since the finding of NGRI, her insight into the situation, and her future violence risk using a formal risk assessment. Again, expert witnesses need to consider her treatment needs as well as her safety and that of the community and what constraints could be put in place to ensure these (e.g., structured group home, ankle monitor).

Case Conceptualization: Asking Questions in the Forensic Evaluation

In the tables presented in this section, we outline broad areas for inquiry and suggest possible questions to explore the key issues and complexity of experiences that may be operating for the mother in order to ultimately elicit motive. These questions are not necessarily intended to be asked directly of her, nor are they intended to be used as a checklist. In some cases, the questions contain specialist words (e.g., attachment, dissociation) and would have to be reworded or explained if one is speaking directly to a defendant. We give examples from medicolegal reports to illustrate the kind of information that may be relevant and suggest places where corroborating information may be available.

As a reference guide for expert witnesses, the tables here provide the following suggestions to explore: early upbringing and attachment (Table 11–1); psychosocial/sexual development (Table 11–2); prior relationship history (Table 11–3); previous pregnancy history (Table 11–4); previous labor, delivery, and postnatal and parenting outcomes (Table 11–5); psychiatric and medical history with particular reference to pregnancy and the perinatal period (Table 11–6); substance abuse and offending history (Table 11–7); index pregnancy history—neonaticide/filicide (Tables 11–8 and 11–9); index labor, delivery, and postpartum outcomes—neonaticide/filicde (Tables 11–10 and 11–11).

Careful exploration of motive is required, and a table using Resnick's (1969, 1970) classification has been included (Table 11–12), with questions that help elicit motive from the history and collateral information. The cultural component of filicide cases must also be considered in the evaluation. In framing interview questions, sensitive language is helpful (Friedman 2008), such as asking "when he died" rather than "when you murdered him" or "when you smothered him." Also, women who have committed neonaticide should logically be posed different questions than mothers who have perpetrated infanticide or filicide, based on attachment and life stage, as described in Tables 11–8, 11–9, 11–10, and 11–11.

In summary, the forensic evaluation should be comprehensive but relevant. The parent may be reluctant or avoidant at the interview. Be aware of the powerful dynamics exerted by guilt and shame but also be alert to malingering. Be prepared to go back—initial interviews are often about building rapport and piecing together historical context. Particular attention should be paid to symptoms of mental disorder, whether they predate the alleged offense; their presentation in the ante-, peri-,

TABLE 11–1. Early upbringing and attachment

Possible questions	Medicolegal report examples	Potential findings
From her account, other informants (parents, siblings, wider family, friends), and agency records (health, child welfare), what was her own experience of early attachment and concept of mothering?		
What is her family background (e.g., parents, stepparents, grandparents)?	She did not know her paternal grandparents, and her step-paternal grandmother showed her little affection during their infrequent contact.	Own mother was physically and/or emotionally absent
Who else is in the family—siblings, step- or half-siblings? Any adoptions? Interventions by child welfare agencies?	Her parents separated when she was a toddler. She stayed with her mother until her early teens, when she argued with her mother and went to live with her father, stepmother, and two younger stepsiblings.	Received inconsistent parenting (discipline, availability, attachment) Experiences of state care, with poor family support and lack of a positive support system
Any history of childhood trauma?	She and her three half-siblings were placed in the care of child welfare services, where they were all abused by the same foster parent.	
What is her mother's pregnancy history? Pregnancy losses, such as miscarriage, termination, sudden infant death syndrome?	Her mother had a miscarriage and a stillbirth, and her sister's baby died from sudden infant death syndrome.	Consider maternal family medical history of pregnancy, obstetric and post parturition medical complications, and pregnancy/infant deaths
Any other close female relatives with pregnancy complications/loss?		

TABLE 11–1. Early upbringing and attachment *(continued)*

Possible questions	Medicolegal report examples	Potential findings
Was her mother's pregnancy with her a healthy pregnancy and uneventful delivery?	She was an unplanned pregnancy, conceived during her mother's affair with an older man who was physically and sexually violent toward her mother. Her mother had depression and comorbid substance use.	Victim of intrafamilial abuse, including by her own mother
Was she breastfed?		
Did she reach her expected developmental milestones? Any significant childhood illnesses or injuries?	Her mother was 15 when she became pregnant and could not care for her. She was placed in the care of different family members.	Some cultural and religious mores may be strongly associated with shame and expectations of their daughters' behavior; migrant families in westernized cultures may have different ways of parenting
What were the circumstances of her own pregnancy?		
How were her intrafamilial attachments and relationships growing up? Any significant attachment issues/enforced separations?	Her stepfather had strong religious beliefs and influenced her mother. He favored his own children and was emotionally and physically abusive to her. Her mother worked during her childhood and was a pragmatic, private woman who could appear emotionally distant.	

TABLE 11–2. Psychosocial/Sexual development

Possible questions	Medicolegal report examples	Potential findings
From her account, other informants (parents, siblings, wider family, friends) and agency records (school, health, child welfare, justice), how was she socialized?		
What is her educational history/attainment level?	She left school at age 15, with no educational qualifications.	Low education levels
Any adjustment difficulties moving into and through the school system?	As a teenage migrant from a small underdeveloped country, with a poor command of English, she had no peers at school to whom she could relate.	Disadvantaged background
		Removal from cultural roots in early teens to a first-world country, leading to social and cultural isolation.
Did she have any difficulties socializing/making friends at school?	She was an average achiever at school, but her performance dropped off in her early teens when she began to socialize with the "wrong crowd."	
Did she have any hobbies or extracurricular activities while at school?	She had no close friends at school and was teased because of her weight.	
	She was a quiet, shy child who found it difficult to socialize. Her self-esteem was low.	
How old was she when she started her periods? What is her menstrual history?	Her stepmother did not prepare her for the start of her periods. Her menstrual cycle was irregular.	Unprotected sex common for girls just becoming sexually active
What was her experience of sex education?	She was sexually active from an early age, when drinking, and did not think about contraception or possible pregnancy.	Emotional immaturity and failure to appreciate long-term consequences of actions
What is her preferred sexual orientation?	She was heterosexual and first became interested in boys in her mid-teens when she was at college.	

TABLE 11–3. Prior relationship history

Possible questions	Medicolegal report examples	Potential findings
From her account, other informants (parents, siblings, wider family, friends), and agency records (health, child welfare, police family violence reports), what was her experience of relationships?		
When did she first become sexually active? Use contraception?	She was raped as a teenager. She had been drinking at a party and did not tell anyone of this.	Possible pattern of unstable relationships
Has she had any prior intimate relationships (male or female)?	She had four heterosexual intimate relationships in two years and one brief relationship with another woman after two of her male partners were violent toward her.	
What were the circumstances of each relationship (how old were they when they met? Where? Sexually active?	She was in receipt of social welfare benefits that her partners appropriated for their own use.	
	They met as teenagers at college and were still living at home. They were quickly sexually active, including while at his parents' house. She kept this a secret from her parents.	
What were their living circumstances? Partner with mental health issues? Live together?	He was verbally abusive to her and emotionally controlling, even after he moved back to live with his mother. He pushed her when she suggested taking a break and she was seen to hit him back, for which she received court diversion to attend an anger management course.	Primary victim of intimate partner violence and abuse
Any history of trauma/violence in relationships?		

TABLE 11-3. Prior relationship history (*continued*)

Possible questions	Medicolegal report examples	Potential findings
When, why, and how did each relationship end?	She was nearing the end of her first pregnancy when she met an older, unemployed man who moved into her apartment and subsequently looked after her and her baby. They used cannabis together. However, he was unfaithful and was frequently in trouble with the law. They separated acrimoniously, and he threatened her with child welfare services. The relationship ended when his drinking escalated and he started becoming jealous and possessive of her.	Financial instability Impoverished social circumstances, lack of support from family and social welfare agencies

TABLE 11–4. Previous pregnancy history

Possible questions	Medicolegal report examples	Potential findings
From her account, other informants (parents, siblings, wider family, friends), and agency records (health, child welfare, police family violence reports, parenting assessments for family court proceedings), what was her prior experience of pregnancy?		
Has she ever been pregnant before? Pregnancy outcomes (miscarriage, stillbirth, termination, full-term delivery—baby kept, adopted, taken into foster care)?	She had four pregnancies with three different partners. The first, in her midteens, ended in miscarriage, unknown to anyone. She felt a sense of relief. She missed two periods shortly after but had no other signs of pregnancy. She did a home pregnancy test that was positive. She and her	Possible pattern of unstable relationships
For *each* pregnancy, what were the circumstances of conception? Ask about paternity, nature of relationship, response of putative father. What was the relationship status at likely time of conception? Was she aware of being pregnant? How and when? Did anyone else notice or comment on any physiological changes?	boyfriend agreed to a termination, which they kept secret. However, she felt guilty afterward and became moody, and the relationship ended. She started drinking heavily. She forgot to take the oral contraception regularly, and when she felt sick, she did a home pregnancy test that was negative. The sickness persisted, and her periods were "a bit weird." A second pregnancy test was positive. Her boyfriend	Uncertain paternity and absence of a consistent parenting partner
Who knew about her pregnancy? Did she want anyone to know? If not, how did she attempt to manage this?	questioned paternity when she refused to terminate and moved away. She was anxious about telling her parents and concealed the pregnancy with baggy clothes until shortly before delivery. She had no prenatal care. Her parents were	
Did she conceal or deny pregnancy?	shocked and disappointed but supported her. She did not disclose her previous pregnancies. Her fourth baby was the	
Did she plan for the birth? Did she attend antepartum/prenatal care?	victim of the alleged offense.	

TABLE 11–4. Previous pregnancy history (*continued*)

Possible questions	Medicolegal report examples	Potential findings
Was it a healthy pregnancy (physical health antepartum, delivery, puerperium)?	There were serious obstetric complications during the delivery of her first baby, from which she recovered, with no sequelae for the baby. She and her teenage boyfriend felt in no position to care for the baby, who was adopted shortly afterward. She became pregnant again very quickly but concealed this from her new boyfriend, who was abusive and violent. She had no antenatal care and made no plans for the birth.	May be the primary victim of intimate partner violence and abuse
Did her health-related behaviors change (smoking, drinking, substance misuse)?		Financial instability and impoverished social circumstances
Any complications during pregnancy?		Inconsistent mothering/ insecure or disorganized attachment
Ask about the psychological impact of *each* pregnancy. How did she feel about being pregnant? Did pregnancy present any difficulties for her (including religious, cultural, parental/intrafamilial difficulty?) Did she fear for her safety? Did she consider termination or adoption? Did she consider harming herself or the fetus?	She did not realize she was pregnant until the second trimester, despite having morning sickness and gaining a little weight. She put it out of her mind and carried on as usual, drinking on weekends with friends.	
If a pregnancy miscarried, what were the circumstances and how did this affect her?		
If a pregnancy was terminated, how was this arranged? How did this affect her?		
Did she experience any trauma or violence during the pregnancy?		

TABLE 11–5. Previous labor, delivery, postnatal, and parenting outcomes

Possible questions	Medicolegal report examples	Potential findings
From her account, other informants (parents, siblings, wider family, friends), and agency records (health, child welfare, police family violence reports, parenting assessments for family court proceedings), what was her prior experience of delivery and parenting? Exploration of attachment needs to take account of her age/life stage.		
Ask about the circumstances of going into labor. Where was she? What did she experience, and how did she account for her physiological presentation? Was she aware of what was happening? Was anyone else aware?	She concealed the pregnancy from her abusive partner. They had sex just hours before she gave birth in the park, alone. She was found in a distressed state with the baby and was taken to the hospital. The baby was placed with child welfare services, and she agreed to closed adoption.	Precarious social circumstances Absence of supportive partner Social isolation Emotional immaturity
Ask about the circumstances of the delivery. Where was she? Was anyone else at the delivery?		
Ask her to describe the delivery. Any evidence of dissociation? Any other states of altered consciousness? How did she deliver? Was it a traumatic delivery?	Uncertain of paternity, she concealed the pregnancy from her parents, with whom she was living. She went into labor during the night, in her bedroom. Frightened by the pain, she called out for her mother, who realized what was happening and took her to the hospital. She delivered a full-term infant of low birth weight. Although shocked and disappointed, her parents accepted the baby, who was brought up in the family home primarily by her mother.	
What was the outcome of that delivery? If stillbirth, what was the likely cause? If live, were there any congenital/hereditary abnormalities?		
Did she breastfeed or have skin-on-skin contact?		

TABLE 11–5.   Previous labor, delivery, postnatal, and parenting outcomes *(continued)*

Possible questions	Medicolegal report examples	Potential findings
Have child welfare agencies or family court proceedings been involved? What arrangements did she make for the future care of her baby? Adoption (open/closed)?	Her first pregnancy in her midteens ended in open adoption at the request of her parents. Her second unplanned pregnancy at 17 was a healthy delivery. She moved away from her parents with the baby to live with a new partner. He was violent toward her and "rough" with the baby. She told him to leave. She coped for a short period as sole caregiver for her baby, in rental accommodations, but was chronically depressed and traumatized. She had a number of short-term partners move in with her. She began to neglect her son, including not taking him to school regularly. Her parents notified child welfare services, and he was placed in their care.	Unprepared for motherhood Struggled with independent living Unsupported in day-to-day parenting and neglectful of child's needs

TABLE 11–6. Psychiatric and medical history, with particular reference to pregnancy and the perinatal period

Possible questions	Medicolegal report examples	Potential findings
In addition to the history that would be taken in any forensic assessment, there needs to be a particular exploration of mental and physical health during the index and previous pregnancy and perinatal periods. In addition to her own account and that of other informants (parents, siblings, wider family, friends), agency records (health, child welfare, police family violence reports, parenting assessments for family court proceedings) may provide additional information as to her mental state, physical health, and capacity to attach during pregnancy and in the perinatal period.		
Has she ever had any contact with mental health services? Has she ever been treated by her primary care physician for mental health problems?	She has a history of extensive contact with mental health services for a major psychotic disorder, partially responsive to antipsychotic and antidepressant medication. She had an acute relapse within days of the birth of her first baby, whose newborn jaundice she delusionally interpreted as indicating the infant was the devil's spawn, sent to poison the world, and needed to be "exterminated."	Mentally ill mothers are often older when they kill their baby, and they may attempt to kill all their children, particularly if the children are very young, at the same time. Many planned to kill themselves at the time, but their filicide-suicide was unsuccessful.
Has she ever been detained for treatment under mental health legislation? What treatment interventions has she received?		
What is her relevant medical history (e.g., epilepsy, head injury, diabetes mellitus, thyroid dysfunction, hypertension, autoimmune disorders, systemic lupus erythematosus)? Include gynecological disorders such as menstrual disorders, polycystic ovarian syndrome, and obstetric history.	She was hospitalized with preeclampsia/eclampsia during her first pregnancy, which if untreated can result in fetal (and maternal) death.	It is not uncommon for women to have a history of menstrual dysfunction, miscarriage, ectopic pregnancy, stillbirth, or previous obstetric complications with traumatic deliveries.

TABLE 11–6. Psychiatric and medical history, with particular reference to pregnancy and the perinatal period *(continued)*

Possible questions	Medicolegal report examples	Potential findings
Take a history of episodes, particularly relating to pregnancy, puerperium, and the postnatal period (including the index pregnancy).	She was low in mood, stressed, and anxious during the pregnancy. Her mood deteriorated when she was no longer able to conceal the pregnancy from her partner. He was physically abusive toward her for the first time, and her mood deteriorated further. She experienced symptoms of traumatic stress and suicidal ideation. She stated, "I remember the baby and having these thoughts that he would be better off, safe and in a better place away from me. I held him next to me and put my hand over his mouth. I can't remember how long until he stopped breathing." She then overdosed on her prescribed antidepressant and was found by her partner. She tearfully denied any malevolent feelings toward the baby or that her actions had been influenced by any psychotic phenomena.	

TABLE 11–7. History of substance abuse and offending

Possible questions	Medicolegal report examples	Potential findings
From her account, other informants (parents, siblings, wider family, friends), and agency records (health, child welfare, police family violence reports, parenting assessments for family court proceedings, criminal and traffic history, addiction service providers), what is the role of addictive behaviors in the alleged offending? Are there previous convictions for homicide or violent offending, particularly against children (including concealment of the body of an infant or failure to provide the necessaries of life to a child)?		
Take a history of alcohol use/misuse and abuse of any other psychoactive and prescribed or nonprescribed substances.	She was socially isolated and estranged from her family and drank excessively on weekends.	Women may use psychoactive substances as a coping mechanism that enables them to bear the overwhelmingly difficult circumstances in their lives, such as trauma.
Has she ever had any contact with addiction services? Has she ever been treated by her primary care physician for addiction problems?	She described "blackouts" and episodic amnesia, sometimes finding herself in vulnerable and potentially dangerous situations.	Addictions can lead to death by failure to provide the necessaries of life. Family, friends, and state services are often aware of the neglect and risk but frequently fail to intervene and support.
What treatment interventions has she received?	When her younger child was 12 months old, her partner's mother contacted child welfare services because the subject was sniffing spray paint. Both children were removed from her care and placed with her partner's mother. She was referred to the addiction service again for her binge drinking, marijuana use, and sniffing spray paint.	

TABLE 11–7.   History of substance abuse and offending (continued)

Possible questions	Medicolegal report examples	Potential findings
Did she change her pattern of use when she became pregnant? What was her use of alcohol/psychoactive substances postpartum? In the index pregnancy?	Her drinking behavior of up to four glasses of wine during the week and binge drinking on weekends continued during her pregnancy. She drank heavily the evening before the baby's birth. She continued to binge drink in the week after the baby's death, until the body was discovered, in order to cope with the intolerable stress she was feeling.	Substance-misusing women may avoid seeking help during pregnancy if they fear that this disclosure will inevitably lead to statutory agencies removing their child.
Has she ever come to the attention of police or the criminal justice system? Are there any convictions related to substance abuse; violent offending, particularly against children; neglect; or concealment? How have these been addressed?	Review of psychiatric records revealed a history of assaultive behaviors when mentally ill and when using psychoactive substances, for which she has not been prosecuted.	
	She has a history of acquisitive offending (e.g., shoplifting, theft, social welfare fraud), possession of cannabis, and one conviction for common assault. She has been given primarily community-based sentences and a brief remand in custody.	
Was she under the influence of psychoactive substances at the time of the offense?		
When and how was the baby found?	She had one previous conviction, which was for concealing the dead body of a child. She was sentenced to 18 months' supervision/probation and counseling.	

TABLE 11–8. Neonaticide: index pregnancy history*

Possible questions	Medicolegal report examples	Potential findings
From her account, other informants (parents, siblings, wider family, friends), and agency records (health, child welfare, police family violence reports, parenting assessments for family court proceedings), what was her experience of this pregnancy? Was the baby wanted?		
What were the circumstances of conception? Ask about paternity, nature of relationship (including cohabiting), response of putative father (if he is aware).	She had sex with a man she had just met through an online dating site, after her boyfriend ended their relationship.	Most women accused of neonaticide are young and single; younger age range, <25 years old
		Pregnancy often unwanted
	She was the victim of incest by her adoptive father, to whom she was related.	Not in committed relationship with father of baby
Was she aware of being pregnant? When did she become aware of being pregnant? Look for evidence of denial of pregnancy. Did she notice any physiological changes, such as secondary amenorrhea, weight gain, breast tenderness? When did these occur?	She experienced bleeding, which she attributed to her periods continuing, despite it sometimes being lighter than her usual menstrual bleeding and her stomach feeling hard. She did not gain much weight and was still able to fasten her trousers, although she did wear loose-fitting jerseys.	May fear telling father because of fear he will end relationship
		Emotionally immature
		Not usually mentally ill/psychotic
		Denial of pregnancy
	She appeared to know at an intellectual level that she was pregnant, but not at an emotional level. She stated, "I didn't really want to think about it. I didn't want to think about anything. I wanted to push everything aside."	Concealment of one pregnancy associated with greater risk of subsequent concealment, with harmful outcomes for baby

TABLE 11–8. Neonaticide: index pregnancy history* *(continued)*

Possible questions	Medicolegal report examples	Potential findings
How did she feel about being pregnant? Did pregnancy present any difficulties for her (e.g., religious, cultural, parental or intrafamilial difficulties)? Did she fear for her safety? Did she consider termination or adoption? Did she consider harming herself or the fetus?	She recognized she was pregnant at 5 months because she had missed two periods and her clothes were becoming tight. It was too late for a termination.	Termination seldom sought because it requires prompt action when mother is avoidant or in denial
	She did not think about what would happen, but although "I put a smile on my face, inside I was stressing out."	Adoption requires acceptance of pregnancy and action; processes complex
	She was past the date of termination and did not even consider this. She said that she had considered adoption now and again.	Concealment may be response to incest, intimate partner violence, or fear of separation from the baby, e.g., in substance misuse
Did her health-related behaviors change (e.g., smoking, drinking, substance misuse)?	She forced herself to continue her usual routine.	Most live either with parent(s), guardian(s), or other family and/or are financially dependent on them
Did she share the information about her pregnancy with anyone?	She took little interest in her appearance, wearing the same clothes over and over, and told no one of how depressed she was feeling or of the baby's existence.	Afraid of being ostracized by parents with strong traditional social, cultural, or religious values who disapprove of extramarital sex and teenage pregnancy
Did she attend antepartum/prenatal care?		
Did she try to conceal the pregnancy? If so, how did she do this?	She told no one because she was scared of her parents' reaction, and another baby would add more stress to the family.	May fear for her life if seen to bring shame on family
Did anyone notice or comment on her changing body?	Her father was described as watchful and protective of his daughter. His attitude was in keeping with his non-Western culture.	Family and friends may be in a state of denial and not notice the pregnancy or feel too awkward to comment, reinforcing strategy of denial and passivity

*Although this occurs across all sociodemographic groups, there are underlying similarities.

TABLE 11–9. Filicide: index pregnancy history*

Possible questions	Medicolegal report examples	Potential findings
From her account, other informants (parents, siblings, wider family, friends), and agency records (health, child welfare, police family violence reports, parenting assessments for family court proceedings), what was her experience of this pregnancy? Was the baby wanted?		
What were the circumstances of conception? Ask about paternity, nature of relationship (including cohabiting), response of putative father (if he is aware).	Her second pregnancy was unplanned. They had been living with her partner's mother for 2 years. She was happy to have a baby close in age to the first, but he wanted a termination. The pregnancy was traumatic. He became violent toward her for the first time, knocking out her teeth. She was hospitalized twice with antepartum bleeding.	From a broad range of backgrounds

More likely to be married or living with a partner than those who commit neonaticide

Often have more than one child

Socially isolated |
| Was she aware of being pregnant? When did she become aware of being pregnant? Look for evidence of denial of pregnancy. Did she notice any physiological changes, such as secondary amenorrhea, weight gain, breast tenderness? When did these occur? | The pregnancy was unplanned and from a casual liaison. Her psychotic illness was partially responsive to treatment, and she was unable to mother her three children, who were in the care of her aunt. She was supported by the community mental health team to live in rental accommodations. She chose to continue the pregnancy. She reduced her substance abuse. She was referred to the high-risk pregnancy team, and child welfare services were notified. | Those with psychotic disorders often have little or no concept of mothering, poor personal experience of being mothered (mothers emotionally or physically absent or abusive)

Often a complex interplay between vulnerability to mental illness and social isolation.

Failure of social support agencies |

TABLE 11–9. Filicide: index pregnancy history* *(continued)*

Possible questions	Medicolegal report examples	Potential findings
How did she feel about being pregnant? Did pregnancy present any difficulties for her (e.g., religious, cultural, parental or intrafamilial difficulties)? Did she fear for her safety? Did she consider termination or adoption? Did she consider harming herself or the fetus?	She was helped to attend her antenatal appointments by her community psychiatric nurse. She was pleased when the scan showed she was expecting a girl. She prepared for the baby's birth and was excited that she was being helped to continue mothering postdelivery, with oversight by child welfare services. Her mental state prior to delivery was described as stable but with established cognitive impairment.	Most are primary caregivers for their children

Experience stressors such as failed relationships, financial strain, or abuse

Most women financially dependent on partner or social welfare |
Did her health-related behaviors change (e.g., smoking, drinking, substance misuse)?		
Did she share the information about her pregnancy with anyone?		
Did she attend antepartum care?		
Did she try to conceal the pregnancy? If so, how did she do this?		
Did anyone notice or comment on her changing body?		

*Although this occurs across all sociodemographic groups, there are underlying similarities.

TABLE 11–10. Neonaticide: index labor, delivery, and postpartum outcomes

Possible questions	Medicolegal report examples	Potential findings
From her account, other informants (parents, siblings, wider family, friends), and agency records (health, including records of antenatal attendance or failure of attendance and psychiatric records; child welfare; police family violence reports; parenting assessments for family court proceedings), what was her experience of this birth?		
Ask about the circumstances of going into labor. Where was she? What did she experience? How did she account for her physiological presentation? Was she aware of what was happening? Was anyone else aware?	She had had a number of casual relationships and was in a state of emotional denial of her third pregnancy. Her first conscious awareness of imminent delivery was pain, with no further memory until she awoke in her apartment 2 days later to find herself in bed with a baby dead beside her. She concealed the body in a shoebox. She unknowingly became pregnant again shortly afterward.	Usually living with parents or other relatives Social and emotional isolation Pregnancy ending in neonaticide may not be mother's first; there may have been other neonaticides or living children Assaults to the newborn occur in extreme emotional crises, including rage, panic, and desperation, which may be accepted as mental disturbances but not as mental illness. They may or may not be planned. Common methods include suffocation to stifle crying, drowning after delivering into the toilet (common in pregnancy denial), strangulation, head trauma if delivery occurs while crouching or standing, and exposure.
Ask her to describe the delivery. What were the circumstances? Where was she? What did she experience?	She remembered feeling dizzy and watching herself "going through the motions, like you are not actually there, like a slowed-down movie which then jumps to the next scene."	

TABLE 11–10. Neonaticide: index labor, delivery, and postpartum outcomes *(continued)*

Possible questions	Medicolegal report examples	Potential findings
Any dissociation or other states of altered consciousness during delivery? How did she deliver? What did the baby look like? Did the baby cry? How did she respond?	She told her mother she had period pains. She went to the bathroom, ran the shower, and gave birth to a baby therein, with her family a few rooms away. She could not recall the sex. The baby was a mottled purple and started to cry. She wrapped it in a towel, covering its face, and the crying quickly stopped. She cleaned up the	When the reality of contractions and labor occurs, most can no longer deny or conceal. Some present to the hospital for delivery or, in partial recognition, complain of abdominal pain. Some women with intellectual disability may not associate this with pregnancy.
When did she think her baby had died?	shower, carried the baby into her bedroom, and put it on the bed. There was no movement. In a	Women try to avoid detection and deliver alone, often at home on the toilet while others are also home. They make little or no noise, followed by
How did she manage, thinking her baby had died, and with the situation in which she found herself (i.e., what did she do with the baby and placenta, how did she clean up)? Did she seek help from anyone?	state of panic, she put the baby and the placenta in a bag, which she put in the closet. She put the towel in her laundry basket and fell asleep, exhausted, on the bed. The baby was found by her mother a week later while hanging clothes. If she finds events, thoughts, or feelings too painful to remember, she "blocks it out, so things are a black space in my head." Consistent with her	either exhaustion or panic. They often experience intense cramping and stomach pains and interpret these as a need to defecate. After delivery, they may be surprised by or not fully cognizant of what has happened. They may panic or be in a state of mental confusion that renders them unable to take appropriate action. If they understand the reality of the baby, they may respond in a panic to silence the baby's cry.
What did she do in the days after the birth?	verbal account, her scores on the Dissociative Experiences Scale were in a range that suggests "a higher tendency to dissociate."	Without a scale for malingering, high self-reported rates on the Dissociative Experiences Scale of dissociative phenomena and intermittent
When/how was the baby found?	She returned to work a few hours after her baby was born but felt "lousy, numb, anxious." She continued to work despite her low mood and difficulty concentrating.	amnesia during the delivery and homicide could be exaggerated as attempted exculpation.

TABLE 11–11. Filicide: index labor, delivery and postpartum outcomes

Possible questions	Medicolegal report examples	Potential findings
From her account, other informants (parents, siblings, wider family, friends), and agency records (health, child welfare, police family violence reports, parenting assessments for family court proceedings), what was her experience of this birth and her subsequent attachment? Exploration of attachment needs to take account of her age and life stage.		
Ask about the circumstances of going into labor. Where was she? What did she experience, and how did she account for her physiological presentation? Was she aware of what was happening? Was anyone else aware?	This was her fourth delivery after a gap of 6 years. It was planned that her baby would be induced, but she underwent an emergency cesarean section at term under general anesthetic, for fetal distress.	There is often a complex relationship between the vulnerability to mental ill-health, particularly postpartum, and social isolation.
What were the circumstances of the delivery? Where was she? What did she experience?	She was understandably anxious. She awoke to the baby being in the special-care unit/neonatal intensive care unit with breathing difficulties.	Some women are cognitively or intellectually impaired.
Ask her to describe the delivery. Any evidence of dissociation? Any other states of altered consciousness? How did she deliver? What did the baby look like? Did the baby cry? How did she respond?	Although the infant's condition stabilized, she was not able to hold her for 3 days. She struggled to express breast milk and became increasingly agitated: "Why did I have a sick baby?" Her sleep pattern was disturbed. Long-acting injectable antipsychotic medication was restarted. Convinced the baby was going to be removed from her care, she became more paranoid, restless, and preoccupied and barricaded herself and the baby in the room.	Faced with the challenges of mothering, some women may be rendered more vulnerable to filicide by their histories of abuse and associated low self-esteem, poor impulse control, depression, anxiety, and antisocial behavior, including aggression and substance abuse. This is compounded by social isolation and financial precarity.

TABLE 11–11. Filicide: index labor, delivery and postpartum outcomes *(continued)*

Possible questions	Medicolegal report examples	Potential findings
How was she cared for after the delivery? Did she seek or receive help from anyone?	She had a number of small bleeds antepartum and had an emergency cesarean section at term after the fetal heart rate dropped. The baby was small for due date. Her abusive partner did not attend the birth, nor did his mother, who was looking after their toddler. Her partner resumed his abusive behavior. She avoided the midwife because she was scared that her bruises would be seen.	Explore possibility of child abuse
How long did the baby live? What was her attachment to the baby?		Consider whether any recent relationship or marital problems could provide a motive for partner revenge filicide
How was the baby found to be dead?	She left the father, taking the 8-week old baby, and moved in with an older man who offered her accommodation and appeared to care about her and the baby. She saw bruising on the baby after he had been babysitting. He said this had occurred accidentally, but she witnessed further violent handling, particularly when the baby cried. She became increasingly stressed and angry with the baby's "deliberate" crying, afraid that they would be kicked out. She held a pillow over the baby's face one evening until he quieted. He was dead when she went to his cot/crib in the morning.	Women with psychosis may express delusional beliefs about the baby. They may present with depression and suicidality.
	She smashed up the room, and the baby died from head injuries. She was floridly psychotic and later said she had flashbacks of her last baby being taken from her at birth.	

TABLE 11–12. Motive

Possible questions	Medicolegal report examples
From her account, other informants (parents, siblings, wider family, friends), and agency records (health, child welfare, police family violence reports, parenting assessments for family court proceedings, criminal and traffic history, addiction service providers), what is the likely motive for the killing? Consider classifications of motive such as those originally developed by Resnick (1969, 1970), including unwanted child, altruistic, acutely psychotic and partner revenge.	
What are the sociodemographic characteristics of the offender (i.e., age, relationship/marital status, level of education, socioeconomic status, ethnicity, pregnancy history)?	She began a new relationship in her early twenties, when her baby was a few months old. She was emotionally immature, and her new partner was in his late teens. He moved in with her but continued to go out and party with friends. The baby was fractious and difficult to settle. She was unable to find a babysitter and resented having to stay at home. She and her partner both believed the baby was deliberately "playing up" by crying and handled him roughly. One evening, she slapped the baby's face "to teach him a lesson" and shook the infant until he went quiet and limp. She left him in his cot, where her partner found his lifeless body in the morning.
Was the pregnancy denied or concealed?	The pregnancy was an unwanted threat to her future. She and her boyfriend were in their early teens; both were becoming sexually active, but she had not expected to become pregnant. She did not realize she was pregnant initially but started gaining weight. Her boyfriend ended the relationship, and her parents attributed her weight gain to unhealthy eating in response to this breakup. She concealed the pregnancy with baggy clothing, began skipping school, and gave birth in her bedroom at home while her parents were asleep in the next room. Afraid they would hear the newborn's crying, she smothered the infant and hid the body in a cupboard.
Did she act alone or in concert with a partner?	The pregnancy was healthy, but her history of intrafamilial childhood sexual abuse rendered her emotionally fragile. A traumatic delivery triggered flashbacks of the abuse, which she did not divulge to her midwife or to her partner. The recurrence of traumatic nightmares prevented her from sleeping, and she became increasingly concerned that her baby would also be abused.

TABLE 11–12. Motive (*continued*)

Possible questions	Medicolegal report examples
Is there a history of mental disorder? If so, what is the nexus between this and the offending behavior? Does it meet the jurisdictional threshold for an insanity defense or infanticide?	She became hypervigilant around the infant and did not want her partner to be involved in any intimate care, such as washing and diaper changing, fearful that he might abuse the baby. Midwifery records described her as being an anxious and overprotective but very caring first-time mother. However, she perceived her own mothering to be inadequate and became depressed. When her partner and his family offered to help with the baby, she developed the delusional belief that the baby's abuse was inevitable. Feeling increasingly powerless to prevent this, she altruistically smothered the baby with a pillow and made an unsuccessful suicide attempt by overdose. She had a longstanding history of psychosis and comorbid substance misuse. Her three previous children had been taken at birth by child welfare services, after which she stopped using psychoactive substances.
	Her symptom control improved on long-acting injectable antipsychotic medication. The index pregnancy was unplanned and from a casual relationship, but she wanted to keep the baby and was managed by the specialist high-risk pregnancy team. Against advice, she discontinued her medication in the third trimester. Some mild mood instability was evident prior to delivery, and she was closely monitored. The delivery was uneventful, but her mood state became changeable and rapidly deteriorated within a few days postpartum. Acutely psychotic and believing her baby to have special powers from God, she acted on command hallucinations and threw the infant from the hospital window, believing she would fly like an angel. The infant was fatally injured.
	The divorce and child custody proceedings were particularly acrimonious. She had devoted herself to her husband and their 3-year-old daughter and had not suspected her husband's infidelity. She felt socially stigmatized by his behavior and embittered by her changed personal circumstances. She unsuccessfully opposed the contact/visitation arrangements imposed by the child custody process and could not reconcile herself to her daughter having any contact with her ex-husband's new partner. She drowned her daughter in the bathtub the evening before the first court-ordered contact.

and postnatal periods; and their nexus to the alleged offense. It is important to remember that the mental disorder may not be directly connected to the motive for the offending, or it may not reach the threshold for an insanity defense. As for any other forensic evaluation, when exploring motive, try not to ask leading questions and avoid lists of possible mental symptoms.

In this chapter, we provide material for the first-time expert and add some tips for those more used to requesting or providing expert reports for mothers accused of killing their child. Professionals wishing to act as expert witnesses must be duly qualified in their area of practice and have a thorough knowledge of both perinatal and forensic psychiatry. This is a serious role; experts should be familiar with the role, responsibilities, and potential conflicts inherent in acting as an expert witness and adhere to good practice guidelines as issued by their regulatory/ governing authority. The roles of the treating practitioner and expert witness practitioner are different, although they do overlap at times. Unless necessary, the two are best kept separate, but if situations arise in which this is not possible, then any conflict or potential bias must be thoroughly considered and made explicit to stakeholders, particularly the court.

Reports should be written carefully and objectively and should include appropriate collateral information, the source of which should be recorded in the report. Forensic experts should guard against their own biases and be careful in their use of language in reports. There are several types of report, and we have detailed what needs to be considered in providing expert testimony for a competency/fitness report, Infanticide Act report, NGRI evaluation, mitigation report, disposition, or conditional release eligibility report. Each type of report will have the same basic structure, but the nuances of each have been detailed to avoid unnecessary pitfalls.

Better outcomes are gained when psychiatrists, psychologists, and lawyers work respectfully with each other. Counsel can assist in providing clear instructions and prompt delivery of collateral material; if the expert is needed to give testimony in court, then as much notice as possible is helpful for clinicians who may have other clinical duties to which they must attend. Expert witnesses need to understand that legal counsel's role is different from theirs. They are not "in charge," as they would be in a clinical role. Respect for the legal process and court is paramount.

Gaining experience as a trainee by shadowing seniors who are conducting assessments, attending court to observe the court process, and attending training courses can demystify and help assuage some of the anxiety when first starting as an expert witness. Working as an expert witness is a privilege and an extremely rewarding experience, and we hope that we have provided you with the necessary tools to start on this journey.

Core Competencies

1. Expert witnesses must ensure that they are an expert in the field and adhere to the relevant (national body's) expert witness code of practice. What defines an "expert" has been the subject of regulatory investigation proceedings against practitioners who offered opinions to the court in areas outside their expertise and had poorly reasoned their opinions (Rix et al. 2015). It would be prudent to have the requisite experience in both perinatal and forensic work (Friedman and Sorrentino 2012). Although the reasons for miscarriages of justice (unsafe convictions) are complex, experts must be mindful of potential pitfalls when acting as expert witnesses, for example, by not commenting directly on the "ultimate issue" and culpability, to safeguard against falling afoul of the expert role (Hallet 2020). If giving direct evidence in court, experts need to be familiar with court processes and protocols and with some of the strategies and techniques used by counsel when cross-examining experts (Allnut et al. 2007; Casey 2003).

2. An important task of the expert witness is to help the court make sense of psychiatric issues in this context. Expert witnesses in neonaticide and filicide cases must understand the literature and phenomenology of both of these unique types of cases and be able to explain perinatal mental health issues and the characteristics of neonaticide or infanticide so that the layperson judge or jury can make sense of what may be perceived as a nonsensical event. Language used by the general public versus medical and legal professionals may mean different things, have several definitions, be used interchangeably (e.g., for infanticide and neonaticide), and be confusing for the court. Psychiatric literature may be specific to issues in a particular culture, country, or region, and laws will differ depending on where the expert witness is practicing.

3. Expert witnesses must be aware of the mental illnesses that can arise in the perinatal period and be confident in describing current understanding of these disorders to the court. Sound knowledge of postpartum (puerperal) psychosis, a severe mental illness that requires urgent medical attention, is important. PPP occurs in about 1 of 1,000 (0.1%) women who give birth (VanderKruik et al. 2017). There is an increased risk of PPP if the mother already has a psychiatric illness,

such as schizophrenia, but more so if she has a past history of schizoaffective disorder or bipolar disorder (DiFlorio et al. 2018; Wesseloo et al. 2016). If a mother has had an episode of PPP, there is a 50% chance she will have another episode when she has another child (DiFlorio et al. 2018). Hospitalization is usually required in a psychiatric unit, preferably a mother-and-baby unit where skilled staff can help the mother recover while keeping the infant safe. Presentation may differ from other psychotic presentations more familiar to a general psychiatrist, particularly regarding the cognitive symptoms, such as confusion or a delirium-like presentation sometimes referred to as a "cognitive disorganization psychosis" (Isik 2018; Monzon et al. 2014; Wisner et al. 1994). Experts must assess for PPP and key differentials such as an organic disorder, depression, catatonia, malingering, factitious disorder, and anxiety disorders such as OCD.

4. Good collateral information and detailed questioning at the interview is important. Collateral records are obtained in any forensic evaluation, but additional records may particularly assist in understanding the nature of the relationship between the mother and the child in filicide cases (Friedman et al. 2012). Prenatal care and delivery records may be useful regarding her statements about whether the pregnancy was desired or not. Pediatric records for the child may additionally give information about bonding, parenting, and abuse. If the child had previously been reported to child protective services, these records should also be sought. Additionally, lack of appropriate pediatric visits may be noted. School records for the child may also be useful. If collateral records can be reviewed prior to the psychiatric evaluation, the expert may be aware of specific behaviors or inconsistencies between the records and the mother's account that can be clarified in the interview (Friedman et al. 2012). See tables for details regarding collateral information.

MAIN CLINICAL/LEGAL POINTS AND CULTURAL PERSPECTIVES

- The forensic expert role is distinct from the role of the treating clinician, with responsibility to the court and the interests of justice rather than to the interests of a patient.
- Forensic reports must be logically written and able to stand alone. Forensic reports utilize collateral sources of information, rather than merely self-report.

- Various types of reports may be requested of the expert witness in a maternal filicide case, and one must also be aware of the law in one's locale.
- Understanding the mother's motive for taking the life of her child is critical in writing court reports.
- The forensic expert witness in a maternal filicide case should be able to explain maternal mental health concepts to laymen and the court.
- Forensic expert witnesses should carefully examine their cultural and gender biases when evaluating any parent who has committed filicide.

Practice and Discussion Questions

1. Review these four examples of notable common errors in perinatal forensic reports that we have come across in our forensic experience. Discuss how to specifically remedy and mitigate against such errors. Use the learning points provided as well as Grisso's (2010) discussion of the main errors found in forensic reports as discussed in the chapter.

   A. "I would want to rule out an organic condition such as delirium in this patient because she presents with confusion, delusions, and hallucinations."

      A medicolegal report is different from a clinical report in which the diagnostic sieve is still wide. Expert witnesses should be able to make a definitive diagnosis or, at the very least, a provisional diagnosis. They should not write what they wish to rule out. All of the documents needed to make a diagnosis and write a report should be made available, ideally before the expert sees the evaluee.

   B. "This poor woman deserves mercy from the courts; the loss of her child is punishment enough" and "I cannot believe they missed this postpartum psychosis diagnosis; how this doctor can call himself a specialist is a joke!"

      Overly emotive language and unprofessional language should be avoided.

C. "It is clear this lady infanticided her child, and therefore the infanticide defense holds true. She had diminished responsibility for her actions."

> Using colloquial terms such as "this lady" and confusing or mixing up concepts should be avoided. Experts should be familiar with the legal concepts (e.g., the infanticide defense) in the legal jurisdiction where they practice.

D. "This woman has schizophrenia; therefore, she is insane by definition. She killed her child, which is an insane act, and therefore she should be given the insanity defense."

> Experts must explain the nexus between the mental illness and the act and provide coherent reasoning rather than circular logic.

2. You are asked to provide an expert witness report for a 32-year-old woman accused of killing her 6-week-old baby. Her husband came home from work to find the baby face down in the bath and the mother lying in bed, asleep. She was arrested and taken to prison. You have a copy of some of the prison records, which describe her as oppositional and not following the prison officers' orders. She appeared to be confused, laughing one minute and crying the next if she did not get her way. All you know about her past history was that she delivered the baby at 38 weeks after a difficult labor. She has had two previous terminations and used cannabis when she was a college student. The defense team has raised the issue of infanticide. You have been instructed by the prosecution's legal team to provide a report, questioning this. They have also asked you to comment on whether the prison records would confirm she may have been high on illicit drugs and if that is why she may have killed her baby and acted in an oppositional manner in prison.

> As an expert witness you should respectfully but firmly ask that all documents relating to this case be sent to you, ideally before you see the defendant, including family doctor records, general and psychiatric hospital records if there has been any prior psychiatric history, obstetric records, prison records, postmortem records, and, if applicable, school records. Previous criminal history records are also helpful. Any screening physical examination, blood tests, or urine

sample results taken at prison reception or soon after would be helpful.

You should ask the legal team for a clear written letter of instruction. Agreeing to a fee schedule is best completed at the beginning of a case so that both parties are clear about what is expected in terms of time spent, timelines, costs, and remuneration. You would then arrange to see the defendant. Allow time for this, because if she is still in prison, you will have to adhere to a security clearance procedure and may need to schedule with the prison and show identification to gain access.

A forensic report is really an excellent psychiatric assessment report, plus a bit more. Extra care should be taken to develop a detailed and thorough psychiatric assessment, which may take several hours in one session or over several sessions. This needs to be completed with great sensitivity, but objectively. The defendant should be appropriately informed and give consent before going ahead with the assessment. Upon gathering the information, practitioners' actions differ, but a common step is to compile necessary background and detail on record and start filling out sections of a psychiatric history, which will make up the body of the report. This gives you more time to consider your opinion and recommendations. The case here, although exaggerated in part, is not atypical, and including a detailed analysis of how a postpartum psychosis may differ from other psychotic states should be explored to help the court make sense of the mother's behavior. Form your opinion and any potential counterarguments or flaws in your deductive reasoning when you write your opinion and recommendations.

Go back and read the original letter of instruction to see if you have answered all the questions. Correct any grammar or spelling errors. Securely deliver the report in a timely manner. Be prepared: there may be a time lapse between delivering the report and appearing in court, so your report should be a stand-alone document that is detailed and easily referred to when under cross-examination.

3. You are asked to provide a report on an 18-year-old woman who left her baby under a bridge who later died. She was arrested and claims

she didn't know she was pregnant and panicked when she had "stomach pains." You have been asked to write a report for the court. You and your partner have been struggling with infertility and feel angry when you read the transcripts from the police interview.

It is important to be aware that these cases are highly emotionally charged, and it is important to take care of one's own mental health. The expert must be as objective as possible, and you may decide not to take the case on.

References

Allnut S, Samuels A, O'Driscoll C: The insanity defence: from wild beasts to M'Naghten. Australasian Psychiatry 15:292–298, 2007

American Academy of Psychiatry and the Law: Ethics Guidelines for the Practice of Forensic Psychiatry. Bloomfield, CT, American Academy of Psychiatry and the Law, 2005. Available at: https://aapl.org/ethics-guidelines. Accessed September 3, 2020.

American Psychiatric Association: Diagnostic and Statistical Manual of Mental Disorders, 5th Edition. Arlington, VA, American Psychiatric Association, 2013

Bartels L, Easteal AM: Mothers who kill: the forensic use and judicial reception of evidence of postnatal depression and other psychiatric disorders in Australian filicide cases. Melbourne University Law Review 37(2):297–342, 2013

Berger SH: Template for quickly creating forensic psychiatry reports. J Am Acad Psychiatry Law 36:388–392, 2008

Brown P, Stahl D, Appiah-Kusi E, et al: Fitness to plead: development and validation of a standardised assessment instrument. PLoS ONE 13:e0194332, 2018

Casey P: Expert testimony in court. 2: in the witness box. Adv Psychiatr Treat 9:183–187, 2003

Cox J: Postnatal mental disorder: towards ICD-11. World Psychiatry 3:96–97, 2004

DiFlorio A, Gordon-Smith K, Forty L, et al: Stratification of the risk of bipolar disorder recurrences in pregnancy and postpartum. Br J Psychiatry 213:542–547, 2018

Friedman SH: After the murder: mothers who have killed. Correctional Mental Health Report 10:55–56, 2008

Friedman SH: Realistic consideration of violence in women is critical. J Am Acad Psychiatry Law 43:273–276, 2015

Friedman SH, Resnick PJ: Child murder by mothers: patterns and prevention. World Psychiatry 6:137–141, 2007

Friedman SH, Sorrentino R: Postpartum psychosis, infanticide and insanity: implications for forensic psychiatry. J Am Acad Psychiatry Law 40:326–332, 2012

Friedman SH, Hrouda DR, Holden CE, et al: Child murder committed by severely mentally ill mothers: an examination of mothers found not guilty by reason of insanity. J Forensic Sci 50(6):132–136, 2005

Friedman SH, Cerny C, West S, et al: Reel forensic experts: forensic psychiatrists as portrayed on screen. J Am Acad Psychiatry Law 39(3):412–417, 2011

Friedman SH, Cavney J, Resnick PJ: Child murder by parents and evolutionary psychology. Psychiatr Clin North Am 35(4):781–795, 2012

Friedman SH, Cavney J, Resnick PJ: Mothers who kill: evolutionary underpinnings and law. Behav Sci Law 30:585–597, 2013

Friedman SH, Prakash C, Nagle-Yang S: Postpartum psychosis: protecting mother and infant. Current Psychiatry 18(4):12–21, 2019

Glancy GD, Ash P, Bath E, et al: AAPL practice guideline for the forensic assessment. J Am Acad Psychiatry Law 43:S3–53, 2015

Grisso T: Guidance for improving forensic reports: a review of common errors. Psychiatry Publications and Presentations 2:102–115, 2010

Hallet N: To what extent should expert psychiatric witnesses comment on criminal culpability? Med Sci Law 60:67–74, 2020

Isik M: Postpartum psychosis. East J Med 23(1):60–63, 2018

The Law Commission: Murder, Manslaughter, and Infanticide. Project 6 of the Ninth Programme of Law Reform: Homicide. London, The Law Commission, 2006. Available at: http://www.lawcom.gov.uk/app/uploads/2015/03/lc304_Murder_Manslaughter_and_Infanticide_Report.pdf. Accessed September 3, 2020.

McKee GR, Shea SJ, Mogy RB, Holden CE: MMPI-2 profiles of filicidal, mariticidal, and homicidal women. J Clin Psychol 57(3):367–374, 2001

Monzon C, Lanza di Scalea T, Pearlstein T: Postpartum psychosis: updates and clinical issues. Psychiatric Times, January 15, 2014. Available at: http://www.psychiatrictimes.com/special-reports/postpartum-psychosis-updates-and-clinical-issues. Accessed September 3, 2020.

Mossman D, Noffsinger SG, Ash P, et al: AAPL practice guideline for the forensic psychiatric evaluation of competence to stand trial. J Am Acad Psychiatry Law 35(suppl 4):S3–S72, 2007

New South Wales Law Reform Commission: Partial Defences to Murder: Provocation and Infanticide (Report No 83, 114 [3.29]). Sydney, Australia, New South Wales Law Reform Commission, 1997

Oberman M: A brief history of infanticide and the law, in Infanticide: Psychosocial and Legal Perspectives on Mothers Who Kill. Edited by Spinelli MG. Washington, DC, American Psychiatric Publishing, 2003, pp 3–18

Parameshwaran S, Chandra PS: Will the DSM-5 and ICD-11 "Make-over "really make a difference to Women's Mental Health? Indian J Soc Psychiatry 34:S79–S85, 2018

Resnick PJ: Child murder by parents: a psychiatric review of filicide. Am J Psychiatry 126(3):325–334, 1969

Resnick PJ: Child murder by parents: a psychiatric review of neonaticide. Am J Psychiatry 126(10):1414–1420, 1970

Resnick PJ, Soliman S: Planning, writing, and editing forensic psychiatry reports. Int J Law Psychiatry 35:412–417, 2012

Rix K, Eastman N, Adshead G: Responsibilities of Psychiatrists Who Provide Expert Opinion to Courts and Tribunals (CR 193). London, Royal College of Psychiatrists, 2015

Rogers T, Blackwood N, Farnham F, et al: Fitness to plead and competence to stand trial: a systematic review of the constructs and their application. Journal of Forensic Psychiatry and Psychology 19:576–596, 2008

Spinelli MG: A systematic investigation of 16 cases of neonaticide. Am J Psychiatry 158:811–813, 2001

Strasburger LH, Gutheil TG, Brodsky A: On wearing two hats: role conflict in serving as both psychotherapist and expert witness. Am J Psychiatry 154(4):448–456, 1997

VanderKruik R, Barreix M, Chou D, et al: The global prevalence of postpartum psychosis: a systematic review. BMC Psychiatry 17(1):272, 2017

Wesseloo R, Kamperman AM, Munk-Olsen T, et al: Risk of postpartum relapse in bipolar disorder and postpartum psychosis: a systematic review and meta-analysis. Am J Psychiatry 173:117–127, 2016

West S, Friedman SH: To be or not to be: treating psychiatrist and expert witness. Psychiatric Times 24(6), 2007

Wieck A, Davies RA, Hirst AD, et al: Menstrual cycle effects on hypothalamic dopamine receptor function in women with a history of puerperal bipolar disorder. J Psychopharmacol 17(2):204–209, 2003

Wisner KL, Peindl K, Hanusa BH: Symptomatology of affective and psychotic illnesses related to childbearing. J Affect Disord 30:77–87, 1994

World Health Organization: International Classification of Diseases, 11th Revision. Geneva, World Health Organization, 2019

Young G: Psychiatric/Psychological forensic report writing. Int J Law Psychiatry 49:214–220, 2016

FOUNDATION IV

Sociocultural Considerations and Feminist Approaches to Prevention and Treatment

CHAPTER 12

Maternal Filicide in Canadian News

A DECADE IN REVIEW

Kimberly Rock, M.C.

Amy Corkett, M.C.

Nancy Shekarak Ghashghaei, M.C.

Gina Wong, Ph.D.

On March 15, 2019, a mother in Spain was accused of killing her 3.5-year-old son and 5-month-old daughter. Several Spanish articles were published in national and local newspapers in response, with varying descriptions of what happened. Two striking similarities in reporting were 1) the slanderous tone of the articles and 2) the absence of discussion about maternal mental illness and how it may have played a role in the perpetuation of maternal filicide. All media reports in Spain (five in our search) portrayed the mother with crucifying intent. One article, seething with vitriol, was headlined "Deranged Mother Arrested After Killing Her Infant Children in Valencia" (*Murcia Today* 2019), another "The Parricide of Godella Confessed That [S]he Had Killed H[er] Children 'Because They Had Lost Their Soul'"[1] (TellerReport.com 2019), and another "Mother Who Killed Her Own Children Was Found in a Jar" (NewsBeezer.com 2019).

---

[1]Due to translation of the articles from Spanish to English, errors in pronouns were present in headlines and the term "parricide" (killing of parent or close relative) was used instead of "filicide" (killing of one's child).

In the opening paragraph of the "Deranged Mother" article (*Murcia Today* 2019), reporters detailed the "ruined house" in which the family lived, closely followed by information that social services had visited the family only a few days before the event. Statements such as "the parents lived a 'hippie-like' existence" and "were obsessed with paranormal phenomena and alien abductions," and that the mother had been found "naked and incoherent inside a plastic container" were woven into the narrative. In "Parricide" (TellerReport.com 2019), the reporters noted the mother's "creepy" confession in relation to how her "children had lost their soul" and the "macabre crime," with no mention of the mother's mental health status. The instances of the mother's paranoia, nudity, and memory loss that were described would be recognizable to professionals trained in mental health as being consistent with a disturbed state of mind, possibly psychosis. Resnick's (1969) original typologies of motives behind why mothers perpetrate filicide included acute psychosis.

Negative media portrayals of the filicidal mother, coupled with cultural and religious beliefs, may reify stigma and falsehoods about maternal filicide and close people down to understanding or examining the incident further. Without accurate knowledge of the facts or an understanding of the psychiatric underpinnings of maternal filicide, incensed media reports act as judge and jury and incite public revulsion against these mothers. Mothers are particularly denigrated in the media as viewpoints amass that portray them as failures in upholding the coveted maternal role the public holds dear. In response to the news articles about the Spanish mother, the European Institute of Perinatal Mental Health (2019) published a manifesto decrying sensationalist media reports. Their goal was to reduce the spread of misinformation and vilification of mothers who may have severe mental illness and perpetrate filicide. They underscored the need for balanced and responsible media reporting. An excerpt from the manifesto is as follows:

> We, the undersigned, vehemently oppose misrepresentation and sensationalizing of maternal filicide in media reports and take this opportunity to invite greater awareness and prevention by working with the Spanish media to restore the human rights of this mother in demonstrating responsible media reporting. The wellbeing [sic] and lives of children, families, communities, and our nations will thrive as a result. (European Institute of Perinatal Mental Health 2019, para. 7)

By June 2019, more than 350 mental health professionals and 9 mental health entities from across the globe had signed the manifesto in support of responsible media reporting of maternal filicide in Spain.

Media shapes how the general public, as well as any potential jurors, lawyers, judges, and those involved in the care of these mothers, understand and perceive the "crime." In turn, judicious sentencing and access to timely psychiatric treatment is advanced. Indeed, a powerful source of information for lay audiences is the representation of maternal filicide in the news media. This research is the first of a series over the next 5 years in which we investigate media reports of maternal filicide in various countries. Such research serves to generate comparative data and possibly to compel a global manifesto on responsible media reporting.

In this chapter, we share results of the first analysis of maternal filicide coverage in three prominent Canadian newspapers—*The Globe and Mail*, *National Post*, and *Toronto Star*—over more than a decade (January 1, 2008 to August 1, 2018). Ethnographic content analysis (ECA; Altheide and Schneider 2013) was applied to 95 news articles utilizing NVivo 12 software. This Canadian research team included the four authors of this chapter.

Maternal Filicide Background

In 2015, Dawson published the most comprehensive facts about the prevalence of maternal filicide in Canada. Dawson collated data between the years 1961 and 2011 from Statistics Canada's annual homicide survey, collected yearly from police departments across Canada. Findings revealed that 693 women were accused of filicide in that 50-year period, receiving charges of first-degree murder (136), second-degree murder (265), manslaughter (51), or infanticide (83). The remaining 158 cases were cleared either as suicide (136 women) or other reasons (22 mothers), such as mental illness or police discretion. Dawson estimated these numbers to be higher given underreporting of filicide crimes. Since Dawson's article, no comprehensive data on maternal filicide in Canada have been published, leaving nearly a decade of missing data.

General characteristics of those who commit maternal filicide have been elucidated in studies. Mothers who perpetrate filicide are more likely to be under the age of 30 (Kauppi et al. 2010; Mariano et al. 2014; McKee and Egan 2013; Sidebotham and Retzer 2018), to have mental health disorders (Flynn et al. 2013; Gowda et al. 2018; Kauppi et al. 2010; McKee and Egan 2013; Sidebotham and Retzer 2018), and to lack social support systems (Gowda et al. 2018; Kauppi et al. 2010; McKee and Egan 2013). Additional factors identified included marital/intimate partner discord (Gowda et al. 2018; McKee and Egan 2013), high levels of stress (Kauppi et al. 2010), and domestic violence (Sidebotham and Retzer

2018). Several theories have been proposed to substantiate why mothers kill their young (Ciani and Fontanesi 2012; Daly and Wilson 1988; Minocher and Sommer 2016), and classification systems for mothers who commit filicide have been proposed (Friedman and Resnick 2007; West 2007).

Maternal Filicide in the Media

However, an understanding of public perceptions of maternal filicide is less explored. Little and Tyson (2017) researched how parents who commit filicide are portrayed in the Australian media. They found that media promulgated mothers' and fathers' failure to uphold the commonly accepted parental roles ubiquitous in our culture. Women who have killed are disadvantaged in the media and face unrelenting stereotyping for two reasons: 1) becoming a criminal, and 2) violating the accepted gender role of passive femininity (Collins 2016; Whiteley 2012). When women kill or are otherwise violent, it destroys the widely held fixed belief that women are gentle, nurturing individuals incapable of dominance and aggression (Whiteley 2012).

Negativity toward women is magnified in the media when a mother is accused of taking the life of her child. Reverberations from American media tend to be strong, far reaching, and long lasting (Easteal et al. 2015). Behavior viewed as opposite to gentle and nurturing is exemplified in the press through unflattering pictures, the language used to describe the mothers, and critical narratives. Any psychosocial, cultural, or mental health factors are often glossed over in these reports. Furthermore, Easteal et al. (2015) asserted that the media is stunting the public's ability to understand underlying motivations behind filicide and possibly reducing prevention efforts by reporting on mothers in this manner.

From an international perspective, Cavaglion (2008) examined 19 articles about six high-profile cases of maternal filicide in Israel between 1992 and 2001. Within Israeli culture, a dominant assumption is that a mother who kills her child "must be insane" (Cavaglion 2008, p. 272). Cavaglion found that reporters biased their representation of the Israeli mothers based on their marital status, socioeconomic position, and ethnicity. For instance, poor, young, uneducated, and otherwise marginalized mothers were more likely to be labeled with negative characteristics than were more affluent mothers. Mothers who were married and perpetrated filicide were treated with more compassion, in that reporters more likely inferred mental illness as the underlying culprit. Cavaglion also revealed that the ethnic background of the mothers impacted how reporters portrayed them. For instance, Arab immigrant mothers were described with negative attributes. Reporters humanized the mother if she articulated any remorse or regret related to the filicide (Cavaglion 2008). Data regarding media reports of maternal filicide in Israel underscore the value in such investigations. A dearth of research regarding Canadian reporters' portrayal of mothers who commit filicide substantiated our research.

NEWS MEDIA IN CANADA

Reporters have an ethical responsibility to accurately represent and objectively convey the news without sensationalism (Crawford 2008). They play a pivotal role in shaping both positive and negative perceptions, forming values and attitudes that sway public opinion (Baun 2009; McCombs 2014; Rajiva and Khoday 2014; Zollmann 2019) and creating discourses within the sociocultural landscape (Bandes 2004; Baun 2009; Little and Tyson 2017; McCombs 2014; Rajiva and Khoday 2014). Media has been used to demonize groups or individuals through actions such as name calling and sensationalizing atrocities without a balanced focus on possible mitigating factors (Zollmann 2019), as was noted in the case of the Spanish mother described earlier.

When examining the impact of media, Statistics Canada indicated that 60% of Canadians followed the daily news in 2013 (Statistics Canada 2016), and 80% followed digital or print newspaper on a weekly basis in 2015 (Vividata 2016). We forecasted increased percentages with the explosion of social media platforms and other electronic news outlets in recent years. News media is most certainly a primary source of information for many Canadians and has influence in shaping criminal justice policy (Beale 2006).

Studies have affirmed the idea of "trial by media," whereby sensationalistic reporting practices unduly bias the public against the accused (Chagnon and Chesney-Lind 2015; Greer and McLaughlin 2011; Middleweek 2017). Rajiva and Khoday (2014) argued that media is integral to the framework of "governing and disciplining of populations in advanced liberal democracies" (p. 179). In this vein, researching media portrayals is critical to understanding narratives that abound. For instance, the local and national press flagrantly (and inaccurately) portrayed Andrea Yates, the Texas mother who drowned her five children in 2001, as a "traitor" (Barnett 2005, p. 15), a woman who had not only betrayed her family role(s) but also her female gender. The second narrative was "the quest" (p. 19)—the drive to hold Yates accountable and sentenced to the fullest extent of the law.

The Yates case exemplified how mothers are admonished and re-buked in the media and how mental health can be used against them. Singh (2017) discussed "tropes" (p. 515), such as the failure to uphold the beloved mother archetype, despite the fact that the mothers were victims of domestic violence. Similarly, Easteal et al. (2015) suggested that media reporters constructed a "flawed mother narrative" (p. 34) to denounce maternal filicide. They portrayed the mothers as being "mad, bad, and sad" (p. 39) and framed them as deviant. Additionally, these authors in-dicated that news media reporters intentionally excluded relevant facts that could provide compassionate insight into the crime and the mother.

FREEDOM OF THE PRESS

Freedom of the press is ingrained in the Canadian Constitution. How-ever, this freedom does not permit every act of maternal filicide to fall into media clutches. Publication bans are ordered in some cases (Craw-ford 2008). Judges may order a publication ban to maintain the privacy of the accused, uphold the right to a fair trial, or alleviate the fears of any witnesses who may be required to testify (Government of Canada 2015). More specifically, under section 672.5(6) of the *Criminal Code* (1985), a ban may be issued if it is "in the best interests of the accused and not contrary to the public issue" (p. 811). Furthermore, under section 486.5(1), a judge can order a publication ban to protect the identity of the victim or wit-ness of a crime. These conditions can be met in cases of maternal filicide because mothers' privacy rights are important to uphold and the identi-ties of any surviving children may need protection. As such, many cases of maternal filicide are not exposed to the media. Nevertheless, examina-tion of maternal filicide in Canadian media is vital given that cultural understanding and representations are impactful.

Infanticide in the Canadian Criminal Code

The British Infanticide Act of 1922 reduced the punishment for mothers who took the lives of their children, which was originally death by hanging (Friedman et al. 2012). The Infanticide Act (discussed in depth in Chapter 4) was amended in 1938 and served as a model for which Canada and many other commonwealth countries translated their law (Friedman and Resnick 2007). Currently, 50 countries in the world pos-sess some version of infanticide provisions within their respective crim-inal codes, including Austria, Israel, New Zealand, Denmark, Hungary, Ireland, and Canada (Malmquist 2013).

Our Research

We reviewed the Canadian Newsstream database for articles between January 2008 and August 2018 from three major newspapers with the greatest readership according to the Newspapers Canada 2015 Circulation Report. These included 1) *The Globe and Mail*, with a daily average readership rate of 336,487; 2) *Toronto Star*, with a daily average readership rate of 318,763; and 3) *National Post*, with a daily average readership rate of 186,108. The Canadian Newsstream database was used to search articles given its accessibility to full-text versions. Researchers were able to set detailed search parameters to include a specific date range and precise word search terms.

Initial search terms applied were "neonaticide," "filicide," and "infanticide" and yielded 336 articles. However, these search terms did not capture our target subject of mothers who kill their children. The search was expanded to include "child murder by mother," which yielded an additional 3,747 articles. Overall, our initial data set included 4,083 articles. Given the focus on cases of maternal filicide and the need to further sort the data, we narrowed the search to include only cases involving biological mothers, child victims under the age of 6, cases in which the death was not resultant from ongoing neglect or abuse, and cases that occurred in Canada. This yielded a total of 95 articles for detailed review (see Table 12–1 for a summary).

TABLE 12-1. Breakdown of analyzed articles, according to newspaper

Newspaper	Articles
National Post	37
Toronto Star	32
The Globe and Mail	26
Total	**95**

ANALYSIS AND INTERPRETATIONS

Altheide and Schneider's (2013) ECA methodology involves systematic analysis of documents focused on the "process, meanings, and emphases reflected in the content" (p. 2). Discovering meaning in content is achieved via ongoing comparison of news articles to discern nuanced patterns and styles (Altheide 1987; Altheide and Schneider 2013).

We analyzed the data set utilizing NVivo 12, a qualitative research software, to facilitate coding of data into nodes, which were then refined into frames and themes. According to Altheide and Schneider (2013), *frames* have a broad focus on the "how" and "why" an issue is presented, whereas *themes* are ideas continually presented within the body of work. Coding occurred between and within articles, which meant that a single article could yield numerous frames and themes. Altheide (1987) noted that information could be coded "conceptually" (p. 69), meaning the same sentence could be coded in different ways, allowing for both overarching categorical data and specific thematic data.

This process identified two dominant frames: *criminal justice* and *descriptive narrative*. Three themes were identified within each frame, elucidating narratives and discourses presented to the Canadian public via the articles. The criminal justice frame involved themes of 1) criminal proceedings, 2) infanticide law, and 3) mental health considerations. The descriptive narrative frame encompassed themes involving 1) details of the filicide incident, 2) details of the accused mother, and 3) details of mental illness. These findings are presented in the sections that follow.

CRIMINAL JUSTICE FRAME

It was clear that news reporters focused on law enforcement and the maternal filicide case as it proceeded through the court system. Segments of news articles reflecting this frame focused on cases in relation to criminal prosecution and factors relevant to the court case as put forth by defense and prosecution, such as the infanticide law and mental health. Reporters commonly quoted judges, recounted submissions to the court, and provided in-depth coverage of the debate surrounding Canada's infanticide law (Figure 12–1).

Criminal Proceedings Theme

This theme within the criminal justice frame reflected statements made by judges and comments about various court rulings, such as verdicts, sentencing decisions or conditions imposed, and proceedings of the active trial. Regarding criminal proceedings, 89 (94%) articles were identified, with 331 segments that referred to various criminal proceedings. Within these 89 articles, 32 included 75 direct quotes from judges. These quotes were most often in relation to conditions imposed on the mother, such as being detained, attending counseling, or no-contact orders. A legal condition levied to monitor or inhibit future reproduction was apparent in seven articles, as well as an edict to limit sexual activity in one instance. For example, a news article written by Fraser (2010) for the *Na-*

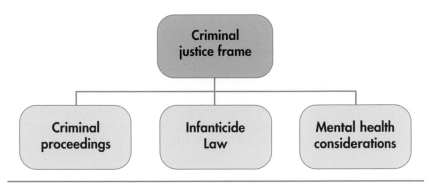

FIGURE 12-1. **Themes within criminal justice frame.**

tional Post shared how a judge declared that a mother who had committed filicide could not have sexual intercourse until the court removed the condition. In fact, four mothers had conditions placed on their sexual activity and reproductive rights.

In addition to judges' statements and rulings, news coverage often followed the proceedings of the active court trial. Attention to prosecution and defense lawyer court submissions were prevalent in 42 (44%) of Canadian news articles reviewed. In 75 instances, reporters closely followed submissions to the court during trials and reported on lawyers' arguments in detail. The defense position involved generally positive and compassionate attitudes, as evidenced in this excerpt published in *The Globe and Mail*: "[I]n his closing statement Friday, defense lawyer Richard Fowler urged the jury to convict his client, 28-year-old Sarah Leung, of infanticide rather than of two charges of second-degree murder" (Burgmann 2014, p. S4).

Conversely, the prosecution's position involved mostly negative or condemning attitudes:

> At a trial that began in Wetaskiwin Court of Queen's Bench on Monday, Crown prosecutor Gordon Hatch said there is no question that Ms. McConnell killed her children. The only questions, Mr. Hatch said, are why, and whether she had the intent required to be convicted of murder in her sons' deaths. (Pruden 2012a, p. A7).

Submissions to the court also encompassed victim impact statements. Impact statements were noted in four (4%) of the articles, for a total of eight mentions. Two of the references noted were in relation to a judge allowing individuals to present their victim impact statements in court, whereas six instances included direct quotes from impact statements.

The poignancy of these statements was highly emotional. For example, a father conveyed the following about the loss of his son:

> What God allows this evil to be perpetrated on our children?...Which God heard his silent cry for help while this monstrosity was set on him and didn't allow him to be saved? What God allows such an angel to be surrounded by so much hate and evil until it suffocates him? It breaks my heart to know that after four months of being denied access to my son by his mother, it was at a funeral home that I gave him his last hug. (Williams, as cited in Mitchell 2011, p. GT.1)

Victim impact statements are an integral part of the Canadian criminal justice system, although they can also serve to promote condemning biases against mothers. This is not to say that every victim impact statement recorded is reproachful of the mother; however, our search yielded no victim impact statements describing the mother either compassionately or through the lens of mental illness.

Infanticide Law Theme

The infanticide law in the *Criminal Code* is a source of contention in the Canadian criminal justice system. A significant number of articles ($n=22$ [23%]) had 63 sections that discussed or debated whether the infanticide law was still relevant in the *Criminal Code* because our social norms have shifted since its inception in 1948. Canadian newspaper reporters predominantly discussed three high-profile cases in Canada that had occurred over the past decade:

1. In 2011, the Ontario Court of Appeal challenged the interpretation of the infanticide law in the Canadian *Criminal Code* in relation to a mother known as L. B. She had been initially charged with two counts of first-degree murder and subsequently convicted of two counts of infanticide for smothering her two children, one in 1998 and another in 2002. The decision rendered continued to support the application of an infanticide conviction when a charge of murder is laid.
2. In 2011, the Alberta Court of Appeal overturned a murder conviction (replacing it with a charge of infanticide) for Katrina Effert, who strangled her newborn son shortly after his birth.
3. In 2016, the Alberta Crown appealed a conviction of infanticide in favor of a second-degree murder charge. The Supreme Court of Canada dismissed the appeal by a 7–0 margin. The mother, Meredith Borowiec, had been charged with infanticide in 2013 after her third newborn had been found alive by the father and she confessed to putting her two previous newborn babies in a dumpster.

Other mothers captured in the 22 articles about the infanticide law debate included one from Ontario, another known as L.G., Jennifer Sinn, and Elaine Campione. Three additional news articles discussed the infanticide law in general and how it factored into the *Criminal Code*.

In 2011, the Ontario Court of Appeal upheld the necessity and use for the infanticide law in the *Criminal Code* as was intended by Parliament when it was enacted. The arguments for or against the infanticide law were staunchly rooted in the culpability and criminal intent of the mothers. Prosecuting lawyers framed the arguments against the infanticide law as an unacceptable and obsolete defense against a higher-level charge of murder. Brean (2016), a reporter for the *National Post*, wrote that the Alberta government claimed the infanticide law was "vague, outdated and rife with problems" (p. A3). In contrast, the defense argued in favor of the law, providing the rationale that a mother can be in a disturbed state of mind given the complex myriad of social, economic, biological, and psychological stressors in early motherhood. Legal counsel representing Meredith Borowiec argued that the biological imperatives influencing a woman's state of mind after childbirth have not changed, and thus, the law did not require modernization. Our media analysis shows that the infanticide law debate was an important theme in Canadian newspapers during our period of review and provided insight that mothers who commit infanticide may be viewed in the Canadian court system with compassion.

Mental Health Considerations Theme

The criminal justice frame included mental health concerns as referenced by both Crown and defense during trials, for opposing reasons. Twelve (13%) articles had 16 segments discussing mental health from a condemning stance and asserting mental illness as either irrelevant to the crime or an excuse to avoid culpability. Conversely, 11 (12%) articles captured 14 instances in which mental illness was provided as a reasonable rationale underlying maternal filicide. Condemning and supportive arguments diverged regarding how much, if at all, mental health was attributable to the crime. For instance, *The Globe and Mail* ran an article about L.B. in which prosecuting lawyer Jennifer Woollcoombe stated the following about mental health as a mitigating factor: "it is a mockery of a child's death for his or her killer to be spared a life sentence for murder. She argued that an out-and-out psychopath could murder her infant and get off with a relative slap on the wrist simply by exaggerating her 'baby blues'" (Makin 2010, p. A7).

Alternatively, the *National Post* published an article titled "Saving Women and Children From Postpartum Psychosis" written by Hajara

Kutty (2010), a Postpartum Support International coordinator in Toronto, Canada. Kutty wrote from a compassionate lens focused on the realities of postpartum psychosis (PPP), including the possibility of filicidal behavior:

> A smaller percentage of women who give birth, 1 in 500, can expect to suffer from postpartum psychosis, a serious illness considered a life-threatening medical emergency. Afflicted women with this condition fall prey to delusions, hallucinations and severe paranoia, all of which cause these mothers to lose touch with reality. Women afflicted with this illness function in a reality of their own, which bears no relation to their ordinary personalities. This is why women who have committed infanticide in the postpartum period typically have no prior run-ins with the law, and why they are frequently supported in the aftermath by spouses and family who depict them as the epitome of gentleness. (Kutty 2010, p. A16)

This news article was among very few that published factual information about postpartum mental illness and PPP. Of those few, this article was the most educative and descriptive. More frequently, articles referenced mental illness as something the mother had, but with no other information provided. For example, "Peng suffered depression after her daughter's birth and was diagnosed with bipolar disorder in 2002. The defence is considering an appeal" (Powell 2008, p. A12).

DESCRIPTIVE NARRATIVE FRAME

The descriptive narrative frame encompassed news articles, or sections in articles, that offered narrative details about the incident, mother, or mental illness. These accounts were typically described via quotes from individuals such as law enforcement officials or family and friends of the mothers shortly after the incidents occurred. Descriptive narratives were also pervasive in news articles in which reporters shared detailed information regarding an active trial. Mental illness was referenced as a diagnosis with which the mother had been labeled or as a rationale for previous suicide attempts. Three key themes of descriptive narrative were noted in these articles: 1) details of the filicide incident, 2) details of the accused mother, and 3) details of the mental illness (Figure 12–2).

Details of Filicide Incident Theme

Reporters often included descriptive narratives that captured the *what* and *how* of the filicide incident, presented in 90 (95%) of our articles, in 459 instances. Overwhelmingly, Canadian reporters relayed information in a neutral tone, conveying the facts objectively in 77 (81%) articles and 179 instances. Unbiased reporting was frequently noted when the inci-

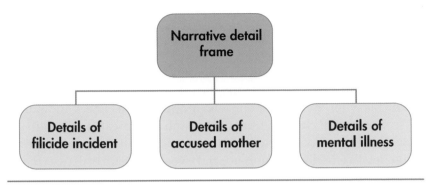

FIGURE 12–2. **Themes within narrative detail frame.**

dent had just occurred and police were providing the public factual information through a press release. For example, the following excerpt was written the day after Nadine Bernard was charged with first-degree murder in the death of her infant son: "Peel Regional Police were called at about 8 A. M. to the Mississauga Executive Centre's underground lot, about a block from the Square One shopping mall in the city's core. They discovered the infant's body with his mother, Ms. Bernard, nearby" (McDonald and Jowett 2009, p. A14).

Canadian reporters also wrote about maternal filicide in a fact-based manner when providing specific court details. For example, "Court was told that the two met in high school in their native China where Peng trained to be a civil engineer. When Peng moved to Canada, Scarlett remained with her grandmother before coming to Canada" (Powell 2008, p. A12). Conversely, 12 (13%) articles had used provocative language on 32 different occasions to describe a filicide event, including "providing baby killers with an easy out" (Makin 2010, p. A7), "she killed them, held their heads under water until those beautiful little girls were dead" (DiManno 2010a, p. A2), or the *National Post* headline "Killer Mom Wants More Children After Prison" (Rook 2008, p. A8). Such descriptions were intended to incite judgment, negative emotion, and anger. Also noted was the journalistic technique of providing visual or auditory details to depict a macabre crime, which serves to sensationalize the filicide event. For instance, featured in the *Toronto Star* on September 29, 2010, Rosie DiManno wrote how the accused mother presented her deceased daughters after drowning them in the bathtub:

> Tinker Bell pyjamas for 19-month-old Sophia, a pretty violet nightgown for 3-year-old Serena—and arrange the girls in a poignant tableau on her

own big bed, dry and comb their silky hair, adorn them with necklaces of gold, force their cold fingers together in a sibling clasp, assemble separate piles of clothing and toys for their burial, even place a fan nearby to dispel the odour of decomposition. (DiManno 2010b, p. A2)

The following short excerpt from the *National Post* detailed how Allyson McConnell's husband found their two boys drowned in the bathtub by his wife: "he was the one who dropped to his knees and pulled his 'cold and stiff' children from the bathtub after breaking through the locked bathroom door" (Pruden 2012b, p. A3). The inclusion of such evocative details (childhood innocence and sweetness amid evil) casts mothers as demons, which contributes to negative bias.

Details of the Accused Mother Theme

Articles in which journalists included details of the accused mother's behavior or appearance fit this theme. Reporters remarked on how the accused mother appeared in court or her behavior leading up to the filicide event or in the aftermath. For example, "Now 35, Ms. Campione, slender and pale, is a wraith in the prisoner's box, frequently pulling tissues from a box and weeping" (Blatchford 2010, p. A8). Most articles in the data set focused solely on the details of the accused mother in the context of the filicide event. However, six reporters relayed comparisons with other mothers who had perpetrated filicide:

> Ms. Yates was originally convicted of capital murder and sentenced to life in prison, but a jury overturned the verdict on appeal in 2006, ruling she was not guilty by reason of insanity. In 2008, an Ontario Superior Court jury found Xuan Linda Peng guilty of second-degree murder for drowning her four-year-old daughter Scarlett in the bathtub of her family's Toronto home four years earlier. She had originally been charged with first-degree murder. (Kenyon and Lodge 2010, p. A6)

More prominent in this theme were details from family and friends and contextual information about the accused mother's life challenges. The frequency with which family and friends portrayed the mother with a positive and compassionate lens or a negative or condemning lens was about the same: 16 (17%) articles published 26 compassionate phrases, whereas 17 (18%) articles published 24 negative phrases. An article from *The Globe and Mail* published a compassionate quote from a neighbor of accused mother Nadine Bernard: "She was an amazing mother, I'm in shock. They're a part of a close-knit neighbourhood. This is inconceivable" (Alphonso 2009, p. A15). Conversely, *The Globe and Mail* published a condemning outburst made in court by the father of one of L.B.'s deceased children: "The father of the seven-week-old stared coldly at the accused before he read a victim impact statement. After the woman was sentenced, he cried out: 'You'll always be a baby killer. Baby killer!'" (Oliveira 2008, p. A7).

Lastly, reporters relayed information to the Canadian public about life challenges the mothers faced. Specific occurrences were noted in 24 (25%) articles in 31 different instances. Quotes included Sarah Leung being "raised by an abusive and controlling father" (Burgmann 2014, p. S4), Allyson McConnell being "sexually abused by her father and first attempting suicide as a teenager while pregnant with her father's baby" (Pruden 2012a, p. A7), or details about Sivananthi Elango that included, "a sad childhood in Sri Lanka, where she was sickly and lived in poverty, before [moving] to Canada at age 14. As an adult, she felt ugly, clumsy and stupid,…telling psychiatrists she tried to kill herself earlier" (Edwards 2008, p. A7). No descriptions of mothers by reporters were found to admonish the mother due to her past history. Our analysis indicated that several Canadian journalists showcased the hardships mothers endured in their lives, which humanized them to the public.

Details of Mental Illness Theme

The descriptive narrative frame involved discussion of mental illness in relation to mothers and filicide. Specific maternal mental illnesses were referenced in these articles and included postpartum depression (PPD) and generalized depression, PPP, and baby blues. Additional mental illness coverage included bipolar disorder, schizophrenia, and PTSD. Multiple articles referenced more than one mental illness; however, the most frequently discussed were PPD and generalized depression in 35 (37%) articles. In these 35 articles, 57 instances were found that noted PPD and generalized depression. Canadian reporters predominantly wrote about mental illness without offering contextual or educational information to the public. For example, one quote from *The Globe and Mail* discussed Allyson McConnell's mental health: "Ms. McConnell, who is originally from Australia, drowned the boys in the family home in Millet, Alta. just south of Edmonton, two years ago when she was severely depressed, suicidal and possibly affected by alcohol and prescription drugs" (Purdy 2012, p. A10). This statement lacked any further description of mental illness's potential role in filicide. Overall, 72 statements in 39 (41%) articles written during a 10-year period spoke to mental illness in relation to filicide within the parameters given.

Overall, maternal filicide in Canadian news articles during that decade was discussed in a neutral and fact-based manner. Reporters generally relayed information about the mothers and the filicide event in a nonbiased fashion, allowing members of the public to reach their own conclusions in relation to moral blame and culpability. However, two specific reporters, Christie Blatchford, who wrote for *The Globe and Mail*, and Rosie DiManno, who wrote for the *Toronto Star*, were outliers. They wrote nine articles altogether attacking Elaine Campione, an Ontario mother who drowned her two young daughters in the family bathtub in 2006. Other articles by these reporters as well as others were found to represent balanced perspectives. In Ms. Campione's trial, two forensic psychiatrists agreed that she had borderline personality disorder, depression, psychosis, and paranoia. However, one believed these mental disturbances had no bearing on her ability to know right from wrong, whereas the other report stated she had been in a delusional state. Spousal revenge was the alleged motive.

The *National Post* also covered the Elaine Campione case, but with much less emotionally charged language, although it was not devoid of sensationalism. Perhaps the shocking facts overshadowed people's ability for compassion. These included Ms. Campione's recording of vengeful statements to her estranged husband following the drownings. The defense presented evidence for a charge of not criminally responsible; however, the jury found her guilty of two counts of first-degree murder. Campione currently remains in federal prison (as of August 2020).

A deficit noted in relation to Canadian reporting on maternal filicide was the minimal contextual information presented about maternal mental health issues. Mental illness was referenced only in relation to what lawyers raised in their arguments or occasionally if mental health experts were called to testify. Given the significant role mental illness can play in maternal filicide, it is essential to provide education and awareness to the public whenever possible.

Barnett (2005) highlighted the importance of challenging and advocating against dominant narratives of motherhood in her analysis of news reports about the Andrea Yates case. Rather than crucifying mothers, media reporters could inform the public about risk factors for filicide, such as maternal mental illness; create space for dialogue about the many burdens of motherhood; and deconstruct the ideology of the perfect mother (Barnett 2005). Cavanagh (2018) conveyed a need for advocacy in relation to maternal filicide to "progress rapidly from knowledge to social action" (p. 203). Such advocacy would support prevention and awareness efforts and encourage mothers experiencing mental illness to seek help. Encouraging reporters to include information about mental illness to reduce stigma as well as promote awareness to mothers with mental illnesses would facilitate meaningful discussion, reduce stigma and negative bias, and advance advocacy work.

Future Research Directions

Our research findings build on existing knowledge of maternal narratives revealed by media analysis in other countries, such as Australia and the United States (see Barnett 2005; Little and Tyson 2017). Researchers in both countries revealed that mothers who committed maternal filicide were portrayed in various negative ways. The 2019 case described at the beginning of this chapter of maternal filicide in Spain, a country that has no research to date on how maternal filicide is portrayed, highlights the need for further country-specific research to be completed. Gathering these data will allow us to compare and contrast findings and elucidate trends as well as differences that may translate to legal outcomes. Furthermore, our research may compel further studies investigating other forms of media, such as books, television, radio, or social networking sites and their impact in shaping public perception of maternal filicide.

Conclusion

ECA (Altheide and Schneider 2013) revealed that reports in the Canadian Newsstream in the decade between January 1, 2008 and August 1, 2018 from three prominent newspapers (*The Globe and Mail*, *National Post*, and *Toronto Star*) demonstrated two dominant frames: criminal justice and descriptive narrative. Most articles (77 [81%, $N=95$]) included sections in which maternal filicide was reported in a neutral and fact-based manner, whereas 12 (13%) articles had pieces that conveyed sensationalizing and condemning language and had been written predominantly by two female reporters. Twenty-two (23%) news articles addressed the infanticide law in Canada. The findings of this research highlight the relative neutrality as well as an overall lack of nuance pertaining to psychiatric and mental health considerations within Canadian news articles.

Media representation of maternal filicide is essential to monitor when considering dominant narratives of mothers and filicide and how members of the public form biases. Media is a platform that shapes public opinion, which may directly influence legal outcomes in juried trials as well as influence policy. Canadian publication standards that limit editorializing and sensationalism have been effective. Newsprint media can be an opportunity to provide the public with credible education and awareness about maternal mental health, including perinatal mood and anxiety disorders. Focusing in the media on awareness and education about perinatal mental illness would decrease stigma, increase utilization of resources, and enhance compassion and prevention of maternal filicide.

MAIN CLINICAL/LEGAL POINTS AND CULTURAL PERSPECTIVES

- The Canadian media has implications in forming public opinion and biases.
- Overwhelmingly, reporters from *National Post*, *The Globe and Mail*, and *Toronto Star* tended to write in a neutral, unbiased, and fact-informed approach; however, some admonishing portrayals were published, particularly in relation to Elaine Campione, and were predominantly written by two female reporters.
- Infanticide law application and interpretation has been challenged and upheld in Canada's highest court, the Supreme Court of Canada, affirming its importance and relevance with the Canadian *Criminal Code*.
- Canadian news articles did not provide an association between mental health and maternal filicide that would educate readers.
- Although several relevant mental illnesses were mentioned, depression and postpartum depression were the most widely raised. Postpartum psychosis also serves as an important factor to consider in maternal filicide and should be taken into careful consideration when reporting about mothers who have committed filicide.
- Further research involving other media formats (e.g., social media, other newspapers, television shows, books) is necessary, as well as research examining maternal filicide within media in other countries.

Practice and Discussion Questions

1. Reflect on your thoughts toward mothers who have taken the lives of their children. What sort of biases do you possess? How were these biases formed?

2. Discuss the case involving Elaine Campione and your thoughts about the verdict and sentencing when mental illness was confirmed, as well as her vindictiveness toward her husband, with whom she was involved in an acrimonious divorce (including alleged domestic violence against her husband) and custody battle. Describe the impact to the verdict, if any, of no news reports offering the counter perspective of mental health involvement and culpability in the crime.

3. When you read news articles, do you question the language used by the reporters who convey the accounts or the biases that reporters may hold?

4. Similar to Question 2, when reporters choose to provide accounts of maternal filicide with sensationalism, how could this impact criminal justice proceedings more generally in your view?

5. Discuss a global manifesto on responsible media reporting in maternal filicide cases. What are barriers and facilitators to this reality? What countries would be next to investigate media reports, and why?

References

Alphonso C: Mother charged in baby boy's death. The Globe and Mail, March 28, 2009

Altheide DL: Reflections: ethnographic content analysis. Qual Sociol 10(1):65–77, 1987

Altheide DL, Schneider CJ: Qualitative Media Analysis, 2nd Edition. Los Angeles, CA, Sage, 2013

Bandes S: Fear factor: the role of media in covering and shaping the death penalty. Ohio State Journal of Criminal Law 1(2):585–597, 2004

Barnett B: Perfect mother or artist of obscenity? Narrative and myth in a qualitative analysis of press coverage of the Andrea Yates murders. Journal of Communication Inquiry 29(1):9–29, 2005

Baun K: Stigma matters: the media's impact on public perceptions of mental illness. Ottawa Life, February 2009, pp 31–33. Available at: https://ontario.cmha.ca/wp-content/files/2012/07/olm_stigma_matters_200902.pdf. Accessed August 27, 2020.

Beale S: The news media's influence on criminal justice policy: how market-driven news promotes punitiveness. William and Mary Law Review 48(2):397–481, 2006

Blatchford C: Accused in girls' death called a model mother. The Globe and Mail, September 28, 2010

Brean J: The baby killer case: Supreme Court to review infanticide law. National Post, January 15, 2016

Burgmann T: Woman who got rid of bodies of newborns feared parents. The Globe and Mail, April 5, 2014

Cavaglion G: Bad, mad or sad? Mothers who kill and press coverage in Israel. Crime, Media, Culture 4(2):271–278, 2008

Cavanagh J: What can professionals and families do? Missed opportunities to protect: sharing knowledge to inform practice change for identifying risks and enabling safety, in When Parents Kill Children. Edited by Brown T, Tyson D, Arias P. Cham, Switzerland, Springer Nature, 2018, pp 201–218

Chagnon N, Chesney-Lind M: "Someone's been in the house": a tale of burglary and trial by media. Crime, Media, Culture 11(1):41–60, 2015

Ciani ASC, Fontanesi L: Mothers who kill their offspring: testing evolutionary hypothesis in a 110-case Italian sample. Child Abuse Negl 36(6):519–527, 2012

Collins RE: 'Beauty and bullets': a content analysis of female offenders and victims in four Canadian newspapers. J Sociol 52(2):296–310, 2016

Crawford MG: The Journalist's Legal Guide. Scarborough, ON, Thomson Carswell, 2008

Criminal Code, R.S.C. 1985, c. 46, s. 233

Daly M, Wilson M: Evolutionary social psychology and family homicide. Science 242(4878):519–524, 1988

Dawson M: Canadian trends in filicide by gender of the accused, 1961–2011. Child Abuse Negl 47:162–174, 2015

DiManno R: Mom's video shakes insanity plea. Toronto Star, November 6, 2010a

DiManno R: A morbid exchange, a macabre vigil. Toronto Star, September 29, 2010b

Easteal P, Bartels L, Nelson N, Holland K: How are women who kill portrayed in newspaper media? Connections with social values and the legal system. Women's Studies International Forum 51:31–41, 2015

Edwards P: Mother not criminally responsible in drownings. Toronto Star, May 21, 2008

European Institute of Perinatal Mental Health: Declaration on the media treatment of filicide case in Godella, Spain, June 11, 2019. Available at: https://eipmh.com/wp-content/uploads/2019/06/FILICIDE-MANIFEST-JUNE-2019_EIPMH_logos.pdf. Accessed August 27, 2020.

Flynn SM, Shaw JJ, Abel KM: Filicide: mental illness in those who kill their children. PLoS One 8(4):1–8, 2013

Fraser K: Mother accused of killing babies gets bail: do not have sex, judge orders. National Post, June 28, 2010

Friedman SH, Resnick PJ: Child murder by mothers: patterns and prevention. World Psychiatry 6(3):137–141, 2007

Friedman SH, Cavney J, Resnick PJ: Mothers who kill: evolutionary underpinnings and infanticide law. Behav Sci Law 30(5):585–597, 2012

Government of Canada: Victims' Rights in Canada, 2015. Available at: https://www.justice.gc.ca/eng/cj-jp/victims-victimes/factsheets-fiches/publication.html. Accessed August 27, 2020.

Gowda GS, Kumar CN, Mishra S, et al: Maternal filicide: a case series from a medico-legal psychiatry unit in India. Asian J Psychiatr 36:42–45, 2018

Greer C, McLaughlin E: 'Trial by media': policing, the 24–7 news mediasphere and the 'politics of outrage.' Theor Criminol 15(1):23–46, 2011

Kauppi A, Kumpulainen K, Karkola K, et al: Maternal and paternal filicides: a retrospective review of filicides in Finland. J Am Acad Psychiatry Law 38(2):229–238, 2010

Kenyon W, Lodge E: Mother guilty of drowning her little girls: gets 25 years. National Post, November 16, 2010

Kutty H: Saving women and children from postpartum psychosis. National Post, September 17, 2010

Little J, Tyson D: Filicide in Australian media and culture. Oxford Research Encyclopedias: Criminology and Criminal Justice (website), May 2017. Available at: https://oxfordre.com/criminology/view/10.1093/acrefore/9780190264079.001.0001/acrefore-9780190264079-e-182. Accessed August 27, 2020.

Makin K: Postpartum-despair defense for baby killers to be tested. The Globe and Mail, September 11, 2010

Malmquist CP: Infanticide/neonaticide: the outlier situation in the United States. Aggress Violent Behav 18(3):399–408, 2013

Mariano TY, Chan HCO, Myers WC: Toward a more holistic understanding of filicide: a multidisciplinary analysis of 32 years of US arrest data. Forensic Sci Int 236:46–53, 2014

McCombs M: Setting the Agenda: Mass Media and Public Opinion. Cambridge, UK, Polity Press, 2014

McDonald C, Jowett C: Mother charged in infant son's death: 18 months old. National Post, March 28, 2009

McKee A, Egan V: A case series of twenty one maternal filicides in the UK. Child Abuse Negl 37(10):753–761, 2013

Middleweek B: Dingo media? The persistence of the "trial by media" frame in popular, media, and academic evaluations of the Azaria Chamberlain case. Feminist Media Studies 17(3):392–411, 2017

Minocher R, Sommer V: Why do mothers harm their babies? Evolutionary perspectives. Interdiscip Sci Rev 41(4):335–350, 2016

Mitchell B: Mom gets life in boy's killing. Toronto Star, January 15, 2011

Murcia Today: Deranged mother arrested after killing her infant children in Valencia. Murcia Today, March 15, 2019. Available at: https://murciatoday.com/deranged-mother-arrested-after-killing-her-infant-children-in-valencia_875124-a.html. Accessed August 27, 2020.

NewsBeezer.com: Mother who killed her own children was found in a jar. NewsBeezer.com, March 19, 2019. Available at: https://newsbeezer.com/portugaleng/mother-who-killed-her-own-children-was-found-in-a-jar-cm-ao-minuto. Accessed August 27, 2020.

Newspapers Canada: Daily Newspaper Circulation Report 2015. Available at: https://nmc-mic.ca/wp-content/uploads/2016/06/2015-Daily-Newspaper-Circulation-Report-REPORT_FINAL.pdf. Accessed December 28, 2018.

Oliveira M: Woman receives six years for suffocating two infant sons. The Globe and Mail, September 27, 2008

Powell B: Mom jailed for killing child: husband and mother of mentally unstable woman claim she's innocent of drowning autistic daughter. Toronto Star, March 15, 2008

Pruden JG: No question woman killed her children: Crown; yung sons drowned. National Post, March 13, 2012a

Pruden JG: 'Unspeakable tragedy': suicidal Alberta mother convicted of manslaughter in her children's deaths. National Post, April 21, 2012b

Purdy C: Family angry over mother's 'ridiculous' sentence. The Globe and Mail, June 5, 2012

Rajiva M, Khoday A: Peddling the margins of gender-based violence: Canadian media coverage of honour killings, in Within the Confines: Women and the Law in Canada. Edited by Kilty JM. Toronto, ON, Women's Press, 2014, pp 174–202

Resnick PJ: Child murder by parents: a psychiatric review of filicide. Am J Psychiatry 126(3):325–334, 1969

Rook K: Killer mom wants more children after prison. National Post, September 27, 2008

Sidebotham P, Retzer A: Maternal filicide in a cohort of English serious case reviews. Arch Womens Ment Health 22(1):1–11, 2018

Singh S: Criminalizing vulnerability: protecting 'vulnerable' children and punishing 'wicked' mothers. Soc Leg Stud 26(4):511–533, 2017

Statistics Canada: The use of media to follow news and current affairs, in Spotlight on Canadians: Results From the General Social Survey, February 15, 2016. Available at: https://www150.statcan.gc.ca/n1/pub/89-652-x/89-652-x2016001-eng.htm. Accessed August 27, 2020.

TellerReport.com: The parricide of Godella confessed that he killed his children "because they had lost their soul." TellerReport.com, May 9, 2019. Available at: https://www.tellerreport.com/news/—the-parricide-of-godella-confessed-that-he-killed-his-children-%22because-they-had-lost-their-soul%22-.B1QbjaW2N.html. Accessed June 1, 2019.

Vividata: Daily newspaper brands still reach 8 out of 10 Canadians, June 15, 2016. Available at: https://nmc-mic.ca/news/vividata-daily-newspaper-brands-still-reach-8-10-canadians. Accessed August 27, 2020.

West SG: An overview of filicide. Psychiatry (Edgmont) 4(2):48–57, 2007

Whiteley KM: Women as victims and offenders: incarcerated for murder in the Australian criminal justice system (doctoral dissertation). Brisbane, Australia, Queensland University of Technology, 2012. Available at: http://eprints.qut.edu.au/59597/1/Kathryn_Whiteley_ Thesis.pdf. Accessed August 27, 2020.

Zollmann F: Bringing propaganda back into news media studies. Crit Sociol 45(3):329–345, 2019

CHAPTER 13

Trauma and Attachment

PREVENTING MATERNAL FILICIDE THROUGH THE GENERATIONS

Nora L. Erickson, Ph.D.

Megan M. Julian, Ph.D.

Jonathan E. Handelzalts, Ph.D.

Gina Wong, Ph.D.

Maria Muzik, M.D., M.S.

Within the extant literature on the predictors of maternal filicide, prior studies have identified numerous individual and psychosocial risk factors. As discussed elsewhere (see Chapters 5 and 6), mothers who commit filicide are more likely to have existing mental health concerns (e.g., depression, psychosis); greater demographic risk (poverty, younger maternal age, lower educational attainment); and ongoing relational stress (single parenthood, intimate partner violence, social alienation). In the broader population, however, this constellation of risk factors is not necessarily uncommon. Up to 18% of women experience depression during the postpartum (Hahn-Holbrook et al. 2018). Furthermore, a substantial subset of reproductive-age women identifies as young, low-income, single mothers. Given similar personal and life circumstances, it is unclear why some mothers commit filicide and others do not. The difficulty in accurately predicting which women may be at risk for filicidal behavior (Friedman et al. 2005; Mugavin 2008) underscores the ongoing need to identify distinguishing features or experiences that differentiate mothers at risk from those who are not.

Among the list of factors associated with maternal filicide, previous researchers and authors in this volume (see Chapters 7 and 8) indicate that many perpetrating women had a history of abuse and maltreatment in their own childhoods (Amon et al. 2012; Brewster et al. 1998; Crimmins et al. 1997; Haapasalo and Petäjä 1999; Krischer et al. 2007; Smithey 1997). For example, in a cluster analysis of motivation for neonaticide, infanticide, and filicide, two primary variables associated with filicidal behavior were a mother's history of depression and of lifetime physical or sexual abuse (Krischer et al. 2007). Consistent with a cumulative risk model—wherein co-occurring risk factors for filicide are considered simultaneously rather than individually (Friedman et al. 2005)—it is likely that a mother's own history of trauma and abuse interacts with other variables to increase the risk of filicidal behavior. Nevertheless, a primary aim of this chapter is to highlight how maternal trauma and attachment patterns may be *critical factors* to consider within a constellation of filicide risk.

In general, people who experience trauma and stress in their childhood are at an increased risk for a range of negative physical and psychological sequelae that persist across the lifespan. Trauma can have an especially deleterious effect on an individual's psychological functioning when the traumatic experiences 1) are interpersonal in nature, 2) are chronic in duration (i.e., complex trauma), and 3) occur early in development (i.e., in their first decade of life) (van der Kolk et al. 2005). Among mechanistic explanations for the associations between early life trauma and maladaptive outcomes in adulthood is significant empirical support for the role of altered brain structure and function. Replicated findings indicate that abuse and maltreatment in early childhood can yield both hyper- and hyporesponsiveness of brain regions that are crucial to emotional health (i.e., limbic system and medial prefrontal cortex, respectively) and alter pathways involved in stress regulation, including those involving the hypothalamus and hippocampus (for review, see Thomason and Marusak 2017). When the perpetrator of child abuse is a family member or a caregiver, this subset of interpersonal trauma can further disrupt the formation of secure attachment (Cook et al. 2005). Disrupted attachment patterns in early childhood can detrimentally affect a person's capacity to form healthy relationships across the lifespan, including subsequent formation of parent–child relationships (Bartholomew and Horowitz 1991). Ultimately, the well-replicated associations among trauma, neurobiology, attachment, and parenting have potential implications for the prevention of maternal filicide.

In the current chapter, we adopt a trauma- and attachment-informed approach to understanding maternal filicide. We explore how intergenerational cycles of abuse and disrupted attachment patterns may pre-dispose people to filicide and how preventative interventions focusing on parent–child relationships may help mitigate filicide risk. We offer a rationale for conceptualizing mothers' adverse childhood experiences (ACEs), history of complex trauma, and disrupted attachment in early childhood as critical risk factors, discussing ways these interrelated experiences may inhibit brain development and healthy maternal functioning and increase propensity toward maternal filicide. While we do not focus on a specific subtype of filicide per Resnick's (1969) typologies, we assert that a mother's early trauma history can yield developmental and relational cascades that may predispose her to a range of filicidal behavior, from altruistic to psychotic or accidental filicide (see Chapter 7).

As clinician researchers in the fields of psychiatry and both clinical and counseling psychology, we have expertise in perinatal mental health, early childhood development, attachment, and parenting in the context of trauma and stress. We aim to contribute to existing filicide research—and literature on filicide risk factors—by integrating relevant research on trauma and attachment. Because every author in this group is a clinician, we believe clinical case material has the power to highlight psychological concepts and phenomena across the lifespan. Our clinical work inspires us to thoughtfully explore conceptual and developmental models, with the hope of understanding risk and resilience factors that potentially lead to filicide. Clinical work is also where we examine and apply the relevance of our models via therapeutic conceptualization.

With this in mind, we begin with a clinical case as the basis for further elaboration of theory, using this as a model for understanding and appreciating the importance of early caregiving experiences in general and early attachment relationships with a parent in particular. We then discuss relevant research and theory on disruptions in the parent–child relationship within the context of trauma and abuse, focusing on effects of trauma on secure attachment formation. Following this background and summary, we place existing filicide research within the broader attachment and trauma-informed literature. Whenever possible, we relate back to the case study in order to bridge research, theory, and clinical material. Finally, we offer information on preventative interventions and describe several evidence-based treatments that focus on healing intergenerational trauma via the parent–child relationship and attachment.

CASE STUDY

LR was a 21-year-old woman who grew up exposed to multiple family stressors and complex trauma associated with abject poverty, brief periods of homelessness, and repeated sexual abuse during her childhood and adolescence. LR's grandmother and mother were also victims of sexual abuse when they were growing up, and there was a pattern of alcoholism on her father's side of the family. LR's father was incarcerated the year she was born and for several years was not part of her life. LR was raised by distant relatives starting at the age of 3. There were seven or eight other children living in the home at one time, and her caregivers were dismissive and emotionally unavailable to her. LR yearned to reunite and live with her biological parents, but it was not possible. She felt rejected and abandoned by her parents, yet simultaneously idolized and idealized them, particularly her mother. When asked about memories of her childhood, LR could not recall any specific relational moments of warmth and connection with caregivers, nor could she recall direct negative experiences. Nevertheless, she revered her mother and believed she could do no wrong. LR believed that one day they would be very close. Her mother continued to reject LR, criticizing her whenever they spoke, telling LR she was "no good" and blaming LR for her own misery. The verbal abuse furthered LR's longing to be accepted and seen as "good" in her mother's eyes. LR's first suicide attempt occurred when she was 15 years old. She began hearing voices when she was 17, and she believed they were helping her to be "good" even though they taunted her, sometimes telling her to end her life.

As a mother herself, LR looked after her children and did what she could to ensure that their basic needs were met. Her eldest was almost 2 years old, and her youngest was 5 weeks old. Her partner, who was the children's father, relegated childrearing to LR. Within their own relationship, he was physically abusive toward LR, very controlling, emotionally unavailable, and rejecting. LR suffered in unspeakable ways—retraumatized by her partner's abuse and unavailability, as well as his cruelty as a father to their children—yet she longed for his love. LR also believed she was a bad mother and that her children would grow to hate and despise her because she believed she was unlovable. Leading up to the day of the filicide, stressors were mounting: LR's mother was diagnosed with a terminal illness, there were threats of homelessness to the family, and the interpersonal violence in the home had escalated. LR was experiencing visual and auditory hallucinations and had periods of extreme confusion. One evening, LR stabbed her children and herself. She believed ending her life was the only way out and that her children were suffering. She felt she needed to save them from the lifelong pain of rejection, neglect, and abandonment that she had endured. LR and her eldest child survived; the infant died.

The reality of LR's case, although devastating and tragic, shows how early relational disruptions, trauma, and adversity may alter attachment patterns across development, disrupt subsequent maternal health and functioning, and potentially yield fatal outcomes for children. Viewed through a trauma-informed lens, numerous factors that may have increased LR's risk for filicide could be identified, including a history of poverty, sexual abuse, younger maternal age, and ongoing intimate partner violence. From a cumulative risk perspective, we acknowledge that such factors are potentially important in LR's case. In subsequent sections of this chapter, however, we hope to underscore the critical role of LR's attachment relationships within the context of complex trauma and adversity, which likely increased her risk for filicide by altering her ability to separate her own painful childhood experiences and disrupted relational history from her current relationship with her young children. We apply and discuss relevant theory and research on attachment, early parent–child relationships, and intergenerational trauma in an attempt to understand risk for filicide, both in the case of LR and more broadly.

Attachment Theory

Attachment theory was primarily developed through the collaborative work of John Bowlby and Mary Ainsworth (Ainsworth and Bowlby 1991; Bretherton 1992). As a construct, *attachment* encompasses the critical role of early caregiving relationships in a developing child's psychological health and well-being. Attachment is not derived from teaching, play, or "quality time" between parents and children but is rather an innate biological motivation to seek comfort and safety from caregivers.

Based on Ainsworth and Bowlby's (1991) seminal work and the ensuant wealth of research supporting the importance of the early caregiving environment, we know that the relationship between a caregiver and a child plays an integral role in healthy development across the lifespan. Attachment not only is important within infancy and early childhood but also has implications for psychological and relational functioning into adulthood (Bartholomew and Horowitz 1991). Typically, developing children establish attachment relationships with all caregivers who regularly provide emotional or physical care, regardless of whether that care is sensitive and responsive or neglectful and abusive. As an innate construct, attachment unfolds and develops across a variety of caregiving contexts; however, the quality of these attachment relationships may differ (Benoit 2004).

ATTACHMENT IN EARLY CHILDHOOD

In her classic work on attachment classification, Mary Ainsworth described three distinct patterns of attachment in childhood: *secure, insecure avoidant*, and *insecure anxious-ambivalent/resistant* (Ainsworth and Bell 1970). Subsequent laboratory research by Main and Solomon (1990) identified an additional classification, *disorganized* attachment. Considerable research now indicates that children who have disorganized attachment are at the greatest risk of a range of maladaptive outcomes. We therefore focus on the characteristics of secure versus nonsecure attachment (with particular emphasis on disorganized), exploring predisposing factors and developmental sequelae associated with each style.

When their interactions with caregivers are consistently and predictably sensitive and responsive, children are most likely to develop secure attachment. The securely attached child uses the parent as a "safe haven" (Bowlby 1969) during times of danger or distress, wherein the parent offers comfort and emotional restoration. The caregiver also becomes the "secure base" from which the securely attached child can learn to explore and practice independence during times of perceived safety (Bowlby 1969). As a critical and foundational factor in early childhood development and social emotional well-being, secure attachment to caregivers is associated with increases in children's emotion regulation abilities (Sroufe 2005), healthier peer relationships (Schneider et al. 2001), decreased risk for internalizing and externalizing problems (Carlson 1998; Lyons-Ruth et al. 1993; Shaw et al. 1997), and better physiological modulation of the infant stress response through the hypothalamic-pituitary-adrenal axis (Lyons-Ruth 2003). The broad developmental significance of early attachment therefore underscores the pivotal role that mothers, fathers, and caregivers play in promoting healthy child outcomes.

Nevertheless, when a secure attachment relationship is not present, this can result in pronounced and prolonged physiological stress, which increases the potential for neurobiological consequences and both behavioral and emotional problems across development (Hertsgaard et al. 1995; Lieberman and Van Horn 2004; van IJzendoorn et al. 1999). Children who experience caregiving that is regularly unpredictable, insensitive, harsh, or neglectful are more likely to develop insecure attachment (Thompson 2006). Specifically, the anxious-ambivalent style of insecure attachment (Ainsworth and Bell 1970) typically develops in the context of caregivers who are not consistently dependable but instead are unreliable or distracted. These caregivers are described as generally capable of sensitive and responsive care, and they provide this care sometimes, but not consistently. Ainsworth et al. (1978) suggested that mothers in this group may be preoccupied by their own changing and sometimes overwhelming feelings and needs, and this can interfere with their ability to recognize and respond appropriately to their infant's signals. Children with an anxious-ambivalent attachment style are less able to use their caregiver as a secure base from which to explore, and when they are distressed, they show high levels of emotion dysregulation and help seeking. When reunited with their caregiver after a stressful event, anxious-ambivalent children are likely to vacillate between clinging to their caregiver and resisting comfort.

In comparison, the avoidant style of insecure attachment (Ainsworth and Bell 1970) is more likely to arise when caregiving is characterized by *consistent* detachment and emotional unavailability. These caregivers are described as providing better care when their children underplay their emotions. Children with this attachment style tend to show little distress and considerable exploratory behaviors when they are separated from the caregiver, and on reunion with the caregiver, these children typically continue exploring and avoid the caregiver. Both secure and insecure attachment represent "organized" attachment patterns, demonstrating consistent and predictable behaviors; children with such attachment styles know what to expect from the caregiver and behave accordingly. In contrast, children who respond unpredictably or inconsistently toward a caregiver may be classified as having disorganized attachment.

Disorganized attachment describes children who present with behavioral and relational patterns characterized by contradictory, disoriented, or fearful responses toward a caregiver, which generally disrupts the development and application of other organized attachment strategies (see Granqvist et al. 2017). For example, within a circumscribed period, a child with disorganized attachment may display variable and turbulent interactions with a caregiver and vacillate from clingy to dismissive to aggressive behaviors (Lyons-Ruth et al. 1999). Attachment disorganization is more likely to occur when caregivers are confusing, hostile, or withdrawing toward their children (Lyons-Ruth and Jacobvitz 2008). For these children, the instinct to pull away or flee from the caregiver—who is associated with a source of danger—directly conflicts with their attachment-related instinct to approach or seek comfort and safety, resulting in a paradoxical push and pull that is difficult for young children to reconcile (Hesse and Main 2000, 2006).

Caregivers who display atypical behaviors associated with disorganized attachment often do so across contexts, and many have their own history of unresolved trauma (e.g., emotional, physical, or sexual abuse) (Bernier and Meins 2008); this is evident in the case of LR, wherein past traumas (e.g., sexual abuse, father incarcerated) impact the attachment system across generations. According to research, approximately 15% of young children exhibit disorganized attachment (van IJzendoorn et al. 1999). For mothers with a history of maltreatment in their own childhood, the rate of disorganized attachment among their children almost triples (44%; Berthelot et al. 2015), and for infants and young children who are the victims of maltreatment, rates of attachment disorganization have ranged from 77% to 90% (Barnett et al. 1999; Carlson et al. 1989; Cicchetti et al. 2006).

This is not to say, however, that maltreatment and trauma are necessary prerequisites for disorganized attachment. As summarized in one review, the "alarming caregiver behaviors" associated with disorganized attachment can take many forms, including intermittent frightening or frightened caregiver behavior, a lack of psychological availability, exposure to domestic violence, or unexpected/prolonged caregiver absences (Granqvist et al. 2017). Regardless of the specific circumstances, it is generally theorized that the erratic behaviors displayed by children with disorganized attachment likely relate to underlying tension and confusion that arise when the child views the caregiver as a source of both safety *and* alarm or danger. Thus, children with disorganized attachment experience simultaneous activation of their attachment and defense motivational systems (Hesse and Main 2000).

In an attempt to explore how these concepts may emerge in clinical or forensic practice, we can apply this information on attachment patterns to the case study of LR. We cannot make a definite attachment classification for LR based on the limited information described in this chapter, yet several components of her history speak to the likelihood that she had a disorganized attachment to caregivers during her childhood. LR's history was marked by frequent and enduring separation from her biological parents, and her case highlights how she simultaneously idolized and felt rejected by her mother. Harkening back to the "push and pull" or tension that children with disorganized attachment may experience in the context of caregiving relationships, it is possible that LR was unable to reconcile her deep longing to be with her mother with her subconscious anger at her mother for abandoning and rejecting her. Ultimately, a disrupted attachment pattern, wherein LR could not rely on either her biological parents or her caregivers for consistent or sensitive care, likely contributed to future difficulties in relationships with both her romantic partner and her children. In the following section, we discuss additional research and theory on the longstanding implications of disrupted attachment in more detail.

ATTACHMENT IN ADULTHOOD: ASSOCIATIONS WITH PARENTING

As adults, attachment patterns from childhood can be transferred onto important interpersonal relationships, including our relationships with romantic partners and children. In particular, early parent–child relationships operate as a template carried forward across the lifespan and form cognitive schemas and affective memory traces of caregiving relationships, known as an *internal working model* (Bowlby 1969). Through the internal working model, relational patterns during formative years become the substrate for the attributions parents make about their own children and the ways in which they interpret their children's behavior, which may influence the quality of parent–child interactions. In this way, attachment behaviors and relational patterns can be transmitted across generations. For a mother whose own parents were sensitive, responsive, and attuned during her childhood, these internalized and positive caregiving experiences help promote benevolent interpretations of her infant's behavior (i.e., a "balanced representational style"), more effective emotion processing, and higher levels of sensitivity and responsivity toward her infant (Dollberg et al. 2010; Rosenblum et al. 2006).

If a mother's early caregiving environment was less optimal, internalized relational patterns may yield more malevolent interpretations of her child's behavior and insensitive and alarming maternal behaviors. As a major transitional time within a woman's life, pregnancy often elicits prior models of maternal behavior and recapitulation of past caregiving experiences. For pregnant women with a history of maltreatment in childhood, this recapitulation is theorized to be triggering and to result in negative attributions toward the fetus (Bonnet 1993). Selma Fraiberg et al. (1980) theorized that caregivers whose own early relational experiences were characterized by helplessness and fear may unconsciously reenact these experiences when parenting their own child. As children, the parents internalized these punitive or neglectful styles of caregiving as an effort toward self-protection, and now enact these harmful parenting behaviors with their own children. When an expectant mother cannot differentiate her own self and her emerging maternal identity from prior abusive or neglectful models of maternal behavior and caregiving, her prior trauma and attachment disruptions are considered "unresolved"; consequently, it is more likely that preexisting interpersonal patterns will reemerge in the developing relationship with her offspring (Giacchetti et al. 2020; Iyengar et al. 2014).

Investigating intergenerational transmission of attachment patterns, Slade et al. (2005) found an association between a mother's attachment style during pregnancy and her infant's later attachment style, measured at 14 months; however, this was largely explained by the mother's ability to understand and conceptualize her child's behavior in relation to underlying feelings and intentions (see section on "Trauma and Reflective Functioning"). Mothers who had secure attachment relationships during pregnancy were better able to make sense of their children's behavior at 10 months postpartum (e.g., needs for proximity and comfort); this invariably increased the likelihood that the child would form a secure attachment to the mother (Slade et al. 2005).

A microanalysis of face-to-face interactions between mothers and infants further identified specific maternal and infant characteristics at 4 months of age that were associated with infant attachment patterns at 12 months of age (Beebe et al. 2010). Observational analyses revealed that mothers of infants who went on to have disorganized attachment did *not* have broad deficits in empathy or difficulties identifying their infant's distress cues. Rather, mothers of future disorganized infants were more likely to exhibit distinct interactional patterns that were notable for 1) more excessive and unpredictable gazes away from the infant, and 2) more discordant responses to infant emotional reactivity (e.g., smiling or surprised facial and vocal responses in reaction to infant distress cues). Instead of viewing these maternal responses as a lack of understanding or inaccurate reading of infant cues, Beebe et al. (2010) hypothesized that the infant's distress cues may evoke maternal distress and dysregulation associated with historical difficulties in intimate relationships and unresolved experiences of trauma and loss. In this way, the behavioral strategies implemented by mothers of future disorganized infants may not necessarily be related to a skill deficit but rather to the mothers' prior experiences of trauma (Beebe et al. 2010).

Applying Beebe et al.'s (2010) findings to our case study, LR did not exhibit global deficits in caring for her children (e.g., she was able to ensure their basic needs were met), nor did she abdicate her role as a mother. Nevertheless, chronic relational traumas within her early caregiving experiences were recapitulated in her relationships with her partner and children and likely remained unresolved. We conceptualize that this unresolved relational trauma disrupted LR's ability to effectively separate her children's experiences from her own past experiences. In the next section, we focus more specifically on attachment and parenting in the context of prior trauma.

Intergenerational Trauma

By adopting a trauma-informed approach, we recognize the pervasiveness of trauma and how prior traumatic experiences can affect individuals' beliefs, behavior, and relationships toward themselves, others, and the world around them. In this way, acknowledging the significant and detrimental impact of trauma requires changing the dialogue from "what is *wrong* with you?" to "what *happened* to you?" (Harris and Fallot 2001). In this chapter, we use *trauma* to describe disturbing events or experiences that involve either actual or perceived threat of death, injury, or bodily harm and result in negative effects on a person's functioning, behavior, and beliefs (American Psychological Association 2020; International Society for Traumatic Stress Studies 2020). The inclusion of "perceived threat" within this definition underscores how appraisals of trauma can be subjective. Memory and cognition play a role in one's appraisal of a traumatic event (Rubin et al. 2008), and objective and subjective ratings of events as "traumatizing" are not always consistent with one another (Boals 2018).

It is well-replicated that specific traumatic experiences in early childhood (e.g., physical or sexual abuse) are generally strong predictors of a broad range of mental health conditions across development, including depression, anxiety, PTSD, substance abuse, eating disorders, and psychotic disorders (Kessler et al. 2010; Read et al. 2014). Maintaining a trauma-informed approach may also involve attention and sensitivity to how cumulative experiences of childhood adversity—known as ACEs—may continue to impact functional and health outcomes across the lifespan. The most common measure of ACEs assesses for 10 experiences of adversity and includes questions about the various forms of abuse, neglect, and household dysfunction a person may have experienced prior to age 18 (Felitti et al. 1998). A growing body of research indicates a dose-response relationship between ACEs and various mental, behavioral, and physical health outcomes, wherein people with four or more ACEs are at the greatest risk for negative outcomes, such as suicide, self-harm, obesity, heart disease, cancer, and perpetrating and/or being a victim of interpersonal violence (Felitti et al. 1998; Noll et al. 2003; Nurius et al. 2015; Roberts et al. 2011).

Unfortunately, many children whose mothers or caregivers have a significant history of trauma or adversity are also at risk of experiencing trauma themselves. *Intergenerational trauma* describes the transmission of trauma from one generation to the next (e.g., from mother to child). A related construct, *historical trauma*, refers to specific intergenerational patterns of trauma experienced by members of certain racial, ethnic, and cultural groups. Historical trauma is passed from generation to generation when an individual's lived experiences of oppression, racism, or violence (e.g., slavery, genocide) continue to psychologically affect their offspring or descendants through genetic, biological, and behavioral mechanisms, as well as large-scale systemic inequities (Sotero 2006). In accordance with Bowen's cycle-of-violence hypothesis, child abuse and neglect within families can emerge from unhealthy family processes being perpetuated across generations (Kerr and Bowen 1988). In general, mothers with a history of trauma exposure have more negative parenting behaviors (Martorell and Bugental 2006; Mills-Koonce et al. 2009; Sturge-Apple et al. 2011). These trauma-related disturbances in maternal functioning can begin as early as pregnancy.

In a study of maternal attachment to the fetus during pregnancy, a mother's history of interpersonal or attachment-based trauma—but not her general trauma history—predicted lower or less-optimal scores on a self-report measure of the maternal–fetal relationship (Schwerdtfeger and Nelson Goff 2007). Schwerdtfeger and Nelson Goff (2007) differentiated nonpersonal traumatic experiences (e.g., accidents, natural disasters) from those that occur within interpersonal relationships, including childhood physical and sexual abuse perpetrated by caregivers, as well as trauma within intimate relationships. Women's experiences of relational trauma are relevant and important not only because of the high rates of differential and gender-based victimization but also because pregnancy marks a period in which many women address and potentially modify their relationships with others as they prepare to have a new baby (Huth-Bocks et al. 2013).

As discussed, when a mother can regularly identify, predict, and respond to her child's needs, this helps promote development of healthy and secure attachment. Unfortunately, parenting behaviors for trauma-exposed women are more often characterized by higher levels of avoidance, intrusiveness, hostility, and controlling/overprotective behavior and by lower levels of sensitivity, responsivity, and emotional availability compared with parents not exposed to trauma (van Ee et al. 2015). For women whose trauma history is unresolved (i.e., they have not consciously processed their trauma history and its effects on their overall functioning), their infants' or children's attachment or distress cues may be triggering (Beebe et al. 2010; Schechter et al. 2004), resulting in maternal dissociation and disengagement from the children (Beebe et al. 2010; Ludmer et al. 2018).

Trauma and Reflective Functioning

Prior literature on mothers with a history of childhood maltreatment and subsequent attachment patterns among their infants has identified a mother's capacity for reflective functioning (RF) or mentalization as an important mediator in the transmission of risk across generations (Allen 2013; Berthelot et al. 2015; Fonagy et al. 1994). Often used interchangeably, the terms *reflective functioning* and *mentalization* describe the capacity to think about ourselves and others as "psychological beings" with mental states and motivations that help determine behavior (Choi-Kain and Gunderson 2008). A parent's capacity for RF can alter the child's resilience and mediate links between parental distress or dysfunction and child psychosocial development (Katznelson 2014). Other studies echo these findings: adults who experienced childhood trauma but exhibit high RF were less likely to develop borderline personality disorder than were trauma-exposed peers with low RF (Fonagy et al. 1995). RF may therefore act as an intergenerational buffer and may promote healthier parent–child relationships by enhancing the caregiver's ability to self-monitor, control impulses, regulate affect, and self-organize while also increasing the caregiver's capacity to predict the child's behavior, distinguish between manifestation and reality, engage in effective interpersonal communication, and encourage and preserve attachment security (Fonagy et al. 1998, 2007).

In his work on the association between mentalization and trauma, Fonagy (1993) described how difficulties thinking about, symbolizing, or mentalizing prior traumatic experiences may predispose parents to align with their former aggressors when their infants become distressed. Limited trauma mentalization can contribute to maternal difficulties, such as regulating one's own distress when confronted by infant distress, ultimately shifting the focus away from the infant's needs. Over time, this interactional pattern is thought to disrupt infant attachment. Among a sample of mothers with a history of abuse and neglect in their own childhood, Berthelot et al. (2015) found a 70% concordance rate between the mothers' level of unresolved trauma/loss (i.e., poor trauma-related mentalization) and their infants' attachment disorganization. Thus, a mother's own history of childhood maltreatment or adult interpersonal trauma can become a risk factor for impairments in her infant's attachment style, especially when her prior trauma is unresolved and she has limited RF. In the next section, we explore how the interrelationship between attachment, parenting, and intergenerational trauma may increase risk for filicide.

Trauma, Attachment, and Maternal Filicide

As mentioned, replicated findings indicate that a large proportion of mothers who complete filicide had a history of abuse and maltreatment (Amon et al. 2012; Brewster et al. 1998; Crimmins et al. 1997; Haapasalo and Petäjä 1999; Krischer et al. 2007; Smithey 1997). Here, we further explore how associations between maternal trauma and disrupted attachment patterns may be a critical risk factor for maternal filicide. From a theoretical standpoint, Mugavin (2008) developed the trauma-focused maternal filicide theoretical framework (MFTF) using data from a combination of 33 narratives and case reports in the existing filicide literature. Mugavin acknowledged how traumatic experiences in childhood may affect women's relationships with their children and ultimately predispose mothers to committing filicide. The MFTF model identifies a number of toxic environmental exposures early in life, deemed "phenotypic vulnerabilities," that may yield filicidal behavior: 1) historical victimization or exposure to physical, sexual, or emotional abuse; 2) a predisposition to mental illness (i.e., one or more caregivers with a psychiatric disorder); 3) exposure to caregiver substance use; 4) inadequate maternal role development (i.e., disruptions in a mother's early attachment experiences); and 5) aversive social environment or constructs (e.g., abject poverty, neighborhood violence) (Mugavin 2008). Viewed through this model, LR had exposure to traumatic early life toxic exposures such as sexual abuse, disruption in secure based parent–child attachment, and poverty.

Regardless of the specific traumatic event in childhood, a mother's history of disrupted attachment has emerged as an important characteristic of maternal filicide (Barone et al. 2014; Debowska et al. 2015; McKee and Egan 2013). Likewise, Debowska et al. (2015) explored a potential intergenerational cascade, wherein a mother's own disrupted attachment history is initially recapitulated in her relationship with her child. She becomes frustrated by the resulting impairments in the parent–child relationship, and this frustration eventually leads to overt aggression and violence (Adshead 2002) and replication of the attachment injuries. Despite the theoretical role that insecure or disorganized attachment may have in motivation for filicide, limited studies have explored maternal attachment styles as a predisposing factor. In one of the few empirical studies to date, Barone et al. (2014) focused on the differential effects of maternal attachment and other descriptive factors commonly linked to filicide risk (e.g., socioeconomic status, psychiatric diagnosis). The authors compared the separate and combined effects of these hypothesized risk factors across three separate groups of mothers: 23 convicted of filicide, 37 with a documented mental health history, and 61 from the normative population. Compared with the normative group, both high-risk groups (i.e., mothers with a history of mental illness and mothers convicted of filicide) had lower socioeconomic status and a higher incidence of prior traumatic events, indicating that these risk factors were not distinctive to the filicide group. Within the group of mothers convicted of filicide, statistical models further indicated that trauma and psychiatric illness (i.e., psychosis or depression) were not predictive of filicide when considered alone; however, strong associations emerged when these variables were considered concurrently with the mothers' attachment style, specifically a hostile-helpless (HH) attachment style (Barone et al. 2014). The HH categorization of adult attachment, basically a specification of the insecure/disorganized typology, was previously developed by Lyons-Ruth et al. (2005) and describes a mother who identifies with a formerly malevolent caregiver (hostile subtype) or abdicates her maternal role (helpless subtype), yet has minimal reflection on these intergenerational patterns. Based on their statistical models, Barone et al. (2014) concluded:

> It was indeed the additive role of the HH attachment states of mind, related to the inability to reflect upon past negative experiences, that significantly increased the probability of filicidal behavior in our sample of mothers....[T]he psychiatric diagnosis was not per se a significant risk factor for being in the filicide group, but its association with an HH state of mind was. (p. 1475)

As shown, although filicide cannot exclusively be predicted by a single vulnerability or event, a disorganized attachment style and a history of intergenerational trauma can have a detrimental effect on parenting cognitions, emotions, and behaviors. In the most extreme cases, coupled with other environmental and personal circumstances, these vulnerabilities can result in tragic circumstances that may include filicide. Earlier we provided one such extreme example in the case study of LR. We hypothesize that it may have been too painful for LR to connect with feelings of anger toward her mother or to process what happened to her as a young child, thereby disrupting her ability to recall explicit relational memories from her childhood. LR's persistent idealization of her mother could be indicative of a limited capacity for trauma mentalization and low parental RF. Ultimately, this limited RF may have shifted the focus away from her own children and contributed to LR's difficulties separating her children's minds and experiences from her own. The interrelated components of disrupted attachment, unresolved trauma, and low mentalization likely perpetuated LR's fear that her children might experience pain and pervasive feelings of longing for a parent similar to her own; LR thereby determined that death was the best escape and the only source of relief for both her children and herself.

In conjunction with the current overview of the critical role of early trauma and attachment relationships, another primary aim of this chapter is to identify and explore preventative interventions that may bolster resilience or protective factors and help mitigate filicide risk. Among the factors that place mothers at risk for filicide, some are unchangeable (e.g., history of childhood maltreatment), whereas others are modifiable (e.g., reflective capacity, processing of traumatic experiences). In fact, while a history of childhood maltreatment is unfortunately common, especially among young children (e.g., 15 per 1,000 children younger than 3 years experienced maltreatment in the United States in 2017; Child Trends 2019); mothers' experience of childhood maltreatment is not universally associated with attachment disturbances in their children (Berthelot et al. 2015; Morelen et al. 2018). It is therefore important to understand that relationships between maternal childhood maltreatment, parenting, and attachment are not deterministic (Berthelot et al. 2015; Morelen et al. 2018). Rather, a mother's psychological symptoms, emotion regulation, and parental RF may play a mechanistic role, and these factors can be important targets for interventions that attempt to ameliorate risk transmission and intergenerational violence and maternal filicide.

Trauma-Focused and Dyadic Interventions

In this section, we discuss several clinical intervention approaches that aim to reduce the risk for disruptions in caregiving and for maternal filicide from the perspective of trauma and attachment theory. Although the list of interventions is not exhaustive, all of the interventions target parenting and mothers' mental representations of their children and aim to enhance parental RF and the capacity to process past trauma and its impact on present-day parenting tasks. These interventions further aim to avert the risk for abusive, aggressive, and hostile mother–child relationships; ultimately, they aim to reduce the occurrence of filicide in our communities. We begin by discussing a trauma-focused intervention that may be beneficial to mothers who have difficulty with emotion regulation, to the extent that it may preclude their engagement in other parent–child treatment. We then shift our focus to several existing dyadic interventions that more explicitly address the parent–child relationship through work with the mother and her young child. These briefly reviewed treatments include Trauma Affect Regulation: Guide for Education and Therapy (TARGET), Mom Power, Circle of Security (COS), Attachment and Biobehavioral Catch-up (ABC), and Child–Parent Psychotherapy (CPP). As clinicians, we recognize that certain factors may impinge upon equal access to such interventions. That is, access to and engagement with treatment programs may be more difficult for some families/individuals due to systemic or situational barriers (e.g., poverty, homelessness, living in a rural community). Individual barriers may also be a factor for many parents, including those with chronic medical concerns or cognitive/developmental delays. These barriers can exacerbate disruptions in caregiving and further limit parental RF. As such, there is a need to understand how such barriers are considered in intervention programs, with specific attention to making treatment accessible and available to all families, regardless of circumstances or abilities.

TRAUMA AFFECT REGULATION: GUIDE FOR EDUCATION AND THERAPY

TARGET (Ford 2015) is an evidence-based, manualized therapy delivered in variable session lengths and adapted for youth and adults in individual, group, or home-based family therapy. TARGET is a framework (rather than a prescriptive model) for strengths-based, client-centered, emotion regulation psychotherapy (Ford and Russo 2006). It is intended for individuals who experienced trauma and developed PTSD, complex PTSD (Ford 2018), and related psychopathology (Dvir et al. 2014). Although TARGET provides manuals with session-by-session guides, it does not require therapists to follow a fixed, formulaic, "one-size-fits-all" protocol but instead offers vocabulary and structure designed to be adapted to each unique client. Thus, TARGET is a user-friendly treatment model and is highly applicable to pregnant or postpartum mothers with trauma histories.

As a central symptom addressed by TARGET, emotion dysregulation is a universal feature of trauma-related disorders, including PTSD and its complex variants involving depression, dissociation, anxiety, substance abuse, personality disorders, suicidality, and nonsuicidal self-injury (Ford 2018). Mothers with emotion dysregulation secondary to traumatic exposures are more likely to present with hostile or aggressive projections/mental representations toward others, including their children. Psychotherapy focused on traumatized mothers' emotion regulation may therefore be important not only to help them recover from traumatic experiences but also to prevent intergenerational transmission of emotion dysregulation, traumatic stress disorders, and violence. A mother's unresolved trauma may limit her ability to maintain emotion regulation during dyadic psychotherapy (i.e., parenting-focused relational treatments, described later) or inhibit her capacity to reflect on and translate the changes achieved in therapy to her day-to-day parenting. Moreover, traumatic stress reactions are prototypically characterized by survival-based hypervigilance—preconsciously scanning one's environment for the smallest sign of impending danger—that is fundamentally incompatible with RF (Ford et al. 2011). Thus, mothers with significant, ongoing, and persistent trauma-related pathology, (including emotion dysregulation and hypervigilance) may initially benefit from a trauma-specific treatment such as TARGET that addresses the individual functioning and maternal symptoms that typically interfere with parenting rather than focusing primarily on the parent–child relationship itself.

This intervention begins with a thorough and sensitive psychosocial and safety assessment and collaborative goal setting designed to establish a strong working alliance between the client and the clinician. Next, psychoeducation helps explain the link between PTSD symptoms and emotion dysregulation by describing how traumatic threats and injuries lead to survival-based biological adaptations. Through this, mothers can learn a new way of understanding their own traumatic stress reactions, which is both destigmatizing and strengths based. TARGET helps traumatized mothers recognize the adaptive purpose of hypervigilance; enables them to become conscious of when and how they are becoming hypervigilant; and supports their attention to feelings, thoughts, goals, and actions that reflect their core values and sense of purpose in life. This helps facilitate a shift from a chronic alarm mode (i.e., PTSD) to a focus on achieving other life goals, including goals related to emotion regulation and parenting (Ford 2018). As such, TARGET aims to enhance the mother's reflective capacity about her own life and foster her reflectiveness toward her children. TARGET is well researched and highly effective with various populations of traumatized mothers, including teen mothers in juvenile detention (Ford et al. 2011, 2012).

MOM POWER

Mom Power is an evidence-supported, multimodal intervention rooted in attachment and trauma theory that aims to enhance mothers' reflective capacity and mental health and promote sensitive, nurturing parenting (Muzik et al. 2015). It is especially well suited for mothers of all ages, including teenagers (Leplatte et al. 2012), who have a history of interpersonal traumatization, as well as mothers who are facing ongoing adversity and stress while parenting children (up to age 6). The 12-week treatment model involves 10 group sessions and 3 individual sessions; individual sessions occur prior to the beginning of group, during the middle of group to "check-in," and at the end of group to discuss referrals and next steps. Each group session begins with a shared meal as a warm-up before mothers and children separate; while mothers attend the parenting group, their children participate in a separate child group focused on one-on-one child-led play. The mother–child dyads are supported by separations and reunions throughout the session. Mom Power offers a conceptual framework for empathic and sensitive parenting and helps mothers with a history of trauma develop balanced mental representations toward their children. It accomplishes this via an integrated focus on enhancing self-care, mindfulness, and mental well-being; improving parenting competence and reflection and positive parent–child relationships; and strengthening social support and access to additional care. Although Mom Power is manualized, it has a flexible focus on assessing each family's individual needs and providing a warm hand-off to other services. The curriculum is highly personalized, interactive, and intended to create a welcoming, trust-building atmosphere for "planting the seed" that relationships can be safe and satisfying.

An initial open-trial study (no control) of Mom Power demonstrated that participation was associated with decreases in mothers' depression, PTSD symptoms, and caregiving helplessness and with increases in parenting confidence, social support, and connection to care (Leplatte et al. 2012; Muzik et al. 2015). A more rigorous randomized controlled trial (RCT) found Mom Power to be associated with improvements in mental health symptoms and parenting stress, with the highest efficacy among mothers with a history of interpersonal trauma (Rosenblum et al. 2017). Moreover, mothers who participated in Mom Power showed increases in "balanced" maternal representations and in maternal reflective capacity (Rosenblum et al. 2018). No significant changes were found in the control group. Finally, mothers randomly assigned to Mom Power exhibited differences in key brain circuits related to social cognition and empathy responses to expressions of positive affect from their own children versus unfamiliar children (Swain et al. 2016, 2017).

CIRCLE OF SECURITY

COS is an attachment-based intervention for parents of children from birth to 5 years old (Powell et al. 2014). COS is centered around a user-friendly graphic that explains the attachment system through two primary modes: 1) in times of distress or threat, parents provide a *safe haven* for their children, and 2) when their safety and security needs are met, children are able to venture out and explore, using the parent as a *secure base*. COS helps parents improve their observational and inferential skills in understanding their children's behavior and teaches parents about ways children can "miscue" or present behavior that appears in contrast to what they actually need (e.g., pushing parents away when they need emotional support). It can help parents recognize ways that their own emotions and reactions may interfere with their ability to meet their children's needs; given the many ways that parenting brings up emotions from one's own childhood, this skill is particularly critical for parents who have a history of childhood maltreatment.

COS can be administered in a 20-week multifamily group format, in a four-session home-based program that uses video-based feedback of caregiver–child interactions, or in an 8- to 10-session DVD-based parenting group format. In a pre/post review, the original 20-session group format was associated with improvements in children's attachment patterns as well as caregiver RF and caregiving representations (Hoffman et al. 2006; Huber et al. 2015). An RCT of the home-based model found that, although no main effect of treatment was found, the program was effective for the most irritable infants (Cassidy et al. 2011). Research on the efficacy of the DVD-based model is emerging; thus far, an RCT has shown that participating mothers provided fewer self-reported unsupportive responses to child distress and that their 3- to 5-year-old children had better observed inhibitory control (Cassidy et al. 2017).

ATTACHMENT AND BIOBEHAVIORAL CATCH-UP

ABC is a home-based 10-session intervention designed for caregiver–child dyads that have experienced early adversity (Bernard et al. 2012). Complementary versions are available for infants (ABC-I; ages 6 months to 2 years) and toddlers (ABC-T; ages 2–4). Based in attachment theory and knowledge of stress neurobiology, ABC uses both in-the-moment and video-based feedback, structured activities, and psychoeducation. Interventionists help caregivers practice more synchronous, nurturing, sensitive, and responsive interactions with their children. They discuss research supporting the importance of sensitive and synchronous care and draw links between the caregivers' early experiences and their ability (or barriers) to provide nurturing care. The key goals of ABC include helping caregivers create a responsive and predictable environment (to facilitate their children's ability to regulate themselves); reduce any behaviors that may frighten or overwhelm the children; follow their children's lead and show delight in them; and coregulate the children in times of distress.

Several RCTs have been conducted on ABC, with promising results for both parents and children. The mothers who participated in ABC-I showed increased sensitivity and decreased intrusiveness in interactions with their children, along with reductions in child abuse potential and parenting stress and accompanying changes in neural circuitry in response to emotional faces (Bernard et al. 2015c; Bick and Dozier 2013; Sprang 2009; Yarger et al. 2016). Children in ABC-I demonstrated improvements in attachment behavior, less negative affect in a challenging task, fewer behavior problems, and improvements in several domains of cognitive skills (Bernard et al. 2012, 2017; Lewis-Morrarty et al. 2012;

Lind et al 2014; Sprang 2009). Evidence is also emerging for lasting effects of ABC-I on children's stress neurobiology. Specifically, children with a history of neglect who participated in ABC-I showed improved diurnal cortisol patterns 3 months after the intervention ended, when they were 5 months to 3 years old, and these improvements persisted at least until ages 4–6 years (Bernard et al. 2015a, 2015b). Children's participation in ABC-T has also been associated with better parent-reported attention and cognitive flexibility relative to children in a control condition (Lind et al. 2017).

CHILD–PARENT PSYCHOTHERAPY

CPP is an evidence-based dyadic treatment model designed specifically for young children (ages 0–5 years) and their caregivers who have been exposed to traumatic events, including abuse and neglect (Lieberman et al. 2015). CPP places explicit focus on the caregivers' own trauma histories and calls attention to the ways these histories can affect their thoughts about and behaviors toward their children. CPP is well suited to treat both families in which the caregiver has significant risk factors but the child has not yet experienced explicit trauma (e.g., perinatal CPP; Cassidy et al. 2010) and families in which the child has already experienced trauma (e.g., physical or sexual abuse, neglect, separation from a caregiver, medical trauma). Families generally attend CPP sessions weekly, with 1-hour sessions either in a clinic or in the family's home, and treatment typically lasts about 1 year.

The clinician works with the caregiver–child dyad to develop a play-based narrative of the trauma, acknowledge the impact of the trauma, and promote positive and pleasurable play that will bolster the dyad's attachment bond. Rather than a predesigned protocol, clinicians use in-the-moment "ports of entry" to provide developmental guidance, draw attention to dynamics within the parent–child relationship, and offer different interpretations of the child's behavior, all with the goal of helping the dyad heal from prior trauma. Safety is a core theme throughout treatment, and the CPP clinician works to ensure that the child is safe physically (e.g., not exposed to domestic violence, has access to needed services) and psychologically (e.g., creating consistency and predictability in relationships). For mothers who have a significant history of childhood maltreatment, a key aspect of treatment is understanding the ways their history shapes their interpretations and attributions of their child's behavior. In other words, clinicians help caregivers explore their "ghosts in the nursery," or the ways that their own early experiences of feeling helpless or fearful in a caregiving relationship can unconsciously lead them to have negative attributions about their child's behavior and to behave in harsh or neglectful ways toward their child. Over time, the clinician helps caregivers regulate their affect in these moments, reframe their understanding of the behaviors, and respond to their child in more sensitive and balanced ways. Clinicians also help caregivers identify and draw upon any memories of "angels in the nursery," or memories of figures from their own childhood who helped them feel understood, loved, and accepted (Lieberman et al. 2005a). Bringing these memories into conscious focus often elicits a sense of hope and self-worth for caregivers and allows for exploration about how the caregiver might create a similar positive experience for his or her own child.

The evidence base supporting the efficacy of CPP is well established, with several prior RCTs. Among mother–child dyads (children ages 3–5) exposed to domestic violence, CPP treatment was associated with improvements in children's behavior problems and traumatic stress symptoms and in mothers' avoidant symptoms and general distress, with effects persisting at least 6 months after treatment ended (Ghosh Ippen et al. 2011; Lieberman et al. 2005a, 2005b). CPP has also been found efficacious among maltreated children, children with anxious attachment styles, and children of depressed mothers; specific treatment outcomes include positive changes in children's behavior and attachment and increases in caregiver empathy and the quality of interaction with their child (Cicchetti et al. 2006; LIeberman et al. 1991; Toth et al. 2002). There is emerging evidence that CPP and other similar interventions can alter the stress neurobiology of young children who have experienced trauma (Cicchetti et al. 2011); further research on the specific effects of CPP on both mothers' and children's biology is currently under way.

OTHER HOME VISITING PROGRAMS

Finally, two similar home visiting programs target high-risk perinatal women and their young children. Minding the Baby (MTB; Sadler et al. 2013) is a 27-month intervention for first-time mothers. MTB follows women from the third trimester of pregnancy through the child's second birthday. It is interdisciplinary and involves alternating home visits from a master's-level nurse and a social worker. The program emphasizes the mother–child relationship to promote more positive interactions that support secure infant attachment and healthy child development. Clinicians work with new mothers to regulate their infant's distress and attend to their child's mental and physical needs, while the mother's own mental health needs are assessed and treated as needed. In their RCT, Sadler et al. (2013) found that participation in MTB was associated with improvement in maternal RF and child attachment security and organization, as well as a higher likelihood of being on track with child immunizations, lower rates of rapid subsequent childbearing, and decreased involvement with child protective services.

A multiyear home-visit intervention for families called Child and Family Interagency Resource, Support, and Training (Child FIRST; Lowell et al. 2011) is offered by a clinician and care coordinator. Treatment includes a combination of trauma-specific treatment (e.g., CPP), parent guidance, and care coordination to help connect families with community resources. An RCT of the effects of Child FIRST demonstrated positive outcomes for mothers, children, and families that included reduced parenting stress, decreased maternal psychopathology, improved child language outcomes, fewer child externalizing problems, less protective-service involvement, and greater access to services (Lowell et al. 2011).

Conclusion

The development of secure attachment relationships in early childhood is beneficial to both healthy development and interpersonal functioning across the lifespan and intergenerationally. Nevertheless, various forms of early adversity can negatively affect attachment formation. We have explored the ways a mother's history of interpersonal and childhood trauma—especially when it is unresolved—may disrupt her attachment style, her internal working model of intimate relationships, and her ability to relate to and safely parent her child. The well-established associations between trauma, attachment, and parenting can help provide a conceptual framework for reducing the risk factors that contribute to filicide perpetration. We hope that understanding the interrelationships between trauma and attachment will help ongoing efforts to identify critical variables within a cumulative risk factor model. In this regard, the many trauma-focused and relational interventions described in this chapter offer specific treatment modalities to help mitigate the perpetuation of intergenerational trauma and attachment disruptions and ultimately help prevent the loss of lives through maternal filicide.

The intervention approaches reviewed here predominately share a focus on the mother–child relationship as an agent of change, with a focus on maternal RF and promotion of nurturing, sensitive, and responsive caregiving behaviors. We have also emphasized the importance of maternal well-being and emotion regulation within the context of dyadic interventions and separately as a correlate of parent–child work. Had LR, the mother in our case study, participated in one of these intervention programs we have highlighted, along with receiving support to safety from the domestic violence she experienced, would it have prevented the filicide-suicide attempt? Although there is no panacea, we believe attention to the attachment relationship, sensitive caregiving, and addressing one's past traumas can make a difference. Perhaps save lives. As the evidence base of these interventions grows, with most programs demonstrating beneficial outcomes for mothers and children, we hope that the trauma- and attachment-informed approaches described herein may continue to inform the field of filicide prevention.

MAIN CLINICAL/LEGAL POINTS AND CULTURAL PERSPECTIVES

- Relational trauma and maltreatment during one's own childhood, especially when it is interpersonal in nature (e.g., physical or sexual abuse perpetrated by a caregiver), is a critical risk factor for maternal filicide.

- Trauma and maltreatment may be perpetuated across generations through various intergenerational mechanisms. Historical trauma may affect generations of marginalized and oppressed racial, ethnic, and cultural groups with lived and historical experiences of racism, systemic and structural inequalities, and violence (e.g., slavery, genocide).

- Abuse or maltreatment perpetrated by a caregiver can disrupt the formation of children's secure or healthy attachment relationships and alter brain structure and function in ways that affect behavior and development throughout the lifespan.

- Attachment relationships during early childhood continue to exert effects on functioning through adulthood. Our internal working models, based on our own childhood attachments, influence how we relate to romantic partners and to our own children.

- Disorganized attachment in childhood occurs at a significantly higher rate among children who have experienced abuse or maltreatment and is associated with the greatest risk of later maladaptive outcomes.

- Reflective functioning is a key mediator between parents' own history of trauma and the likelihood of the parents reenacting those behaviors with their own children.

- A history of maternal trauma or abuse in childhood may act as a precursor for filicide because it disrupts the formation of secure attachments and the mother's relationship with her child that supports stability and normalcy of the hypothalamic-pituitary-adrenal axis in brain development.

- Experiences of trauma and maltreatment are not deterministic, and it is possible to mitigate risk through the promotion of resilience factors.

- Interventions that aim to mitigate risk by focusing on the parent–child relationship are effective in improving parents' reflective functioning, parenting behaviors, and children's outcomes.

- Racial, ethnic, and cultural factors, along with systemic and situational barriers, are important when considering parental access to and engagement with treatment programs; these factors may also exacerbate disruptions in caregiving and parent reflective functioning.

Practice and Discussion Questions

1. This chapter focuses on intergenerational pathways of risk (and resilience). Discuss this idea within the context of filicide. Specifically, how might a mother's own developmental history relate to her possible propensity toward maternal filicide?
2. What developmental questions might you ask to identify a higher risk for filicide in a mother presenting to clinical care and describing general psychological distress (e.g., depression)?
3. Discuss how the concept of trauma-informed care may be applicable to forensic work. In what ways might your professional field or practice strive to become more trauma-informed in the context of filicide work?
4. A trauma-informed perspective in maternal filicide cases is valuable to clinicians for treatment, for general understanding and compassion for these mothers, for support and prevention efforts, and for the purpose of the sentencing in court. However, "trauma" does not inform Canadian and American criminal justice proceedings and decisions about criminal responsibility. Discuss this gap and your thoughts about developmental understanding of the mother versus legal decisions that do not consider this history. What perspectives exist in other countries?

5. How do racial, ethnic, and cultural factors play into experiences of trauma and attachment from an intergenerational perspective? What structural, social, and racial contexts impinge upon individual mothers that must be considered in intervention programs? If intervention programs alone are not enough, what other systems, policies, or support services need to be in place to help address effects of historical trauma on mothers, children, and their families?

6. We offer several examples of evidence-based preventative interventions. In the context of filicide risk, what key factors (e.g., for mothers, children, and the parent–child relationship) might be especially critical targets for intervention?

References

Adshead G: Three degrees of security: attachment and forensic institutions. Crim Behav Ment Health 12(52):S31–S45, 2002

Ainsworth M, Bell SM: Attachment, exploration, and separation: individual differences in strange-situation behavior of one-year-olds. Child Dev 41:49–67, 1970

Ainsworth M, Bowlby J: An ethological approach to personality development. Am Psychol 46:331–333, 1991

Ainsworth MDS, Blehar M, Waters E, Wall S: Patterns of Attachment: Observations in the Strange Situation at Home. Hillsdale, NJ, Erlbaum, 1978

Allen JG: Developments in Psychoanalysis: Mentalizing in the Development and Treatment of Attachment Trauma. London, Karnac Books, 2013

American Psychological Association: Dictionary of Psychology (website), 2020. Available at: https://dictionary.apa.org/trauma. Accessed August 26, 2020.

Amon S, Putkonen H, Weizmann-Henelius G, et al: Potential predictors in neonaticide: the impact of the circumstances of pregnancy. Arch Womens Ment Health 15(3):167–174, 2012

Barnett D, Ganiban J, Cicchetti D: Maltreatment, negative expressivity, and development of type D attachments from 12- to 24-months of age. Monogr Soc Res Child Dev 64:97–118, 1999

Barone L, Bramante A, Lionetti F, Pastore M: Mothers who murdered their child: an attachment-based study on filicide. Child Abuse Negl 38(9):1468–1477, 2014

Bartholomew K, Horowitz LM: Attachment styles among young adults: a test of a four-category model. J Pers Soc Psychol 61(2):226–244, 1991

Beebe B, Jaffe J, Markese S, et al: The origins of 12-month attachment: a microanalysis of 4-month mother-infant interaction. Attach Human Dev 12(1–2):3–141, 2010

Benoit D: Infant-parent attachment: definition, types, antecedents, measurement and outcome. Paediatr Child Health 9(8):541–545, 2004

Bernard K, Dozier M, Bick J, et al: Enhancing attachment organization among maltreated children: results of a randomized clinical trial. Child Dev 83:623–636, 2012

Bernard K, Dozier M, Bick J, Gordon MK: Intervening to enhance cortisol regulation among children at risk for neglect: results of a randomized clinical trial. Dev Psychopathol 27:829–841, 2015a

Bernard K, Hostinar CE, Dozier M: Intervention effects on diurnal cortisol rhythms of child protective services–referred infants in early childhood. JAMA Pediatrics 169:112–119, 2015b

Bernard K, Simons R, Dozier M: Effects of an attachment-based intervention on child protective services referred mothers' event-related potentials to children's emotions. Child Dev 86:1673–1684, 2015c

Bernard K, Lee AH, Dozier M: Effects of the ABC intervention on foster children's receptive vocabulary. Child Maltreat 22(2):174–179, 2017

Bernier A, Meins E: A threshold approach to understanding the origins of attachment disorganization. Dev Psychol 44(4):969–982, 2008

Berthelot N, Ensink K, Bernazzani O, et al: Intergenerational transmission of attachment in abused and neglected mothers: the role of trauma-specific reflective functioning. Infant Ment Health J 36:200–212, 2015

Bick J, Dozier M: The effectiveness of an attachment-based intervention in promoting foster mothers' sensitivity toward foster infants. Infant Ment Health J 34:95–103, 2013

Boals A: Trauma in the eye of the beholder: objective and subjective definitions of trauma. J Psychother Integr 28(1):77–89, 2018

Bonnet C: Adoption at birth: prevention against abandonment or neonaticide. Child Abuse Negl 17:501–513, 1993

Bowlby J: Attachment and Loss: Attachment. New York, Basic Books, 1969

Bretherton I: The origins of attachment theory: John Bowlby and Mary Ainsworth. Dev Psychol 28:759–775, 1992

Brewster AL, Nelson JP, Hymel KP: Victim, perpetrator, family, and incident characteristics of 32 infant maltreatment deaths in the United States Air Force. Child Abuse Negl 22:91–101, 1998

Carlson EA: A prospective longitudinal study of attachment disorganization/disorientation. Child Dev 69(4):1107–1128, 1998

Carlson V, Cicchetti D, Barnett D, Braunwald K: Disorganized/disoriented attachment relationships in maltreated infants. Dev Psychol 25:525–531, 1989

Cassidy J, Ziv Y, Stupica B, et al: Enhancing attachment security in the infants of women in a jail-diversion program. Attach Hum Dev 12(4):333–353, 2010

Cassidy J, Woodhouse SS, Sherman LJ, et al: Enhancing infant attachment security: an examination of treatment efficacy and differential susceptibility. Dev Psychopathol 23(1):131–148, 2011

Cassidy J, Brett BE, Gross JT, et al: Circle of security–parenting: a randomized controlled trial in Head Start. Dev Psychopathol 29:651–673, 2017

Child Trends: Child Maltreatment. Bethesda, MD, Child Trends, 2019. Available at: https://www.childtrends.org/indicators/child-maltreatment. Accessed August 18, 2019.

Choi-Kain LW, Gunderson JG: Mentalization: Ontogeny, assessment, and application in the treatment of borderline personality disorder. Am J Psychiatry 165:1127–1135, 2008

Cicchetti D, Rogosch FA, Toth SL: Fostering secure attachment in infants in maltreating families through preventive interventions. Dev Psychopathol 18(3):623–649, 2006

Cicchetti D, Rogosch FA, Toth SL: Normalizing the development of cortisol regulation in maltreated infants through preventive interventions. Dev Psychopathol 23(3):789, 2011

Cook A, Spinazzola J, Ford J, et al: Complex trauma in children and adolescents. Psychiatr Ann 35(5):390–398, 2005

Crimmins S, Langley S, Brownstein HH, Spunt BJ: Convicted women who have killed children: a self-psychology perspective. J Interpers Violence 12(1):49–69, 1997

Debowska A, Boduszek D, Dhingra K: Victim, perpetrator, and offense characteristics in filicide and filicide-suicide. Aggress Violent Behav 21:113–124, 2015

Dollberg D, Feldman R, Keren M: Maternal representations, infant psychiatric status, and mother–child relationship in clinic-referred and non-referred infants. Eur Child Adolesc Psychiatry 19(1):25–36, 2010

Dvir Y, Ford JD, Hill M, Frazier JA: Childhood maltreatment, emotional dysregulation, and psychiatric comorbidities. Harv Rev Psychiatry 22(3):149–161, 2014

Felitti VJ, Anda RF, Nordenberg D, et al: The relationship of adult health status to childhood abuse and household dysfunction. Am J Prev Med 14:245–258, 1998

Fonagy P: Psychoanalytic and empirical approaches to developmental psychopathology: can they be usefully integrated? J R Soc Med 86(10):577–581, 1993

Fonagy P, Steele M, Steele H, et al: The Emanuel Miller Memorial Lecture 1992: the theory and practice of resilience. J Child Psychol Psychiatry 35(2):231–257, 1994

Fonagy P, Steele M, Steele H, et al: Attachment, the reflective self, and borderline states: the predictive specificity of the Adult Attachment Interview and pathological emotional development, in Attachment Theory: Social, Developmental, and Clinical Perspectives. Edited by Goldberg S, Muir R, Kerr J. Hillsdale, NJ, Analytic Press, 1995, pp 233–278

Fonagy P, Target M, Steele H, Steele M: Reflective-Functioning Manual Version 5: For Application to Adult Attachment Interviews. London, University College London, 1998

Fonagy P, Gergely G, Target M: The parent-infant dyad and the construction of the subjective self. J Child Psychol Psychiatry 48(3/4):288–328, 2007

Ford JD: An affective cognitive neuroscience-based approach to PTSD psychotherapy: the TARGET model. J Cogn Psychother 29(1):68–91, 2015

Ford JD: Trauma memory processing in posttraumatic stress disorder psychotherapy: a unifying framework. J Trauma Stress 31(6):933–942, 2018

Ford JD, Russo E: Trauma-focused, present-centered, emotional self-regulation approach to integrated treatment for posttraumatic stress and addiction: trauma adaptive recovery group education and therapy (TARGET). Am J Psychother 60(4):335–355, 2006

Ford JD, Steinberg K, Zhang W: A randomized clinical trial comparing affect regulation and social problem-solving psychotherapies for mothers with victimization-related PTSD. Behav Ther 42:661–578, 2011

Ford JD, Steinberg K, Hawke J, et al: Randomized trial comparison of emotion regulation and relational psychotherapies for PTSD with girls involved in delinquency. J Clin Child Adolesc Psychol 41:27–37, 2012

Fraiberg S, Adelson E, Shapiro V: Ghosts in the nursery: a psychoanalytic approach to the problems of impaired infant-mother relationships, in Clinical Studies in Infant Mental Health. New York, Basic Books, 1980, pp 164–196

Friedman SH, Horowitz SM, Resnick PJ: Child murder by mothers: a critical analysis of the current state of knowledge and research agenda. Am J Psychiatry 162:1578–1587, 2005

Ghosh Ippen C, Harris WW, Van Horn P, Lieberman AF: Traumatic and stressful events in early childhood: can treatment help those at highest risk? Child Abuse Negl 35(7):504–513, 2011

Giacchetti N, Pancheri C, Williams R, et al: Violence and motherhood: a case study about the personality profile and attachment style of a filicide woman. Deviant Behav 41(5):607–618, 2020

Granqvist P, Sroufe LA, Dozier M, et al: Disorganized attachment in infancy: a review of the phenomenon and its implications for clinicians and policymakers. Attach Hum Dev 19(6):534–558, 2017

Haapasalo J, Petäjä S: Mothers who killed or attempted to kill their child: life circumstances, childhood abuse, and types of killing. Violence Victims 14:219–239, 1999

Hahn-Holbrook J, Cornwell-Hinrichs T, Anaya I: Economic and health predictors of national postpartum depression prevalence: A systematic review, meta-analysis, and meta-regression of 291 studies from 56 countries. Front Psychiatr 8:248, 2018

Harris M, Fallot RD (eds): New Directions for Mental Health Services: Using Trauma Theory to Design Service Systems. San Francisco, CA, Jossey-Bass, 2001

Hertsgaard L, Gunnar MR, Erickson MF, Nachmias M: Adrenocortical responses to the strange situation in infants with disorganized/disoriented attachment relationships. Child Dev 66(4):1100–1106, 1995

Hesse E, Main M: Disorganized infant, child, and adult attachment: collapse in behavioral and attentional strategies. J Am Psychoanal Assoc 48:1097–1127, 2000

Hesse E, Main M: Frightened, threatening, and dissociative parental behavior in low-risk samples: description, discussion, and interpretations. Dev Psychopathol 18(2):309–343, 2006

Hoffman KT, Marvin RS, Cooper G, Powell B: Changing toddlers' and preschoolers' attachment classifications: the Circle of Security intervention. J Consult Clin Psychol 74:1017–1026, 2006

Huber A, McMahon CA, Sweller N: Efficacy of the 20-week circle of security intervention: changes in caregiver reflective functioning, representations, and child attachment in an Australian clinical sample. Infant Ment Health J 36:556–574, 2015

Hughes K, Lowey H, Quigg Z, Bellis MA: Relationships between adverse childhood experiences and adult mental well-being: results from an English national household survey. BMC Public Health 16(1):222, 2016

Huth-Bocks AC, Krause K, Ahlfs-Dunn S, et al: Relational trauma and posttraumatic stress symptoms among pregnant women. Psychodyn Psychiatry 41(2):277–301, 2013

International Society for Traumatic Stress Studies: What Is Traumatic Stress? (website), 2020. Available at: https://istss.org/public-resources/what-is-traumatic-stress. Accessed August 26, 2020.

Iyengar U, Kim S, Martinez S, et al: Unresolved trauma in mothers: intergenerational effects and the role of reorganization. Front Psychol 5:1–9, 2014

Katznelson H: Reflective functioning: a review. Clin Psychol Rev 34:107–117, 2014

Kerr ME, Bowen M: Family Evaluation: An Approach Based on Bowen Theory. New York, W.W. Norton, 1988

Kessler R, McLaughlin K, Green J, et al: Childhood adversities and adult psychopathology in the WHO World Mental Health Surveys. Br J Psychiatry 197(5):378–385, 2010

Krischer MK, Stone MH, Sevecke K, Steinmeyer EM: Motives for maternal filicide: results from a study with female forensic patients. Int J Law Psychiatry 30(3):191–200, 2007

Leplatte D, Rosenblum KL, Stanton E, et al: Mental health in primary care for adolescent parents. Ment Health Fam Med 9(1):39–45, 2012

Lewis-Morrarty E, Dozier M, Bernard K, et al: Cognitive flexibility and theory of mind outcomes among foster children: preschool follow-up results of a randomized clinical trial. J Adolesc Health 51:S17–S22, 2012

Lieberman AF, Weston DR, Pawl JH: Preventive intervention and outcome with anxiously attached dyads. Child De 62:199, 1991

Lieberman AF, Van Horn P: Don't Hit My Mommy: A Manual for Child-Parent Psychotherapy With Young Witnesses of Family Violence. Washington, DC, Zero to Three, 2004

Lieberman AF, Padrón E, Van Horn P, Harris WW: Angels in the nursery: the intergenerational transmission of benevolent parental influences. Infant Ment Health J 26(6):504–520, 2005a

Lieberman AF, Van Horn P, Ghosh Ippen C: Toward evidence-based treatment: child-parent psychotherapy with preschoolers exposed to marital violence. J Am Acad Child Adolesc Psychiatry 44:1241–1248, 2005b

Lieberman AF, Ghosh Ippen C, Van Horn P: Child-Parent Psychotherapy: 6-month follow-up of a randomized controlled trial. J Am Acad Child Adolesc Psychiatry 45:913–918, 2006

Lieberman AF, Ghosh Ippen C, Van Horn P: "Don't Hit My Mommy!": A Manual for Child-Parent Psychotherapy With Young Children Exposed to Violence and Other Trauma. Washington, DC, Zero to Three, 2015

Lind T, Bernard K, Ross E, Dozier M: Intervention effects on negative affect of CPS-referred children: results of a randomized clinical trial. Child Abuse Negl 38:1459–1467, 2014

Lind T, Raby KL, Caron EB, et al: Enhancing executive functioning among toddlers in foster care with an attachment-based intervention. Dev Psychopathol 29:575–586, 2017

Lowell D, Carter A, Godoy L, et al: A randomized controlled trial of Child First: a comprehensive home-based intervention translating research into early childhood practice. Child Dev 82(1):193–208, 2011

Ludmer JA, Gonzalez A, Kennedy J, et al: Association between maternal childhood maltreatment and mother-infant attachment disorganization: moderation by maternal oxytocin receptor gene and cortisol secretion. Horm Behav 102:23–33, 2018

Lyons-Ruth K: The two-person construction of defenses: disorganized attachment strategies, unintegrated mental states, and hostile/helpless relational processes. J Infant Child Adolesc Psychother 2:105–114, 2003

Lyons-Ruth K, Jacobvitz D: Attachment disorganization: genetic factors, parenting contexts, and developmental transformation from infancy to adulthood, in Handbook of Attachment: Theory, Research, and Clinical Applications. Edited by Cassidy J, Shaver PR. New York, Guilford, 2008, pp 666–697

Lyons-Ruth K, Alpern L, Repacholi B: Disorganized infant attachment classification and maternal psychosocial problems as predictors of hostile-aggressive behavior in the preschool classroom. Child Dev 64(2):572–585, 1993

Lyons-Ruth K, Bronfman E, Parsons E: Atypical attachment in infancy and early childhood among children at developmental risk, IV: maternal frightened, frightening, or atypical behavior and disorganized infant attachment patterns. Monogr Soc Res Child Dev 64:67–96, 213–220, 1999

Lyons-Ruth K, Yellin C, Melnick S, Atwood G: Expanding the concept of unresolved mental states: hostile/helpless states of mind on the Adult Attachment Interview are associated with disrupted mother–infant communication and infant disorganization. Dev Psychopathol 17(1):1–23, 2005

Main M, Solomon J: Procedures for identifying infants as disorganized/disoriented during the Ainsworth strange situation, in Attachment in the Preschool Years. Edited by Greenberg MT, Cicchetti D, Cummings EM. Chicago, IL, University of Chicago Press, 1990, pp 121–160

Martorell GA, Bugental DB: Maternal variations in stress reactivity: implications for harsh parenting practices with very young children. J Fam Psychol 20(4):641–647, 2006

McKee A, Egan V: A case series of twenty one maternal filicides in the UK. Child Abuse Negl 37:753–761, 2013

Mills-Koonce WR, Propper C, Gariepy JL, et al: Psychophysiological correlates of parenting behavior in mothers of young children. Dev Psychobiol 51(8):650–661, 2009

Morelen D, Rosenblum KL, Muzik M: Childhood maltreatment and motherhood: implications for maternal well-being and mothering, in Motherhood in the Face of Trauma: Pathways Toward Healing and Growth. Edited by Muzik M, Rosenblum KL. Cham, Switzerland, Springer International, 2018, pp 23–38

Mugavin M: Maternal filicide theoretical framework. J Forensic Nurs 4(2):68–79, 2008

Muzik M, Rosenblum KL, Alfafara EA, et al: Mom Power: preliminary outcomes of a group intervention to improve mental health and parenting among high-risk mothers. Arch Womens Ment Health 18:507–521, 2015

Muzik M, Rosenblum KL, Schuster MM, et al: A mental health and parenting intervention for adolescent and young adult mothers and their infants. J Depress Anxiety 5:3, 2016

Noll JG, Horowitz LA, Bonanno GA, et al: Revictimization and self-harm in women who experienced childhood sexual abuse: results from a prospective study. J Interpers Violence 18:1452–1471, 2003

Nurius PS, Green S, Logan-Greene P, Borja S: Life course pathways of adverse childhood experiences toward adult psychological well-being: a stress process and analysis. Child Abuse Negl 45:143–153, 2015

Powell B, Cooper G, Hoffman KT, Marvin B: The Circle of Security Intervention: Enhancing Attachment in Early Parent–Child Relationships. New York, Guilford, 2014

Read J, Fosse R, Moskowitz A, Perry B: The traumagenic neurodevelopmental model of psychosis revisited. Neuropsychiatry 4(1):65–79, 2014

Resnick PJ: Child murder by parents: a psychiatric review of filicide. Am J Psychiatry 126(3):325–334, 1969

Roberts AL, McLaughlin KA, Conron KJ, Koenen KC: Adulthood stressors, history of childhood adversity, and risk of perpetration of intimate partner violence. Am J Prev Med 40:128–138, 2011

Rosenblum K, Dayton CJ, McDonough SC: Communicating feelings: links between mothers' representations of their infants, parenting, and infant emotional development, in Parenting Representations: Theory, Research, and Clinical Implications. Edited by Mayselses O. New York, Cambridge University Press, 2006, pp 109–148

Rosenblum K, Muzik M, Morelen DM, et al: A community-based randomized controlled trial of Mom Power parenting intervention for mothers with interpersonal trauma histories and their young children. Arch Womens Ment Health 20(5):673–686, 2017

Rosenblum K, Lawler J, Alfafara E, et al: Improving maternal representations in high-risk mothers: a randomized, controlled trial of the Mom Power parenting intervention. Child Psychiatry Hum Dev 49(3):372–384, 2018

Rubin DC, Berntsen D, Bohni MK: A memory-based model of posttraumatic stress disorder: evaluating basic assumptions underlying the PTSD diagnosis. Psychol Rev 115(4):985–1011, 2008

Sadler LS, Slade A, Close N, et al: Minding the Baby: Enhancing reflectiveness to improve early health and relationship outcomes in an interdisciplinary home visiting program. Infant Ment Health J 34(5):391–405, 2013

Schechter DS, Zeanah CH Jr, Myers MM, et al: Psychobiological dysregulation in violence-exposed mothers: salivary cortisol of mothers with very young children pre- and post-separation stress. Bull Menninger Clin 68:319–336, 2004

Schneider BH, Atkinson L, Tardif C: Child–parent attachment and children's peer relations: a quantitative review. Dev Psychol 37(1):86–100, 2001

Schwerdtfeger KL, Nelson Goff BS: Intergenerational transmission of trauma: exploring mother-infant prenatal attachment. J Trauma Stress 20:39–51, 2007

Shaw DS, Keenan K, Vondra JI, et al: Antecedents of preschool children's internalizing problems: a longitudinal study of low-income families. J Am Acad Child Adolesc Psychiatry 36(12):1760–1767, 1997

Slade A, Grienenberger J, Bernbach E, et al: Maternal reflective functioning, attachment, and the transmission gap: a preliminary study. Attach Hum Dev 7(3):283–298, 2005

Smithey M: Infant homicide at the hands of mothers: toward a sociological perspective. Deviant Behav 18:255–272, 1997

Sotero M: A conceptual model of historical trauma: implications for public health practice and research. J Health Dispar Res Pract 1:93–108, 2006

Sprang G: The efficacy of a relational treatment for maltreated children and their families. Child Adolesc Ment Health 14:81–88, 2009

Sroufe LA: Attachment and development: a prospective, longitudinal study from birth to adulthood. Attach Hum Dev 7(4):349–367, 2005

Sturge-Apple ML, Skibo MA, Rogosch FA, et al: The impact of allostatic load on maternal sympathovagal functioning in stressful child contexts: implications for problematic parenting. Dev Psychopathol 23(3):831–844, 2011

Swain JE, Ho SS, Rosenblum KL, et al: Emotion processing and psychopathological risk in the parental brain: psychosocial intervention increases activity and decreases stress. J Am Acad Child Adolesc Psychiatry 55:S320–S321, 2016

Swain JE, Ho SS, Rosenblum KL, et al: Parent–child intervention decreases stress and increases maternal brain activity and connectivity during own baby-cry: an exploratory study. Dev Psychopathol 29:535–553, 2017

Thomason ME, Marusak HA: Toward understanding the impact of trauma on the early developing human brain. Neuroscience 342:55–67, 2017

Thompson RA: The development of the person: social understanding, relationships, conscience, self, in Handbook of Child Psychology, Vol 3, 6th Edition. Edited by Eisenberg N. Hoboken, NJ, John Wiley and Sons, 2006, pp 24–98

Toth SL, Maughan A, Manly JT, et al: The relative efficacy of two interventions in altering maltreated preschool children's representational models: implications for attachment theory. Dev Psychopathol 14:877–908, 2002

van der Kolk BA, Roth S, Pelcovitz D, et al: Disorders of extreme stress: the empirical foundation of a complex adaptation to trauma. J Trauma Stress 18(5):389–399, 2005

van Ee E, Kleber RJ, Jongmans MJ: Relational patterns between caregivers with PTSD and their nonexposed children: a review. Trauma Violence Abuse 17(2):186–203, 2015

van IJzendoorn MH, Schuengel C, Bakermans-Kranenburg MJ: Disorganized attachment in early childhood: meta-analysis of precursors, concomitants, and sequelae. Dev Psychopathol 11(2):225–249, 1999

Yarger HA, Hoye JR, Dozier M: Trajectories of change in attachment and biobehavioral catch-up among high-risk mothers: a randomized clinical trial. Infant Ment Health J 37(5):525–536, 2016

CHAPTER 14

Maternal Filicide in Malaysia

STRUCTURAL INEQUALITY AND CULTURAL DISPARITY

Salmi Razali, M.D., M.Med. (Psychiatry), Ph.D.

Jane Fisher, AO, Ph.D., B.Sc. (Hons), MAPS, FCCLP, FCHP

Maggie Kirkman, Ph.D., B.A. (Hons), MAPS

In this chapter, we summarize the three components of our innovative research conducted in Malaysia: 1) analysis of national data (Razali et al. 2014), 2) interviews with women incarcerated after being convicted of filicide (Razali et al. 2019), and 3) interviews with professionals who work with girls or women who have committed filicide or are at risk (Razali et al. 2020). We chose Malaysia as the site of our investigations in part because one of us (S.R.) is a citizen of that country but also because we could find no previous filicide research in that country. Almost all existing research has been conducted in high-income, predominantly English-speaking countries, which is an artifact of greater resource allocation in these countries for surveillance systems, registries, and maintenance of national records, as well as research funding. In a world that is increasingly global, it is essential to extend one's view beyond the local and familiar. Our results may conflict with what is usually found in

---

Dr. Razali conducted all interviews.

the United States, United Kingdom, and Australia (for example), but they reveal that the meaning of filicide can be transformed by its social context.

The research on filicide (including neonaticide and infanticide) has tended to focus on characteristics of the perpetrators and victims. In his landmark work, Resnick (1969, 1970) classified filicide according to the perpetrator's circumstances or perceived reason for filicide: altruistic, acute psychotic, unwanted child, accidental, or spouse revenge. Other scholars have proposed alternative classifications. Scott (1973), for example, used "source of impulse" as the foundation; his work was elaborated by d'Orban (1979), who classified filicide according to psychiatric characteristics, offense patterns, and "court disposals" (sentencing decisions). Clinical manifestation and diagnostic classification were the primary categories chosen by Bourget and Bradford (1990), Guileyardo et al. (1999), and Bourget and Gagné (2005). Each clinical and diagnostic classification focused on the individual person in the proximal microsystem. Although we set out in a similar vein to understand filicide in Malaysia, our evidence led us to shift our focus to social context, structural inequality, and cultural disparity.

Malaysia

Malaysia is a Southeast Asian country of more than 30 million people that occupies parts of the Malay Peninsula and the island of Borneo. It is multiethnic and multicultural; about half the population is indigenous (often described by the contentious term *bumiputera*: Malays,[1] indigenous people and natives of Sabah and Sarawak such as Dayak, Murut, Kadazan, and Iban), with minorities including Malaysian Chinese and Malaysian Indians. Recent economic progress has encouraged immigration, especially from Indonesia, Bangladesh, and the Philippines. The *bumiputera* live predominantly in suburban and rural areas, whereas the Chinese and Indians tend to live in urban areas. About 60% of Malaysian citizens are Muslim; the other prominent religions are Buddhism, Christianity, and Hinduism. Malays dominate the government and state

---

[1]A Malay is described in Article 60 of the Malaysian Constitution as a person who "professes the religion of Islam, habitually speaks the Malay language, conforms to Malay customs and is the child of at least one parent who was born within the Federation of Malaysia before independence of Malaya on 31 August 1957, or the issue (off-spring) of such a person."

structures, whereas non-Malays (predominantly Chinese and Indians) control the economy.

Despite impressive economic development, Malaysia struggles with high economic, social, and gender inequality. Women's participation in politics, decision making, and managerial positions is low (Ng 2016). Almost all Malaysians complete primary education, but only about two-thirds finish secondary school. Malaysia has relatively free health care facilities, but accessibility to certain health services, including contraception, abortion, and counseling, is limited by attitudes toward sexuality (intolerance of sexual diversity and sexual relationships outside marriage) (Talib et al. 2012) and mental health (disrupted by cultural differences in the meaning of "mental health" and appropriate treatments for mental ill-health) (Chong et al. 2013).

The most recent report on nations' progress toward gender equality scored Denmark as first on the list, Canada as eighth, Australia as tenth, the United Kingdom as seventeenth, the United States as twenty-eighth, and Malaysia in the sixtieth position (Equal Measures 2030 2019). Equal Measures 2030 (www.equalmeasures2030.org), the organization behind the report, was formed to measure progress in achieving the United Nations' Sustainable Development Goals by 2030. Their Gender Index comprises 51 indicators relating to 14 of the 17 official sustainable development goals; it was applied to 129 countries across all regions of the world. There are gender-specific indicators and others that, although not gender specific, have a disproportionate effect on girls and women.

Malaysia's complex legal system combines common law, inherited from its time as a British colony, with Islamic or Syariah law. Civil and criminal matters (e.g., infanticide, murder, rape, and family violence) are subject to common law (Rahim et al. 2012). Syariah law applies to Muslims in relation to personal and family matters such as succession, betrothal, marriage, divorce (and associated settlements), guardianship, adoption, trusts, Islamic religious revenue, and mosques (Shuaib 2012). *Hudud*, or strict Syariah law, is not practiced in Malaysia (Shuaib 2012).

Maternal Filicide in Malaysia

Neonaticide and infanticide came to prominence in Malaysia in the late 1990s with increased reporting in the news media of newborn babies being dumped in sewers, thrown out of buildings, discarded in garbage areas, or abandoned near mosques and temples; it was constructed as a social crisis (Niner et al. 2013; Razali et al. 2016a). Emphasis in the media was on a phenomenon colloquially known as "baby dumping," for which women were held solely responsible (Niner et al. 2013; Razali et al. 2016a). Filicide, commonly limited in public discourse to neonaticide and infanticide (disregarding deaths of children older than 1 year of age), was said to be caused by promiscuous young people (Razali et al. 2016a). In Malaysia, sexual activity is traditionally confined to marriage; it is considered immoral and transgressive to indulge in sexual behavior in any other relationship. Blame is directed particularly at women and girls if sexual activity occurs outside of marriage (Razali et al. 2016a). In public discourse, "immoral" behavior, including nonmarital sex, arises from inadequate parental control, the lack of effective sexual abstinence education, and the lifelong stigma attached to being born ex-nuptially (Razali et al. 2016a).

Malaysia's response to this perceived filicide "crisis" was consistent with the attributed causes, also informed by research from high-income countries (predominantly Christian and socially liberal). Neither local evidence nor rigorous national data collection was sought as a means of understanding filicide in Malaysia. In attempting to prevent filicide, the strongest emphasis was placed on reducing transgressive sexual behavior by reinforcing abstinence via secondary and tertiary education programs (Mutalip and Mohamed 2012; Talib et al. 2012). Ex-nuptial birth as a cause of neonaticide was recognized with the introduction of "baby hatches," which provide safe, anonymous, and legal means for handing over newborn babies for care and adoption (Cochrane and Ming 2013). This apparently nonjudgmental preventive measure was matched by widespread calls (not implemented) for harsh legal sanctions against perpetrators of filicide, including capital punishment (Razali et al. 2016a).

Our Research in Malaysia

The lack of filicide research in Malaysia can be explained, in part, by limited research funding. However, a more fundamental reason is that the subject is associated with "socially, culturally, and politically sensitive matters, including gendered social structures and behaviours, legal and ethical complexity, emotionally arousing topics, a rare phenomenon, and hard-to-reach participants," as we have stated elsewhere (Razali et al. 2017, p. 34). These were among the challenges we confronted in conducting our own research in Malaysia, exacerbated by the country's poor data-gathering practices and inadequate surveillance concerning filicide (see Razali et al. 2014). The limited resources (including mental health professionals) available to support those at risk of committing filicide or who have committed filicide not only restrict the potential for prevention or other mitigation but also reduce opportunities for conducting research on filicide (see Razali et al. 2017).

SECONDARY ANALYSIS OF NATIONAL DATA

In the absence of peer-reviewed evidence about filicide in Malaysia, we set out to describe the prevalence and characteristics of infanticide and illegal infant abandonment in that country and to estimate annual rates for the previous decade (Razali et al. 2014). To achieve these research objectives, we sought and reviewed national police records on infant abandonment and neonaticide and related them to the national registry of live births for the years 1999–2011 (Razali et al. 2014). We calculated the estimated inferred infanticide rate as fluctuating between 4.82 and 9.11 per 100,000 live births, a moderate rate relative to other countries. Rates have been found to vary from 2.4 to 7.0 per 100,000 in industrialized countries (Porter and Gavin 2010), with higher rates in lower-middle income countries (Razali et al. 2014). Malaysia also has moderate human development (United Nations Development Programme 2015) and, at that time, moderate gender development (United Nations Development Programme 2019). Countries with lower levels of human and gender development (e.g., Tanzania and India) have higher estimated infanticide rates, whereas countries with very high human and gender development (e.g., Finland, Austria, and Australia) have low estimated infanticide rates (Razali et al. 2014). Malaysia's moderate rate of infanticide is thus consistent with its moderate gender and human development.

We discovered that substantial data were missing from Malaysian police records, with essential details—including age and sex of the victims, characteristics of the likely perpetrators, and the perpetrators' relationship to the victims—which were undocumented for more than 80% of cases. The paucity of data leads us to be cautious in drawing conclusions. Documented cases identified more boys than girls as victims, with accused perpetrators predominantly Malay women, usually the mother of the victim. It was difficult to avoid wondering whether gender bias could be found in arrest practices; our later interviews with convicted women reinforced this possibility.

It was clear that the police confronted challenges in recordkeeping. A fundamental problem lay in establishing, once a body had been found, whether it was a miscarriage, stillbirth, neonaticide, or infanticide. The forensic pathologist had classified about a quarter of the 1,096 cases on the infant abandonment register as *janin* (fetus, associated with miscarriage or abortion, which is legal in Malaysia), resulting in a likely overestimate of the infanticide rate: these should not have been registered as infants killed or abandoned after being born alive. In our view, Malaysia would benefit from improvements in data gathering and recordkeeping.

INTERVIEWS WITH WOMEN CONVICTED OF FILICIDE

Having examined filicide from a national perspective, we sought to learn firsthand about the lives and perspectives of convicted women (Razali et al. 2019). Our goal was to interview all women who had been convicted of filicide and were, as a result, incarcerated in one of the five prisons and two forensic psychiatric institutions in Malaysia. To ensure that research data could not be sought as evidence and that women would not falsely believe that we could engage in legal matters on their behalf, we chose not to include anyone whose legal process was incomplete. Gaining access to these women entailed lengthy negotiations at several levels of institutional and state bureaucracy. Great care was taken to ensure that participation was voluntary and that the women were capable of giving consent. We received approval for all aspects of our research from the Medical Research and Ethics Committee, Ministry of Health, Malaysia; the Medical Research and Ethics Committee, Universiti Teknologi MARA, Malaysia; and the Monash University Human Research Ethics Committee, Melbourne, Australia.

Ten women were eligible, of whom nine consented to participate. One woman refused because she claimed to have been wrongfully convicted. Each in-depth interview took 3–4 hours. Four of the women had been convicted of neonaticide (despite, in three cases, the baby having been stillborn as far as the women could tell), and five had been convicted of involvement in the death of an infant or child. The women had limited education; had been engaged in poorly remunerated jobs, such as cleaners or factory workers; and had occupied low socioeconomic positions. All came from poor families, and one was an illegal immigrant.

Their life stories revealed that these women had lacked choice and agency throughout their lives and had been victims of violence and adverse control, including rapes, beatings, forced marriages, and restrictions on activity. It was evident that three women had been convicted and were serving sentences for crimes that had been committed by men who were themselves less likely to be convicted. Sal had participated in the beating of her foster daughter by the girl's father, who was not convicted. Tira was interviewed on death row; her 4-year-old stepdaughter had been beaten to death by the child's father, who had been arrested but found not guilty. Tira had been convicted as an accessory because she had been in the house when the killing occurred. The third was Ina, whose story is summarized later. (Details of all the women are provided in Razali 2015, pp. 158–205.)

The following are excerpts of accounts provided by three women involved in our study (for whom we use pseudonyms): Nora, who had been convicted of neonaticide; Liya, convicted of infanticide and the only apparent case of overt psychopathology; and Ina, convicted of filicide. All three women were Malay.

NORA

Nora was a 20-year-old woman who had been brought up by her impoverished grandmother after her parents divorced. To contribute to the household income, She began working as a cleaner when she was a teenager. After a few days at her new job, she was raped by her supervisor: "One day, he gave me a drink. I believe that he put pills in the drink. It was mixed with Coke. I was thirsty, and I drank. I felt as if I was influenced by a devil. I was raped that day." Nora kept the incident to herself.

After a few weeks, she went to the city to look for another job to escape the supervisor. She found a job as a waitress and stayed with other workers in a rented house. Without realizing she was pregnant from the rape, Nora continued working until, one day, she felt tremendous pain and returned to her residence. At midnight, she telephoned her mother, who told her, "Don't call; pray a lot." Nora was shocked when the pain became more severe and felt her "bottom" was stretched. She became frightened and, with no idea what was happening, felt "something" come out of her "bottom." It made no sound. Confused and afraid, she threw "the thing" out of the window. Nora was arrested the next day.

LIYA

Liya was 39 years old when interviewed and, like Nora, had lived with her grandparents after her parents divorced. Her grandparents had died when Liya was 15, leaving her with an uncle. They had no income, and Liya left school to work in a factory, where she met a man she wanted to marry. Because the relationship was not *direstui* (approved) by her uncle, Liya eloped. She described her marriage as happy for only a few months. When her husband lost his job, Liya realized he was addicted to alcohol and illicit drugs. Liya had five children in quick succession and had difficulty caring for them all solely on her inadequate income.

Liya began to experience postpartum symptoms after the birth of her second child. The symptoms became severe with the birth of her fifth child, but she received no treatment. She described hearing intrusive voices demanding that she kill her 10-month-old son, whom she suffocated with a pillow. In her confusion, she took his body to the bank of a river not far from her dwelling. She was arrested within 24 hours.

INA

Ina was 29 years old. Her partner, who was violent, unemployed, and addicted to drugs, frequently abandoned Ina and their three children.

They dreaded his return: "He came back, he beat me. He beat my kids. He scolded me whenever he came back. I was scared! Scared of him. He would kill me!" He forced Ina to relinquish her job at the factory and would lock her in the house. She could neither run away nor seek help, because their nearest neighbor was too far away to hear her cries: "I shouted, but nobody came to help me." One day, her partner beat their eldest daughter, age 2 years, until she died. He then buried her body in their backyard.

For months, Ina was isolated and told no one until her sister visited, learned what had happened, and urged Ina to report the murder to the police. Ina expected and hoped that the police would arrest her partner and put an end to her torment. Instead, she was arrested for abetting the crime by failing to report it immediately. Ina felt deeply the injustice of her incarceration while the murderer remained at liberty: "I hope the police find him. He was the one who killed my daughter. I was too afraid. I was scared. I am not supposed to be here."

COMMON FEATURES OF WOMEN'S ACCOUNTS

Like Nora, Liya, and Ina, the remaining incarcerated women had lived in poverty, had experienced marginalization, had limited access to education and employment, and had little if any family support. All had been victims of violence. Those who had partners were not supported by them; two had been abandoned by their partners during pregnancy. All women demonstrated the harmful effects of living in a patriarchal society. Detrimental features of all accounts included gender-based exploitation, social isolation, and inadequate structural support.

The exploitation, oppression, and control experienced by all nine of these women clearly played a role in their convictions for filicide. Three of the four young and nulliparous women convicted of neonaticide, one of whom disclosed rape although the others had not necessarily participated in consensual sex, had been unaware of the pregnancy until they were in labor. The fourth woman (Ika) concealed her pregnancy. Given the stigma in Malaysia attached to pregnancy outside of marriage and the profound shame and fear accompanying such a pregnancy, it is understandable that women would not want to report sexual assault and might repress knowledge of conception.

Among the women convicted of killing an older infant or child, Ina was not the only one who had been held captive and abused by a drug-addicted partner. It was evident in women's accounts that their partners, families, and employers maintained traditional patriarchal views of gender roles, including that women must submit to men's authority. Some women told of being forced by their parents or guardians to leave school to earn money for the family, which we identified as exploitation. Some women entered forced marriages. In one case, a woman was denied the opportunity to continue developing a promising business she had started. It was evident that the men and boys associated with these subjects were given greater respect and support than the women and girls, from whom more was demanded. The women were left to bear sole responsibility for fertility management under circumstances in which they had no agency or decision-making capacity.

Women's experience of gender-based violence and control took place in a wider context of marginalization and isolation, with inadequate social support for the women and their children. Even when they lived with others—a partner, family members, in-laws, colleagues—they were not embraced by their co-residents, families, neighbors, communities, or employers. This lack of reliable support made the women vulnerable to abuse and decreased the possibility that they would disclose their circumstances and be aided to escape. This extreme and unremitting stress, experienced without empathy or assistance from people around them, is conducive to psychological disturbance that can impair effective coping strategies and capacity to assess appropriate action. These women deserved to be understood and managed in light of such insights.

The women's oppression and lack of interpersonal support was exacerbated by failures in structural support systems. In theory, facilities are available in Malaysia to support women and their children, including free obstetric care at primary health clinics, welfare support, special accommodation, and baby hatches. Nevertheless, women's access was limited. At the most fundamental level, they were frequently unaware that these services existed. Those with violent partners were prevented from seeking help. When they did approach services, women reported experiencing judgmental and punitive attitudes from service providers.

INTERVIEWS WITH RELEVANT PROFESSIONALS

After examining national data and listening to the stories of nine women convicted of filicide, we aimed to elucidate the ways in which relevant professionals explained the causes of filicide in Malaysia and their recommendations for mitigating it (Razali et al. 2019). To achieve this, we interviewed experienced psychiatrists, psychologists, senior nurses, an obstetrician-gynecologist, a social worker, shelter managers, a teacher, a baby-hatch worker, and prison personnel, using the same semistructured interview guide with each subject. The 15 informants worked with girls and women who had committed filicide, had been convicted of filicide, or were at risk of committing filicide.

Analysis of interview data revealed that the opinions of these professionals were consistent with the public discourse of filicide in Malaysia (and elsewhere). Informants primarily identified young women as responsible for filicide. Although those at risk were often described as adolescents and young people, it was clear that girls and women, not boys and men, were the targets of the professionals' comments. Filicide was constructed predominantly as neonaticide and infanticide; professionals attributed these phenomena to women's failure to adhere to Malaysian norms of morality, religion, customs, and traditions. Poor religious practice (e.g., not attending daily prayers and having too little religious knowledge) by girls and young women was claimed to lead to socializing with boys and men, sexual transgression (having sex outside of marriage), and the potential for an ex-nuptial child. They said that girls and women who socialized with men put themselves at risk of rape, which was unlikely to be reported to the authorities; an unwanted pregnancy was a possible outcome. Because the lifelong stigma attached to an "illegitimate" birth is so powerful, the interviewees claimed that children born outside of marriage, whether from consensual sex or rape, were likely to be unwanted and therefore deliberately abandoned or killed by their mothers immediately after birth.

When we asked the professionals about reasons other than women's personal failings that might contribute to filicide in Malaysia, they nominated Malaysian society's strong stigmatization not only of unmarried mothers and their children but also of the services that work with them. They identified as contributory factors poor policy development directed at preventing filicide, limited availability of services to which at-risk girls and women could turn, and restricted access to those services that are available, including sexual and reproductive health and mental health services. Professionals also said that inadequate communication across what should be multidisciplinary teams was a factor in poor prevention of filicide.

Although the professionals suggested some social and political contributors to filicide, potential solutions were directed predominantly at improving girls' and women's behavior and knowledge, with an emphasis on sexual abstinence outside of marriage. Even suggested improvements to services and policies were designed to improve the moral fiber or mental health of girls and women as individuals rather than change social attitudes and develop structural support for women. It was notable that the professionals did not suggest ways of assisting women who were victims of sexual assault, nor did they provide recommendations to help victims of intimate-partner violence. Not one professional discussed the need to stop men from raping girls or women or any means of ending violence against women and children. In light of what women revealed about their lives, these are significant omissions.

Context and Perspective in Understanding Filicide

Our results, varying as they did according to perspective (whether convicted woman or professional), came to us as a surprise. Had we looked only at national data and interviewed the professionals, we could have been persuaded that neonaticide and infanticide are the most usual forms of filicide; that it is mostly women who commit the crime to avoid having an ex-nuptial child; and that women's poor self-control, inadequate fertility management, lack of religious observance, and (occasionally) psychopathology predispose them to kill their children.

However, having heard the perspectives of the nine women in our study, we became attuned to the social circumstances that made women vulnerable not only to playing a role in filicide but also to blame for the crime, even when the primary perpetrator was a man. Their poverty and victimization might have been intellectually accepted by the better-educated and more economically secure professionals, but the meaning and implications of their position in Malaysian society seemed almost to have been beyond imagination. When the dominant discourse of filicide—one consistent with the international literature—is that women who are "not like us" are the perpetrators, it is difficult to challenge without evidence of the kind we gathered from the convicted women themselves. The discourse on filicide widely distributed by the media in that country has not, of course, been constructed by journalists, who are informing the public of views already circulating in the community and among professionals. Acceptance of this discourse leads, as it did in Malaysia, to solutions that focus on "fixing" women. It is not surprising that these solutions appear to have been ineffective.

As a clinician or scholar in North America, the United Kingdom, and Australia (for example), it may be easy to condemn a country with different traditions and culture for its injustices against women. However, we suggest that it is more informative to use this evidence from Malaysia to encourage us to continue questioning dominant discourses of filicide and endeavoring to understand the perspectives of those accused of the crime and their social context. If we allow the construct of perpetrators of filicide to ossify, we risk being further blinded to sociocultural and gendered differences, even within our own countries.

PREVIOUS RESEARCH

Before beginning our investigations, we reviewed the literature on filicide research. Almost all reported research had been conducted in Western, high-income countries, mainly North America, Europe (Austria, Croatia, Denmark, Finland, France, Germany, Hungary, Italy, The Netherlands, Serbia, Sweden, the United Kingdom), Australia, and New Zealand (Razali 2015). Most accounts were published in peer-reviewed journals; a few appeared in widely distributed books (e.g., Alder and Polk 2001; Oberman and Meyer 2008).

We found one example of research (from the United States) in which women incarcerated for filicide reported being victims of violence (Oberman and Meyer 2008), as we had found in our own research in Malaysia. However, in our assessment, most U.S. researchers had adopted a perspective in which filicide is largely explained by the psychopathology of the perpetrator. Spinelli's (2004) important review acknowledged the lack of scientifically generated historical or legal evidence about infanticide; she concluded that the way forward for prevention was improved professional recognition of psychiatric illness and public understanding that mental illness can affect behavior and cognition. Barnes and Brown (2016) also argued that infanticide was usually precipitated by postpartum psychosis. None of these authors commented on the circumstances of women's lives or suggested that these circumstances warrant consideration or should be understood and addressed in prevention strategies.

We are not denying the need for work on the role of mental illness in filicide, but we have been alerted to the dominance of these views by the responses to manuscripts that we have submitted for peer review. Some reviewers seemed, at first, unable to accept that we were being honest in reporting our rigorous recruitment of all eligible women in Malaysia and our accounts of their experiences (Razali et al. 2019). For example, even though we described our analysis of national data (making it clear that more than 1,000 abandoned newborns and infants had been recorded) and the steps we had taken to identify all convicted women whose legal process had been completed, one reviewer wrote: "only 9 filicides in Malaysia and 9 incarcerations in Malaysia during the three years of the study and they are all in this paper. I suspect that this is incorrect."

Other reviewers were unable to appreciate the point we were making about cultural differences and the gendered effects of a patriarchal society. In response to our manuscript describing the professionals' understanding of the causes of filicide, in which comparisons between our findings and our interviews with the women, one reviewer wanted us to draw on a paper associating filicide with mental illness as an explanatory guide to filicide rather than appreciating how the professionals' interpretations were at odds with the histories of the convicted women. Furthermore, although we took great care to describe the women we interviewed as "convicted" and never as "offenders," one reviewer criticized us by saying it was "not acceptable to call them all offenders as some of the women are clearly not." This seemed to reflect the expectation that any woman appearing in a paper about filicide must be an offender. In general, reviewers' comments often revealed the challenge of stepping outside of a European or North American cultural perspective.

What we learned from these women seemed to be too far from the scholarly constructs of filicide held by Western scholars to be comprehended. The systemic explanation for women's conviction and incarceration that we identified was at odds with the more individualistic explanations current in the West. In contrast, our results from interviews with Malay professionals seemed to be too prosaic to be accepted as anything more than what was to be expected, rather than a startling contrast with the women's experiences (Razali et al. 2020). We acknowledge and are grateful for the willingness of reviewers to come to understand this very different perspective on filicide. However, all of us who work in this field must be vigilant against allowing the familiar to blind us to new insights.

THEORETICAL FOUNDATIONS

The theory most relevant to our work is Bronfenbrenner's (1979) ecological framework. In practice, we have interpreted our data using framework analysis (Razali et al. 2016b; Ritchie and Spencer 2002) as well as thematic analysis guided by narrative and discourse theories (Razali et al. 2019, 2020). Bronfenbrenner's (1979) framework enabled us to understand filicide in Malaysia as resulting from interaction among five levels of the social environment, all of which influence human growth and development. The *macro* level (e.g., gendered inequality, economic deprivation, poor structural support, inadequate general and sex education, stigma and shame, injustice) interacts with the *exosystem* (poor neighborhood support, stigmatizing community), the *mesosystem* (lack of support from friends and workmates), the *micro* level (abusive and irresponsible partner, domestic violence, poor family support), and the *individual person* (denied agency, choice, and education; challenges to well-being and mental health; limitations arising from gendered inequality). The ecological framework also helped us to see that directing all preventive measures only to the level of the individual would be unlikely to achieve success. Adjustments at every level, especially attempts to overcome the gendered inequality that is evident throughout, must be made to improve the status of women and thus make their lives and those of their children safer and more secure.

Blaming young people for their sexual behavior and women for allowing themselves to be victims of violence increases the social isolation and exclusion that predispose to filicide. Relying on fear-based education directed solely at sexual abstinence, with threats of harsh punishment (whether women and girls are willing or unwilling participants in sexual intercourse), heightens stigma and further ostracizes sexually active and pregnant women. These approaches make it almost impossible for women and girls to seek help. When a society provides a safe environment, strong support system, and nonjudgmental care, all members of the community are enabled to participate and contribute.

Conclusion

Our groundbreaking research in Malaysia suggests a need to appreciate all levels of the ecological system and their influence on filicide. Understanding filicide in a country so fundamentally different from those in which research is usually conducted can help highlight the significance of perspective and open our eyes to possibilities beyond the familiar. At the most basic level, it can alert us to the potentially different meanings of filicide among immigrants, whose social and cultural experiences and perspectives may be alien to us. As we learned (Razali et al. 2017), researching filicide requires investigators to be open minded and prepare to be challenged and surprised. Filicide prevention will benefit from collaboration among disciplines such as health professionals, scholars, educators, legislators, policymakers, and theologians to ensure that all levels and perspectives are considered. Government and nongovernment organizations must be included in all measures, because they are essential participants in systemic change. As we turn our thoughts to Malaysia, we conclude that interventions promoting social change are essential and that strategies exclusively targeting women serve only to reify structural and gender inequities.

UPDATE ON MALAYSIA

Since we conducted our research, changes have occurred in Malaysia that have implications for women. In May 2018, a new government was elected, with a woman as deputy prime minister—a historical first for the country. Transformational policies have been proposed in health, social care, and education, and implementation has begun. These changes reflect the Shared Prosperity Vision 2030, designed to include women and other vulnerable people in the national social development agenda. Agencies under the governance of the Ministry of Women, Family and

Community Development (e.g., the Social Welfare Department, the National Population and Family Development Board, the Social Institute of Malaysia, and the NAM Institute for the Empowerment of Women in Malaysia) are facilitating the implementation of the National Social Policy, which focuses on including women in the national agenda.

Among changes already evident to Dr. Razali, who lives in Malaysia, where she holds an academic appointment in psychiatry, are the incorporation of sex education into mainstream academic curricula for primary and secondary schools based on the United Nations Educational, Scientific, and Cultural Organization's Comprehensive Sexuality Education (www.unfpa.org/comprehensive-sexuality-education), although the extent of implementation is not yet clear; the increased female participation in the labor force from 50% to 60% of women; the recommendation for amending legal provisions to protect women from sexual harassment and violence (details to be negotiated); and the implementation of improved financial security for women who, as long as they pay RM5 (~$1.20 USD) into the Employees' Provident Fund (EPF), will receive RM40 (~$9.60 USD) monthly from the government in a scheme called i-Suri. According to the government website, "Housewives can now opt in for the EPF contributions via our new government incentive under i-Suri. i-Suri is catered specially to ensure the wellbeing of housewives and acknowledge your contribution to your families and the development of the country" (www.kwsp.gov.my/member/contribution/insentif-suri).

It is still too soon to see any effects of these policies on filicide and women's well-being. Further research and evaluation are essential.

MAIN CLINICAL/LEGAL POINTS AND CULTURAL PERSPECTIVES

- Consider social context (e.g., poverty, polyvictimization, domestic violence, drug abuse, role of women in society) when attempting to understand perpetrators of filicide or those accused of filicide; it may be necessary to think outside the familiar territory of psychopathology.

- Different legal and social systems, especially those that are highly patriarchal, may have different standards of criminal responsibility than high-income English-speaking countries and may reveal gender bias in their policing and judicial systems.

- Filicide research is predominantly conducted in well-resourced countries with adequate surveillance systems and recordkeeping. Maternal filicide research in Malaysia contributes to extending the breadth of understanding in a world that is increasingly global.

Practice and Discussion Questions

1. How might culture influence the construct of filicide, and how might this affect the work of mental health professionals?
2. What are the human rights implications when marginalized and victimized women commit or are charged with filicide?
3. How can mental health professionals approach the care of marginalized and victimized women who commit or are charged with filicide?
4. Interrogate dominant narratives and discourses. How do they frame understanding of maternal filicide?
5. Consider the effects on understanding filicide arising from research evidence that is biased by the unequal distribution of research funding. What might we do to mitigate these effects?

References

Alder C, Polk K: Child Victims of Homicide. Cambridge, UK, Cambridge University Press, 2001

Barnes DL, Brown J: Understanding postpartum psychosis and infanticide. Forensic Scholars Today 1(4), 2016

Bourget D, Bradford JM: Homicidal parents. Can J Psychiatry 35(3):233–238, 1990

Bourget D, Gagné P: Paternal filicide in Québec. J Am Acad Psychiatry Law 33(3):354–360, 2005

Bronfenbrenner U: The Ecology of Human Development: Experiments by Nature and Design. Cambridge, MA, Harvard University Press, 1979

Chong ST, Mohamad MS, Er AC: The mental health development in Malaysia: history, current issues and future development. Asian Soc Sci 9(6):1–8, 2013

Cochrane J, Ming GL: Abandoned babies: the Malaysian 'baby hatch.' Infant 9(4):142–144, 2013

d'Orban PT: Women who kill their children. Br J Psychiatry 134(6):560–571, 1979

Equal Measures 2030: Harnessing the Power of Data for Gender Equality: Introducing the 2019 EM2030 SDG Gender Index. Surrey, UK, Equal Measures 2030, 2019. Available at: https://data.em2030.org/wp-content/uploads/2019/05/EM2030_2019_Global_Report_ENG.pdf. Accessed December 18, 2019.

Guileyardo JM, Prahlow JA, Barnard JJ: Familial filicide and filicide classification. Am J Forensic Med Pathol 20(3):286–292, 1999

Mutalip SSM, Mohamed R: Sexual education in Malaysia: accepted or rejected? Iran J Public Health 41(7):34–39, 2012

Ng C: Positioning Women in Malaysia: Class and Gender in an Industrializing State. London, Springer, 2016

Niner S, Ahmad Y, Cuthbert D: The 'social tsunami': media coverage of child abuse in Malaysia's English-language newspapers in 2010. Media, Culture and Society 35(4):435–453, 2013

Oberman M, Meyer CL: When Mothers Kill: Interviews From Prison. New York, NYU Press, 2008

Porter T, Gavin H: Infanticide and neonaticide: a review of 40 years of research literature on incidence and causes. Trauma Violence Abuse 11(3):99–112, 2010

Rahim AbA, Zainudin TNAbT, Shariff AAbM: Curbing the problems of baby dumping and infanticide: a Malaysian legal perspective. Int J Humanit Soc Sci 2(12):173–178, 2012

Razali S: Understanding Filicide by Women in Malaysia. PhD dissertation, Monash University, Melbourne, Australia, 2015

Razali S, Kirkman M, Ahmad SH, Fisher J: Infanticide and illegal infant abandonment in Malaysia. Child Abuse Negl 38(10):1715–1724, 2014

Razali S, Almashoor SHSA, Yusoff AN, Basri HH: Newspaper analysis on filicide and infant abandonment in Malaysia. Journal of Media and Information Warfare 8:39–70, 2016a

Razali S, Kirkman M, Fisher J: Overlaps and gaps in understanding filicide in Malaysia: framework analysis of the perspectives of convicted women and service providers. Proceedings of the 1st International Conference on Women and Children: Legal and Social Issues, Subang Jaya, Malaysia, October 17–18, 2016b

Razali S, Kirkman M, Fisher J: Research on a socially, ethically, and legally complex phenomenon: women convicted of filicide in Malaysia. International Journal for Crime, Justice and Social Democracy 6(2):34–45, 2017

Razali S, Fisher J, Kirkman M: 'Nobody came to help': interviews with women convicted of filicide in Malaysia. Arch Womens Ment Health 22(1):151–158, 2019

Razali S, Kirkman M, Fisher J: Why women commit filicide: opinions of health, social work, education, and policy professionals in Malaysia. Child Abuse Review 29(1):73–84, 2020

Resnick PJ: Child murder by parents: a psychiatric review of filicide. Am J Psychiatry 126(3):325–334, 1969

Resnick PJ: Murder of the newborn: a psychiatric review of neonaticide. Am J Psychiatry 126(10):1414–1420, 1970

Ritchie J, Spencer L: Qualitative data analysis for applied policy research, in The Qualitative Researcher's Companion. Edited by Huberman M, Miles MB. London, Taylor and Francis, 2002, pp 305–329

Scott PD: Parents who kill their children. Medicine, Science and the Law 13(2):120–126, 1973

Shuaib FS: The Islamic legal system in Malaysia. Pacific Rim Law Policy Journal 21(1):85–114, 2012

Spinelli MG: Maternal infanticide associated with mental illness: prevention and the promise of saved lives. Am J Psychiatry 161:1548–1557, 2004

Talib J, Mamat M, Ibrahim M, Mohamad Z: Analysis on sex education in schools across Malaysia. Procedia: Social and Behavioral Sciences 59:340–348, 2012

United Nations Development Programme: Human Development Report 2015: Work for Human Development. New York, United Nations Development Programme, 2015

United Nations Development Programme: Human Development Reports: Gender Inequality Index. New York, United Nations Development Programme, 2019. Available at: http://hdr.undp.org/en/content/gender-inequality-index. Accessed December 18, 2019.

CHAPTER 15

Postpartum Support International

A LEADING RESOURCE CENTER FOR MATERNAL FILICIDE IN THE UNITED STATES

Jane Honikman, M.S.

Tiffany Ross, M.S.S.W.

Wendy Davis, Ph.D., PMH-C

Postpartum Support International (PSI), the world's largest nonprofit organization dedicated to helping women and families with perinatal mental health disorders, was founded in 1987 by Jane Honikman. Its mission is to increase awareness and to support public and professional communities to address the mental health needs of women and families during pregnancy and postpartum. PSI offers support, reliable information, best practices training, and certification, with more than 450 support volunteers in all 50 U.S. states and more than 40 countries around the world. PSI support volunteers provide local support for families and providers, connecting those in need with trained providers and support groups. In 2019, the organization created a special Postpartum Psychosis Task Force composed of survivors, clinicians, and advocates to improve awareness and understanding of postpartum psychosis (PPP) and resources for addressing it. Working together with volunteers, PSI chapters (representing organized PSI geographic locales), providers, researchers, and other stakeholders, PSI is committed to eliminating stigma and ensuring that compassionate and quality care and treatment are available to all families.

PSI's involvement in criminal justice began in June 1987 at the first PSI conference, titled "Women's Mental Health Following Childbirth," in Santa Barbara, California. The gathering was convened by founder Jane Honikman to start a self-help movement for perinatal mental health that combined the experiences of mothers and families, social support advocates, and medical researchers. The movement originated from Boston Women's Health Book Collective and the American Association of University Women's networks of feminists with roots in the women's movement of the late 1960s and 1970s. In attendance at the 1987 meeting was Angela Thompson, a mother who had drowned her second baby while experiencing PPP. Her presence set the early stages of the advocacy movement for women who committed infanticide and filicide.

In this chapter, we highlight the history and resources of PSI in the areas of criminal justice and advocacy related to maternal filicide. We discuss the dire need for continued education, training, and advocacy in the field of maternal mental illness and criminal justice. We share the content and rationale for several of the resources developed by PSI: the PSI PenPal Network Newsletter for incarcerated women; the Yates Children Memorial Fund Justice and Advocacy program; and the PSI Legal Toolkit, which currently includes the PSI Legal Checklist for Attorneys (Table 15–1) and videotaped excerpts from a training on maternal mental illness and criminal justice.

Although other organizations in support of mothers and fathers in the perinatal period exist internationally, PSI was among the first to focus on support and advocacy for families who have entered the criminal justice system because of the tragedy of crimes committed during an episode of perinatal mental illness. Working with other organizations and educational efforts such as the International Marcé Society for Perinatal Mental Health and Massachusetts General Hospital, PSI is committed to collaborative action to advance best practices for the treatment and defense of women in the criminal justice system for these crimes. We are the founder (Jane Honikman), the Justice and Advocacy Program Manager (Tiffany Ross), and the Executive Director (Wendy Davis) of PSI. We are keenly aware of the need for increased understanding, intervention, and advocacy for families affected by the tragedy of maternal filicide, and we have written this chapter to contribute to the advancement of that cause.

Advocacy for Mothers and Postpartum Psychosis

"Why Mothers Kill Their Babies" (Toufexis 1988) was the title of an article in *Time* magazine on June 20, 1988. It cited a series of recent tragedies, provided medical explanations to understand why they had occurred,

TABLE 15–1. Postpartum Support International checklist for attorneys defending a mother accused of harming or killing her infant/child

Following the death or serious injury of an infant at the hands of a mother:

- ❑ Film client immediately or as soon as possible after arrest or hospitalization.
- ❑ Document client's behavior before client is medicated.
- ❑ Arrange early evaluations by reproductive/perinatal psychiatrists.
- ❑ Research perinatal mood disorders.
- ❑ Review insanity defense laws in the state where the tragedy occurred.
- ❑ Arrange follow-up expert evaluations during course of treatment.
- ❑ Film client after medication takes effect.

Tips from other perinatal psychosis cases:

- ❑ Learn about client's personality and behavior prior to the incident.
- ❑ Do not prejudge the client based on the horrible nature of the infanticide/filicide.
- ❑ Understand perinatal mental illness, including psychosis, as temporary and treatable.
- ❑ Postpartum psychosis can be mercurial in nature, and the mother may appear rational at times.
- ❑ Gather psychiatric history of client, family psychiatric history, obstetric history, evidence of birth trauma, and history of any previous pregnancies with perinatal mood disorders.
- ❑ Find out if the mother has been isolated or lacks a meaningful support network.
- ❑ A psychologist trained in childhood trauma may be useful with defense if the mother was a victim of childhood trauma herself.
- ❑ Be aware of other factors that could be brought up by the prosecution, such as infidelity in the husband or an unwanted pregnancy.
- ❑ Ascertain whether family, neighbors, or friends noticed any changes in behavior.
- ❑ Learn whether there were any recent changes in medications.
- ❑ Determine whether the mother has been under undue stress (e.g., marital stress, loss of financial support [unemployment], buying or selling a home, a recent move, caring for a special-needs child or family member).
- ❑ Evaluate the sleep patterns surrounding the pregnancy and postpartum period.
- ❑ Inquire about social support.
- ❑ Know your local and state mental health resources.

TABLE 15–1.   Postpartum Support International checklist for attorneys defending a mother accused of harming or killing her infant/child *(continued)*

Resources:

❑ Yates Children Memorial Fund—Justice and Advocacy Program. Contact Postpartum Support International at psioffice@postpartum.net

❑ VIDEO: Advice for Lawyers—Postpartum Mental Illness and the Criminal Justice System, https://vimeo.com/253536312

❑ The most recent edition of DSM

❑ PubMed (national U.S. online library of medicine through the National Institutes of Health, www.ncbi.nlm.nih.gov/pubmed).

❑ *Infanticide: Psychosocial and Legal Perspectives on Mothers Who Kill* (Spinelli 2003)

Note.   These guidelines were written in 2015 and updated in 2019 by the Postpartum Support International Justice and Advocacy Committee with help from attorneys George J. Parnham, Guy D. Smith, Po Chau, and Stephen Allen.

and shared details about the prosecutions of the mothers. An outpouring of public sympathy and a natural sense of empathy emerged in response. The powerful stigma attached to postpartum psychiatric illness had come under attack and was starting to lift. Professionals and families began to speak out, write, and advocate for change.

The following year, in March 1989, Pennsylvania State University held a conference on PPP and criminal responsibility. PSI representatives attended the conference and began networking with legal and academic experts. Privately, one psychiatrist expressed a concern about the possible negative impacts on new mothers from public discussion about tragic outcomes related to PPP. Jane countered with the opposite point of view that education and awareness are essential for social advocacy.

That same year, PSI participated in a California State Public Policy Task Force that drafted a resolution on PPP. The resolution directed the California Board of Corrections to assess the mental status of women who had recently given birth and been charged with infanticide. Senate Concurrent Resolution Number 23 passed unanimously in California. Around the same time, widespread media attention fueled a growing understanding that responsibility for these children's deaths lays, in part, with society's failure to recognize the connection between postpartum psychiatric illness and child homicide. Between 1986 and 1990, two couples impacted by infanticide—Angela and Jeff Thompson and Sharon and Glenn Comitz (she was still incarcerated)—made 34 appearances on nationally syndicated television programs and news broadcasts. The details of these cases, when reviewed with an understanding of perinatal mental illness, illustrate just how crucial it is for caregivers and families to understand the symptoms of and proper interventions for severe postpartum mental illness. One of the most important and most misunderstood elements is that PPP is temporary and treatable, distinguishing it from chronic mental illnesses such as psychosis and paranoia.

ANGELA THOMPSON

In 1983, Angela Thompson, a registered nurse in Sacramento, California, who had been in treatment and recovered from perinatal psychosis and depression after her first child, was successfully raising her two young children when she experienced a sudden psychosis and drowned her beloved 9-month-old son Michael in the bathtub. "I started becoming delusional after I stopped nursing Michael. I thought somehow that he represented the devil," Thompson said in a telephone interview. "The morning the baby died, I got a phone call from a woman selling magazines. Right before she hung up, I thought she said, 'All right, Angela.' I had been praying and asking God for guidance, and I thought that was God telling me to drown the baby. I filled the tub, put the baby in the water, and held him down until he drowned....He was an easy baby, a good baby, he was perfect."

Thompson was acquitted of voluntary manslaughter by reason of insanity after four psychiatrists diagnosed PPP. Working with a perinatal psychologist as an expert witness, her attorney, and the court, Angela was able to remain out of prison and was sentenced to supervised probation by state medical personnel and the court. In May 1987, 4 years after losing her son, Thompson gave birth to another son, raised her two children into adulthood, and has gone on to be an advocate and writer advancing the field of perinatal mental health (Butterfield 2006).

SHARON COMITZ

Sharon Comitz was 29 years old when she was sentenced to 8–20 years in a women's prison in Muncy, Pennsylvania, for killing her 1-month-old son, Garret, by dropping him into a mountain stream near Philipsburg in January 1985. Sharon pled "guilty but mentally ill" to a charge of third-degree murder the following June. Her husband and lawyers advocated for her, stating that her mental condition should have prompted a lighter sentence. Sharon served 8 years in prison. Her husband was supportive and fought for her in public. "I was not aware until months later that I was the actual person who did this," said Comitz. Sharon had previously been hospitalized for depression after the earlier birth of a daughter.

Sharon had been advised to wait 5 years to have another child after her first hospitalization. The couple had followed this advice, and just before Garret's birth, Sharon was urged to avoid postpartum depression by her husband and doctor. Such instruction to avoid a mental illness not within one's control likely added pressure and may have contributed to the death of her son, as one psychiatrist testified in court. Although her husband and many advocates lobbied that Sharon was mentally ill, the courts determined that she knew what she was doing when she dropped her son to his death. Sharon had driven to the nearest shopping center and reported that her son had been kidnapped from her vehicle. Her defense team thought she had dissociated the index event and truly had believed Garret was missing.

IMPACT OF STORIES

So much was gained from the courageous decision of these women and their husbands to be public about their cases. They brought awareness that the infanticides had been carried out during the women's postpartum mental illness. Medical professionals and activists affiliated with the postpartum support movement were able to launch an education campaign about the tragic outcome of untreated PPP. PSI has supported this movement and has become a pivotal force for cultural and political change by challenging medical knowledge and practice, mobilizing constituents, changing legal regulations and laws, and fostering public discussion about perinatal mental illness.

Inception of the PSI PenPal Network

Correspondence and calls to PSI came from a variety of sources: women serving time in prison for postpartum-related infanticide and filicide, those who were hospitalized, family members, and the general public. Women and families were asking for information and emotional support, as well as legal and psychiatric assistance. In response, Jane began the PenPal Network for Incarcerated Women in November of 1990 for women in prison due to crimes committed in the throes of a postpartum mental illness. She wished to adopt the model of pen pal friendships she had enjoyed as a child. To start the PenPal Network, Jane wrote a letter of introduction to the imprisoned women; within a month, nine women wanted to be included in the network as pen pals. She generated two lists: 1) noninmates who empathized with the incarcerated women and wished to write directly, and 2) inmates who wished to write to each other. Given prison regulations, however, the traditional pen pal model was not possible because inmates were not permitted to correspond directly with other inmates.

Instead, Jane initiated the *PSI PenPal Network Newsletter*. Incarcerated women wrote to the network coordinator, who summarized their news. The summaries, in turn, were mailed to all the women in the network, whether incarcerated or living in the community. Newsletters provided information about the welfare of network members and the progress of their trials, appeals, and paroles. They also included information about legislative and psychiatric developments related to postpartum illness, infanticide, and filicide and summaries of recently published research. Greeting cards and letters were also sent from supporters to the women in prison, which led to loyal friendships.

Not only did the network benefit its members but it also impacted the lives of those involved. A quote from the PenPal Network coordinator, taken from a July 13, 2000 letter to the PSI board of directors, read:

> I found PSI in March 1996 on the internet as I was searching for help for my sister who was serving a forty-year sentence in a Texas prison. I volunteered to be the PenPal Network coordinator. I've met some wonderful people and I've been able with education and a little hope to help women and families try to ease the pain that my family and I endured for several years. My sister was released in November 1997. (personal communication, J. Honikman)

Furthering the pen pal program, the 2001 annual PSI conference held in Santa Barbara, California, featured life-size cutouts made of black Masonite that represented the incarcerated women in the network. Hanging from a chain around each cutout's neck was that woman's tragic story. This visual project sent a powerful message to the public about the importance of social action and advocacy and demonstrated the success and impact of the network. In an academic paper titled, "From Infanticide to Activism: The Transformation of Emotions and Identity in Self-Help Movements," authors Verta Taylor and Lisa Leitz stated:

> Participation in the PenPal Network allows women the latitude of expressing the guilt, shame, and intense grief they experience as a result of their actions and to overcome their isolation by connecting with other women who have experienced a similar fate. Through supportive communication, often referred to as "a lifeline" or "life-saving," the women in the network develop a sense of "we" that centers around the shared experience of postpartum mental illness that led to what they typically refer to as the "loss" of their children, their negative portrayal in the media, and the injustices they believe they have suffered in the courts and criminal justice system. (Taylor and Leitz 2010, p. 274)

By the end of 1991 there were 17 participants in the PenPal Network, and by 1998 there were 29 members. Six volunteer coordinators served the network from 1990 until 2017, when the newsletter was discontinued (with 24 members at that time). The current coordinator continues to write with a few of the women and occasionally receives an email from women looking for pen pals and connects them with individuals outside the prison system. In June 2018, PSI's executive director and president were notified that the PenPal Network had ended. The PSI Justice and Advocacy Committee is exploring whether there is interest in restarting the network.

Position Paper

The 2004 PSI *Position Paper on Psychosis-Related Tragedies* was written following the 2004 Annual Conference in Chicago, Illinois, and was published on the PSI website (Postpartum Support International 2004). PSI believes defendants with perinatal mental illness deserve a defense that is based on scientific fact, and advocates for diagnostic guidelines to enhance shared knowledge between psychiatry and the law and focus on prevention and treatment in lieu of punishment. PSI advocates for revisions of American legal standards and insanity laws so contemporary neuroscience and psychiatry inform current definitions of sanity and guilt. Scientific and biologically based knowledge must be conveyed to the jury so decisions can be based on informed facts. The position paper outlined four distinct problem areas and presented the PSI's advocacy responses. These problems were 1) DSM diagnostic criteria; 2) American legislation; 3) postpartum mental illness and the law; and 4) early identification, treatment, and prevention. The paper reflected the role that public recognition, awareness, education, and advocacy play in society.

Several years later, a presentation titled "From Infanticide to Activism" was given at the 2010 annual conference in Pittsburgh, Pennsylvania. Based on PSI's 2004 position paper, the presentation's objectives were to share that the worldwide infanticide and infant mortality rates were grossly underestimated and that systematic data on the prevalence of infant murder were rare. In the 2010 presentation, we wanted to convey that sentences for women who committed infanticide vary remarkably because insanity laws differ from state to state as well as from country to country. To date, despite the accumulated knowledge gained over the years, health care and mental health providers continue to miss warning signs of postpartum psychiatric illnesses that can lead to maternal filicide and afflict our most vulnerable populations in health care.

Indeed, postpartum psychiatric illnesses are a major public health problem that is predictable, identifiable, and treatable and therefore preventable. More rigorous and systematic research must be utilized to substantiate a cluster of identifiable symptoms for diagnosis and to pave the way for treatment strategies and rehabilitation. DSM-5 (American Psychiatric Association 2013) does not directly identify the research available to understand the biology, symptomatology, and duration of PPP; thus, courts' understanding is inaccurate and the impact of psychiatric evidence in criminal cases is limited. Although screening for ante- and postpartum illness has increased, more education is needed to ensure consistency and provider competency. There are optimum times to assess risk for puerperal illness and associated potential for infant morbidity and mortality.

PSI Justice and Advocacy Resources

While we have seen improvement in professional education, screening, and treatment for postpartum depression and anxiety, progression has been slower in understanding and developing standards of care for PPP. In particular, women accused of crimes committed during a postpartum mental illness are in urgent need of immediate and informed help. PSI has remained committed to supporting women and families affected by PPP and involved in the criminal justice system. The Yates Children Memorial Fund and the PSI Justice and Advocacy Program were developed out of the need to provide education and awareness about the plight of mothers implicated by the criminal justice system for infanticide or filicide. The goals of the program are 1) providing support to families and 2) providing resources and toolkits for professionals involved with cases concerning perinatal mental illness in the criminal justice system, such as law enforcement, first responders, attorneys, maternal mental health expert witnesses, and psychiatric providers.

PSI JUSTICE AND ADVOCACY PROGRAM

The PSI Justice and Advocacy Program continues to develop over time. The three main components involve resources and outreach, education, and policy and advocacy. All are necessary elements of our goal to ameliorate troubling legal issues for women and to equip legal and mental health professionals with resources to address maternal mental illness in the criminal justice system.

1. **Resources and outreach**: These are important aspects of PSI Justice and Advocacy Program efforts that inform organizations, providers, and community members about the resources PSI can offer regarding legal issues pertaining to women at risk and accused of crimes. PSI has developed an ongoing list of attorneys and expert witnesses for those seeking resources in their states.

2. **Education**: The PSI Justice and Advocacy team furthers the education process for the legal community by holding more continuing legal education (CLE) events that concentrate on maternal infanticide. Currently, no trainings are available from the American Bar Association, among their hundreds of CLE courses, that would help legal professionals to become educated and skilled in representing women accused of crimes committed during perinatal mental illness. A 1-day CLE seminar, "Maternal Mental Illness and the Criminal Justice System," presented in 2015 by PSI and hosted by Sylvia Lasalandra in New Jersey, provided an excellent working model and was used to develop the educational video in the PSI Legal Toolkit.

   Another essential project for the PSI Justice and Advocacy Team is the creation of specifically designed seminars or webinars for qualified mental health providers who are willing to become expert witnesses. These seminars will train licensed perinatal mental health experts to use the most appropriate research and approaches while testifying as expert witnesses in criminal or family law cases. Expert witnesses must learn to clearly explain the abnormality and mental impairment that occur during a psychotic or postpartum episode and defend the condition as a genuine psychiatric disorder. Properly educated maternal mental health professional experts working in tandem with defense attorneys are absolutely vital for educating judges, juries, and court adversaries about the complexities and evolving clinical studies of mental illnesses in cases involving maternal infanticide and filicide.

3. **Policy and advocacy**: PSI collaborates with other advocacy organizations, legal and public health professionals, and psychiatric experts to understand how to improve policies and legal standards and best practices in treatment for perinatal mental illness. The goal of the Justice and Advocacy Program is to research, gather information from experts, and convene discussions about promising legal and legislative initiatives.

PSI LEGAL TOOLKIT

The PSI Toolkit for Legal Professionals outlines best practices and protocols in the recognition, assessment, treatment, and informed legal representation of cases related to perinatal mental illness, especially PPP. PSI has created targeted material for defense attorneys and a program to train expert witnesses from the mental health community. Our goal is to educate the public and the courts that the existence of PPP is a valid mitigating factor in the defense of a woman who commits filicide. It is important to create a climate in which perinatal mental health disorders are represented neither as spousal revenge nor as murder as a result of child custody battles. PSI professional educational materials emphasize that immediate and early engagement of a trained crisis intervention team is critical to ensure proper response to psychiatric symptoms and their impact on rational functioning and judgment. The toolkit describes the importance of pairing a legal defense schooled in the field of perinatal mental illness with a maternal mental health expert witness, emphasizing that PPP is a treatable, temporary, and valid medical condition that is a viable legal defense.

PSI created the Legal Resources Toolkit as part of the education mandate of the Legal and Advocacy Program. The toolkit includes a protocol of best practices and a 17-minute video for attorneys assigned to defend a maternal infanticide case. The educational video includes key points compiled from a live CLE seminar given by experts in the field of maternal mental illness and the law. The day-long seminar provided practical, evidence-based, and case-based information to understand the key elements of perinatal mental illness and the criminal justice system.

The lead faculty member at the recorded seminar was criminal defense attorney George Parnham, J.D., an expert on the defense of individuals with mental illness and a passionate advocate for legal reform of their treatment in the criminal justice system. The video was designed to increase the competence and proficiency of professionals and advocates and discussed key recommendations, including the first and immediate steps attorneys should take when assigned a maternal infanticide case.

PSI CHECKLIST FOR ATTORNEYS

The legal checklist provided in Table 15–1 serves as a guide for attorneys to highlight essential and practical steps for developing an informed defense supported by evidence-based research and best practices.

CONSULTATION WITH LEGAL AND MENTAL HEALTH PROFESSIONALS

In recognition of the importance of making legal resources available to families and professionals, PSI is enhancing its Justice and Advocacy Program by developing a national consultation line for legal and mental health professionals. PSI already operates a national Perinatal Psychiatric Consult Line that offers consultation services to medical and psychiatric providers at no cost. The legal resources line will follow that model and offer legal and mental health professionals an opportunity to speak with experts about legal issues related to maternal infanticide as well as custody cases related to maternal mental illness. The legal resources line will be staffed by attorneys and macrolevel social workers. Macrolevel social workers engage at the community or systems level to improve social policies and practices and play an essential role in raising awareness and sharing resources with families and providers. They will provide available legal resources, including the PSI list of defense attorneys, licensed perinatal mental health professionals trained as expert witnesses, and law clinics at various universities and nonprofit organizations that can provide additional supportive resources.

Next Steps for the Yates Children Memorial Fund Justice and Advocacy Program

In addition to the PSI Legal Toolkit, development of legal resources, initiating a national consultation phone line, and establishing the expert witness training program, a future initiative will be to provide training for front-line community providers, including first responders in law enforcement, emergency medicine, and child protective services. This protocol will follow guidelines of mental health first aid and crisis intervention response teams across the United States; licensed behavioral health professionals will be paired with a trained crisis-intervention team to respond to calls involving mothers in serious mental health crisis. The PSI training for first responders and police officers will provide foundational understanding of the range of maternal mental health disorders, their prevalence, and the signs and symptoms to look for when going on a call pertaining to a mother in a mental health crisis. With the appropriate information, first responders will know better how to deal with various crises and to provide necessary input when working with others who come to the scene. First responders are critical fact witnesses because they are the most immediate individuals who interact with the mother at the scene. Their account of how she presented can make a significant difference in the criminal investigation.

Policy and Advocacy

The next long-term goal for PSI is to establish a stronger presence surrounding legislative advocacy for women with maternal mental illness and PPP by following state and national legislative initiatives. In these efforts, PSI will collect pertinent research and support legislation that improves the proper defense and evidence-based treatment of women with perinatal mental illness. Likewise, we will include a list of past or current legislative initiatives in the United States concerning maternal mental illness and PPP (both passed and failed), gather information concerning other countries' legislative progress, research legislation for the upcoming session, and promote awareness of PSI's legislative advocacy. Our network of support coordinators and chapters and the Postpartum Psychosis Task Force will assist with advocacy and outreach by supporting survivors who wish to speak to legislators and offer testimony on maternal mental health bills. Working with other organizations and advocates, PSI will continue its work to improve access and increase preventive efforts in the proper treatment and legal representation of women accused of filicide crimes related to perinatal mental illness.

MAIN CLINICAL/LEGAL POINTS AND CULTURAL PERSPECTIVES

- Postpartum mental health issues are essential to consider in maternal infanticide/filicide cases. Postpartum Support International (PSI) advocates for revisions of American legal standards and insanity laws so that contemporary neuroscience and psychiatry inform current definitions of sanity and guilt.

- Despite accumulated knowledge gained over the years, health care and mental health providers continue to miss warning signs of postpartum psychiatric illnesses that can lead to maternal filicide, which afflicts our most vulnerable populations in health care.

- The PSI *Position Paper on Psychosis-Related Tragedies*, which is available at www.postpartum.net/professionals/perinatal-psychosis-related-tragedies, was written following the 2004 Annual Conference held in Chicago, Illinois and published on the PSI website.

- The work of the PSI Justice and Advocacy Program is divided into three main components: 1) resources and outreach; 2) education; and 3) policy and advocacy. All are necessary elements of PSI's goal to ameliorate troubling legal issues for women and to equip legal and mental health professionals with resources to address maternal mental illness in the criminal justice system.

- The PSI Legal Toolkit is an excellent guide for legal professionals and advocates taking on cases involving perinatal mental illness. The toolkit contains a checklist for attorneys and a 17-minute informative video to guide them through practical steps to develop an informed defense supported by evidence-based research and best practices.

- PSI professional educational materials emphasize that immediate and early engagement of a trained crisis intervention team is critical to ensure proper response to psychiatric symptoms and the impact of those symptoms on rational functioning and judgment.

- In recognition of the importance of making legal resources available to families and professionals, PSI is enhancing its Justice and Advocacy Program by developing a national consultation line for legal and mental health professionals. The legal resources line will allow legal and mental health professionals to speak with an expert about legal issues related to maternal infanticide as well as custody cases related to maternal mental illness.

Practice and Discussion Questions

1. In your professional practice, what key role do you (or could you) play in cases of maternal infanticide or filicide?
2. What kind of resources do you wish you had to prepare or to fulfill your role successfully?
3. Are you familiar with legal resources related to perinatal mental illness in your area?
4. Are you familiar with case histories pertaining to maternal infanticide or filicide?
5. Do you feel confident that you know the steps it takes to advocate for your client?

References

American Psychiatric Association: Diagnostic and Statistical Manual of Mental Disorders, 5th Edition. Arlington, VA, American Psychiatric Association, 2013

Butterfield J: Blue mourning: postpartum psychosis and the criminal insanity defense—waking to the reality of women who kill their children. John Marshall Law Review 39.2:515–535, 2006

Postpartum Support International: PSI Statement on Psychosis Related Tragedies. Portland, OR, Postpartum Support International, 2004. Available at: https://www.postpartum.net/wp-content/uploads/2014/11/PSI-position-statement-perinatal-psychosis-related-tragedies-2016.pdf. Accessed November 10, 2019.

Spinelli M: Infanticide. Psychosocial and Legal Perspectives on Mothers Who Kill. Washington, DC, American Psychiatric Publishing, 2003

Taylor V, Leitz L: From infanticide to activism: the transformation of emotions and identity in self-help movements, in Social Movements and the Transformation of American Health Care. Edited by Banaszak-Holl J, Levitsky SR, Zald MN. Oxford University Press, 2010, pp 266–284

Toufexis A: Why mothers kill their babies. Time, June 20, 1988

CLINICAL CASES

Application of Foundations and Practical Considerations

CHAPTER 16

Clinical Case 1: The Dark Side of Mother

A CLINICAL CASE IN ITALY

Nicoletta Giacchetti, M.D., Ph.D.

Liliana Lorettu, M.D.

Guido Maria Lattanzi, M.D.

Franca Aceti, M.D.

For 14 years, a service dedicated to perinatal psychopathology has been available at Policlinico Umberto I–Sapienza, University of Rome. In this public outpatient service, which is dedicated to pregnant women and those who have given birth within the past year, two psychiatrists work continuously, supported by residents in psychiatry from the University of Rome and two volunteer psychologists. Each patient is followed up with individual interviews, group therapy, and, if necessary, prescription medication. All women are seen at least once with their child. Furthermore, consultation with a child psychiatrist who is an expert in the early stages of child development is available to assess mother–child interaction. During their periodic visits, mothers are also referred to community psychiatric services and family consultants to ensure continuity of care and intervention even after the first year of the child's life. Dr. Giacchetti and Dr. Lattanzi are enrolled as clinical psychiatrists, and both are involved in research coordinated and supervised by Professor Aceti, our chief psychiatrist. Professor Lorettu is an assistant professor at the University of Sassari who collaborated with our team as a consultant for the medicolegal aspects of the case. We provide this narrative case to share our experience and vertex of observation on an exemplary case of maternal filicide.

In cases in which social difficulties are evident, a social worker from the polyclinic reports the situation to the social services of the local jurisdiction. If the mother or the entire sociofamily context in which she lives does not give sufficient reassurance to protect the safety and well-being of the child, the juvenile court becomes involved to monitor and decide which interventions are the most appropriate.

Theoretical Foundations

OUR RESEARCH IN FILICIDE

Along with clinical work at the University of Rome, we research various issues related to perinatal psychic distress, one of which was the topic of filicide. We found that some women showed high levels of ambivalence toward their own children that was expressed through thoughts of harming and even killing the children, although it was quite rare for the women to act on these thoughts. Data from the literature showed that in industrialized countries the overall rate of filicide ranges between 2 and 10 per 100,000 (Craig 2004; Wolkind et al. 1993) and that a percentage of up to 10% of women with postpartum depression have anticonservative (suicidal) thoughts; moreover, up to 61% of women are tormented in the most serious episodes by thoughts of harming their children (Chandra et al. 2002).

Intrusive thoughts of intentionally harming one's child are present in about half of new mothers (Fairbrother and Woody 2008). These manifestations, while not particularly worrisome for people without psychiatric disorders, are a source of considerable distress for mothers with depression, anxiety, and OCD in the postpartum period. In a sample of healthy women who had recently given birth, an association between a personality feature in which psychoticism was the predominant dimension and the possible onset of thoughts of harming the child was reported (Gutiérrez-Zotes et al. 2013). However, no evidence has proven that the presence of intrusive thoughts of harming represents a specific risk factor for child abuse or neglect (Brok et al. 2017; Fairbrother and Woody 2008; Wisner et al. 2003).

Filicide research stems precisely from the need to detect any common aspects, even in the personality structure, among mothers who commit filicide. These could differentiate them from other mothers, with or without depression, and be defined as a set of risk factors to be used preventively. For this purpose, we interviewed 19 mothers who had committed filicide within the past 10 years. We believe the following case is paradigmatic of the complexity of these clinical situations. Although mothers do not always have relevant psychopathological conditions in the period prior to taking the lives of their children, and the act appears to be unpredictable, the case we share represents a mother who had previously shown some psychic distress features but none that gave rise to suspicion of violent acting out. Some considerations can be made that will encourage clinicians and those involved in the criminal investigation (e.g., judge, jury) to consider carefully the whole history of the patient.

Case Conceptualization

THE FILICIDAL EVENT

After separating from her husband, Greta[1] normally spent New Year's Eve with their son. In 2014, when he was 8 years old, Greta decided she wanted to spend Christmas with him instead. She recalled that she had prostituted herself for the first time in her life, some days before Christmas, to obtain funds to buy her son a gift. She previously had sworn to herself that she would never prostitute herself because she "sought the feeling" (emotional connection) in sexual relations.

On December 24th, after spending the day exchanging wishes with several people, including the parents of her ex-husband, she returned home with her son. Her ex-husband accompanied them, having noticed that Greta was becoming progressively more silent and was smiling less than usual. In recent days the ex-husband had sent a request to the court for exclusive custody of his son due to the explosive behavior Greta had demonstrated in the years since their separation. Greta found out about the request and had become very alarmed and upset, so much so that a psychiatrist from the mental health center had initiated long-acting haloperidol therapy (50 mg) a few days before the crime.

Greta prepared the Christmas Eve dinner, during which the boy insisted on opening his gift early, emphasizing it was "just me and you." After denying him initially, she eventually agreed, but she reported that she could not "stand" the emotional impact generated by the sudden joy shown by the child upon opening the gift. She revealed that, in that moment, she had felt deeply alone and in need of "cuddles." Greta asked

---

[1]A pseudonym for the mother, who provided oral and written consent to the anonymous use of her data.

her son to hug her and to stay close to her, but the child, in the euphoria of the moment, did not pay attention to her. She then went to the kitchen and grabbed the knife; from that moment on, she stated having very confused memories.

Greta only realized what was happening after the last stab, the eighth —a number equivalent to her son's age. She recalled kissing him as soon as he died. "He smiled at me as if he was saying, 'Thank you, Mother. If you hadn't done it, I would have.'" Shocked by what she had done, and in a confused state, she had alerted a neighbor, recognizing herself as perpetrator of the crime. For several weeks after the crime, Greta did not express feelings of guilt for what had happened, claiming she could hear the voice of her son reassuring her, forgiving her, and repeating that if she had not killed him, he would have been killed by his father or would have killed himself.

PATIENT HISTORY

Greta was 3 years older than her sister. Growing up, their father worked as a cook and was often absent from home due to work demands. When he was at home, he was authoritarian and violent with both his wife and his daughters. Greta remembered that he sometimes used "strong" methods (e.g., repeatedly hitting her with the belt of his pants) when she did not want to go to school. Greta's mother, a housewife, came from a wealthy family who was native of another region of Italy, and she had never truly integrated in the new social context. She described her mother as a "regularly" depressed person who spent whole days in bed, in the dark, and could not be disturbed. Greta never understood why her mother had to be secluded. Her mother could also be very unpredictable. One day, when Greta was about 9 years old, her mother threatened her with a knife for a futile reason. Then, when Greta was 10, her mother was hospitalized for a presumable depressive state.

Greta described herself as having poor aptitude for studies. She had stopped going to school when she was 14 years old. She had been a lively child and, even if introverted, loved dancing. She had never used illicit drugs. After Greta dropped out of school, she worked various jobs, first as a saleswoman and later as a pastry chef, bartender, and a go-go dancer in clubs. When Greta was 16 years old and working in one of the clubs, she met a man who was doing his military service, whom she would later marry. She said that she felt very sad at times, especially between the ages of 15 and 16, so much so that she cut her wrists and, another time, planned to ingest a disproportionate number of drugs. In both cases, she stopped herself, fearing death.

At age 17, Greta moved to her partner's city and initially lived at his parents' house. Greta described how tiring her integration in the new social context was and that she had frequent quarrels with her boyfriend's mother. She never felt valued; she was criticized by the mother and felt "exploited" for the housework she had to do. Within a year, Greta finally found a job at the local factory. Then, at the age of 21, she and her partner began living together on their own. They were married when she was 23 years old.

Greta became pregnant when she was 26. During the second month of pregnancy, she received the news that her mother had died by drowning. She was certain it was a suicide, although the dynamic of what happened was never completely determined. She described that period as the most dramatic of her life. She felt extremely sad and apathetic and spent whole days in bed. Greta was aggravated by a sense of responsibility toward the newborn baby and by tension with her spouse and mother-in-law. She perceived her mother-in-law as attempting to replace her in caring for her son. After her own mother's alleged suicide, Greta was less able to rebel and decidedly less able to carry out her usual social and work activities.

Then, at the age of 28 (when her son was 2 years old), she was admitted to a psychiatric ward for the first time due to an anxious-depressive state that was traced to feelings of jealousy toward her husband. Greta was diagnosed with postpartum depression. She remembered that she would sometimes hear the voice of her husband talking to his lover and that his voice sounded as though it were coming from outside, although she admitted being aware it actually came from her inner world. Greta was taking antidepressants, antipsychotics, and mood stabilizers, and she had received many diagnoses over the years: mood disorder not otherwise specified, chronic delusional disorder, major depressive disorder, and schizoaffective disorder.

Around the time of her first hospitalization for mental health, the marital relationship was deteriorating. Greta was having violent outbursts that often would result in quarrels with her husband. During one of these episodes, he threatened to throw her out of the window and hit her so violently that her eardrum was perforated, resulting in permanent hearing loss. On that occasion, she preferred not to go to the emergency department "so as not to ruin her husband"—not only did she not want him to be charged but she was also highly dependent on him and could not stand to be apart.

However, Greta did not tolerate her husband's disparaging attitude toward their son. The child had a motor and language development impairment; he was being followed by a speech therapist and had been assigned a support teacher at school. "My husband wanted a perfect child ....He used to call him an idiot, and he said he was an idiot like me," she said. When she was 31 years old, they separated, and she was given custody of their son, although her ex-husband and his parents often visited.

During the postseparation period, Greta was hospitalized three times in a psychiatric ward due to dysphoric states that resulted in aggression and at times in delusional ideas of jealousy. She did not tolerate the separation from her husband. However, she was able to continue working, with the assistance of outpatient services that facilitated her job placement. The year before the filicide incident, she was hospitalized against her will because she had punched her mother-in-law and destroyed numerous household ornaments. Greta had reacted with violence to a belief that her mother-in-law was interfering in her son's education.

Discussion

After the crime, Greta was admitted to a psychiatric ward. She was later discharged from the ward with a diagnosis of "schizoaffective disorder, multiple episodes, currently in acute episode." DSM-5 indicates "an individual may have pronounced auditory hallucinations and persecutory delusions for 2 months before the onset of a prominent major depressive episode" (American Psychiatric Association 2013, p. 108). This confirmed what was recorded in the expert witness's report.

Without a doubt, Greta's psychopathological debut could be traced back to the period of pregnancy and postpartum (8–9 years prior to the index episode), when she had developed a depressive condition attributable both to the drowning of her mother by presumable suicide and to the birth of her child. Since that period, her life had never been the same. These two "Schlüsselerlebnisse" (key events), as Kretschmer would call them (Kretschmer 1918, p. 138), had trigged her identity fragility. Up to that point, the fragility had lain dormant, managed by defense mechanisms within a psychotic type of functioning. By definition, psychotic functioning is characterized by a deficit in the structure of the self—that is, the person fails to differentiate the self from the other, which is experienced as an integral part of the self in a fusional relationship. This type of functioning cannot differentiate the internal world from the external one, and delirious-hallucinatory realities and fantasies often merge (Scalabrini et al. 2018).

Greta had lived since birth in a context that was not caring (with an absent and chronically depressed mother and a disengaged and rigid father) and had induced her to represent herself as a wary child and a shy teenager while at the same time being a lively person who liked dancing and going out. Her father had responded violently to her provocative refusal to follow his rules (curfews, school attendance), which contributed to the violent, deadly, and neglecting environment. This cycle was persistent: Greta coped by being social and defiant to her father, which triggered his anger, which necessitated Greta's coping.

Greta had always had a good relationship with her mother ("we got along very well"), showing a strong idealization of her. Nevertheless, Greta was unable to provide adequate examples of episodes of maternal care from her mother, and she had emancipated herself from her family very early on, moving to another city (and another family) to follow her husband. Her mother's death had occurred during Greta's pregnancy, which triggered the ambivalence she had likely encapsulated in an area outside her consciousness, leaving her at the mercy of her own "ghosts" (Fraiberg et al. 1999). Several elements of identification with personality traits of her mother emerged. Greta also described, in a more or less conscious way, shared terms and styles in their relationship and their personal stories: both women had not completely adjusted to their social environment; both had unpredictable bursts of anger within the family; both had established highly dependent relationships with their husbands; and both had spent many days in bed due to their low mood.

From a psychopathological perspective, a personal and family history of psychiatric disorders or a personality disorder represents an additional vulnerability (Friedman et al. 2005; Giacchetti et al. 2019; Lysell et al. 2014; Resnick 1969). A psychotic defense mechanism such as denial, splitting, or projective identification is not uncommon in these contexts and was undeniably present in our reconstruction of Greta's history.

PSYCHOMETRIC EVALUATION

Adult Attachment Interview

The Adult Attachment Interview (AAI; Main and Goldwyn 1984) is a semistructured interview designed to assess adult attachment. Greta constantly denied the neglect she experienced in childhood and instead portrayed an idealized view of her parents. She was assessed as having the following attachment profile: unclassifiable, cannot classify, accompanied by failed processing of traumatic and mournful experiences (unresolved with respect to loss and trauma), abbreviated as U/CC/Ds1/E1 (unclassifiable/cannot classify/dismissing 1/entangled 1). The "cannot classify" category referred precisely to the presence of contradictory mental states with respect to attachment (Ds1 and E1) that could not be integrated and thus tended to reactivate in a fragmented manner characterized by dissociated states of mind. The representations of her relationship with her parents emerged in a contradictory manner and were split and difficult to integrate, giving the impression that these disconnected states of mind were fully embodied within her. These fragmented representations of the mind defined the strategies of dissociation and the compartmentalization of some complexes of experiences, representations, and affections. This is the result of traumatic experiences that split consciousness due to their traumatic potential, thus threatening personality integration (Bromberg 2001).

Traumatic Experience Checklist

We administered the Traumatic Experience Checklist (Nijenhuis et al. 2002; see Figure 16–1) to Greta. Her score was 9, which put her within the range (0–12) of "fairly pathological." The categories with the highest scores were those related to bodily threats (BT): BT1 (physical abuse) plus BT2 (threats to life, pain, bizarre punishments) (a total of 10), and emotional neglect (4).

Childhood Trauma Questionnaire

This result was confirmed by the Childhood Trauma Questionnaire (Pennebaker and Susman 1988; see Figure 16–2). Greta showed the highest scores in neglect-related scales, both emotional neglect (13) and physical neglect (11), whereas the scales relating to emotional abuse (7) and sexual abuse (5) were basically within normal range (pathological range between 5 and 25).

Big Five Inventory

Personality tests highlighted Greta's tendency to provide an image of herself as available, pleasant, and reliable toward others despite her own introversion and shyness and a tendency to experience difficulties in impulse and affection control within a fragile identity structure. The Big Five Inventory (John et al. 1991; Figure 16–3) profile was characterized by high levels of openness (score 40) associated with features of neuroticism (34), agreeableness (33), and conscientiousness (31). Extraversion elements were less marked (25).

Temperament and Character Inventory–Revised

The Temperament and Character Inventory–Revised (Cloninger et al. 1993; Figure 16–4) showed high scores on the scales of novelty seeking (120) and cooperativity (116), followed by persistence (108), harm avoidance (107), self-directedness (107), and reward dependence (105). Signifi-

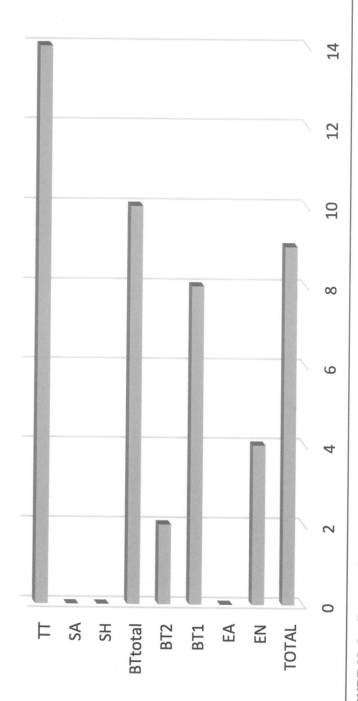

FIGURE 16–1. Traumatic Experience Checklist profile.

BTtotal=total bodily threat; BT1=bodily threat 1 (including physical abuse); BT2=bodily threat 2 (including threat to life, pain, bizarre punishments); EA=emotional abuse; EN=emotional neglect; SA=sexual abuse; SH=sexual harassment; TT=total trauma score.

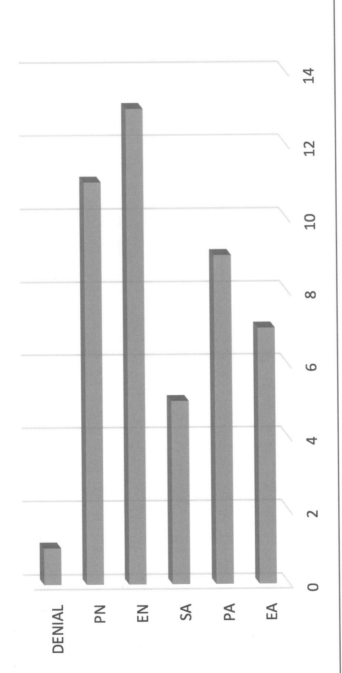

FIGURE 16–2.   Childhood Trauma Questionnaire profile.

DENIAL=possible underreporting of maltreatment; EA=emotional abuse; EN=emotional neglect; PA=physical abuse; PN=physical neglect; SA=sexual abuse.

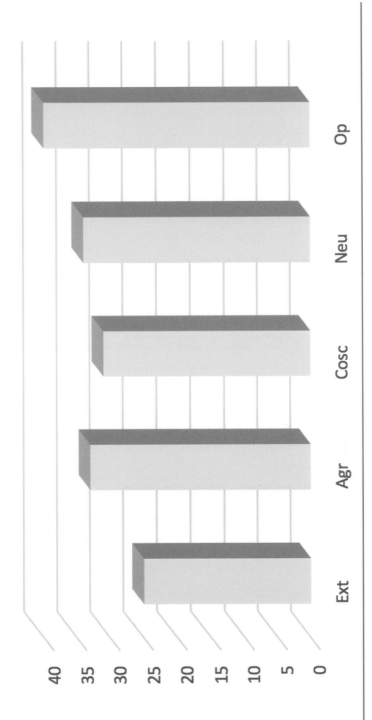

FIGURE 16–3. Big Five Inventory profile.

Agr=agreeableness; Cosc=conscientiousness; Ext=extroversion; Neu=neuroticism; Op=openness.

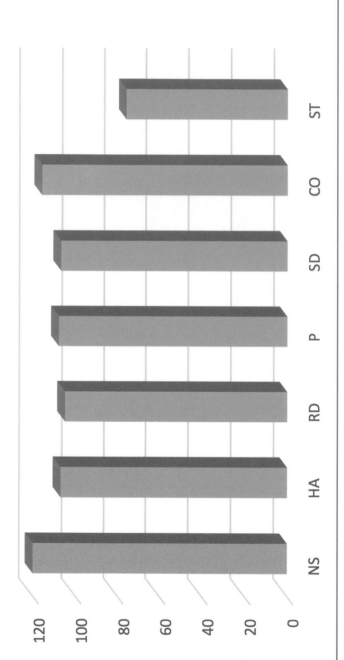

FIGURE 16–4.   Temperament and Character Inventory-Revised profile.

CO=cooperativity; HA=harm avoidance; NS=novelty seeking; P=persistence; RD=reward dependence; SD=self-directedness; ST=self-transcendence.

cantly lower scores were those on the self-transcendence dimension (76). These characteristics could lead to the hypothesis of a borderline type of functioning, in which the high harm avoidance score, associated with the high novelty seeking score, allowed us to differentiate Greta's profile from an antisocial profile. Antisocial profiles most frequently show extremely low scores on harm avoidance. This confirmed her ability to deal with risk, leading to her impulsiveness and aggression (novelty seeking) that led not to anxiety but to acting with coldness. Greta was an impulsive and irritable—but at the same time shy and anxious—person who sought social contact and approval within the relational context, even at the cost of being complacent (reward dependence). She needed others, on whom she depended and to whom she was available (cooperativity), carrying out her commitments with determination (persistence; Greta had always been a hard worker), but she relied mainly on herself, so as to assume rebellious and challenging attitudes toward authority figures when forced to execute an order (self-directedness; e.g., her attitude toward her father and her mother-in-law).

Minnesota Multiphasic Personality Inventory–2

Greta's personality profile was overall represented by the Minnesota Multiphasic Personality Inventory–2 (Butcher et al. 1989). A dysfunctional pattern of a chronic nature emerged on an emotional basis usually found in schizoaffective or bipolar disorders. This picture (Figure 16–5) was characterized by both severe psychopathological elements and outstanding components of Cluster B personality disorder, with elements of antisociality, impulsivity, and poorly controlled aggression. In stressful situations, she could become confusional, with persecutory or grandiose ideas, feelings of unreality, and consequently reduced emotional capacity.

From a psychodynamic point of view, it was possible to hypothesize that the identity reorganization that pertained to the perinatal period had elicited both subjective and relational difficulties. The couple's conflict had been amplified by the transition to having a child (triangularity), causing Greta to experience feelings of loss and loneliness. The difficult relationship with her parents already had led her to leave the family home while still an adolescent and move to the family of her partner. The emotional neglect of her family of origin reappeared in the form of harming fantasies in her acquired family, where the relationship with her mother-in-law was characterized initially by a subjective experience of "exploitation for the housework," then by intrusion in the life of the couple, and finally of exclusion from the management of her child. Her lack of trust in the support of emotional relationships shifted from her primary to her

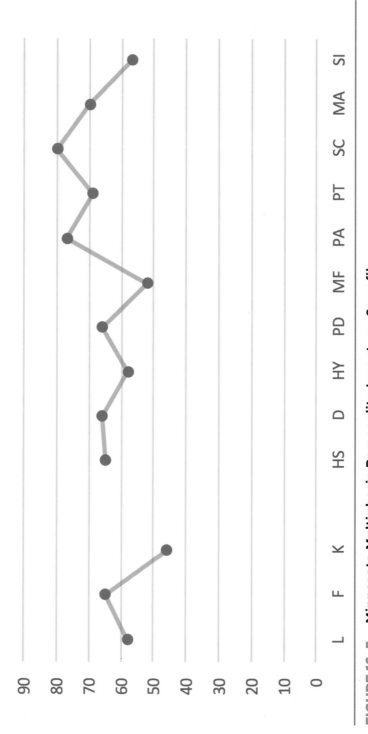

FIGURE 16–5. Minnesota Multiphasic Personality Inventory–2 profile.

D=depression; F=frequency; HS=hypochondria; HY=hysteria; K=correction; L=lie; MA=mania; MF=masculinity/femininity; PA=paranoia; PD=psychopathic deviation; PT=psychasthenia; SC=schizophrenia; SI=social introversion.

current bonds and then declined within the couple. Her jealousy about her husband over time led to an escalation in conflict, including violent acts. Perverse dynamics of insolence with her father to seek his love and attention and feelings of alienation from her mother tended to come back throughout Greta's life. For example, the episode of her eardrum being perforated during a quarrel with her husband was paradigmatic of this victim–perpetrator relational scheme. Greta prostituting herself to buy a Christmas gift for her son also represented an unconscious victimizing behavior that was consciously justified by her need for money.

After spending the afternoon exchanging Christmas wishes with her friends and relatives, Greta had returned home with her son in an atmosphere of profound solitude that was amplified by the anguish aroused by her ex-husband's request for exclusive custody of their child. The joy expressed by the child, along with the frustration caused by his lack of attention to her need for emotional closeness ("lack of cuddles"), was likely experienced by Greta as a traumatic abandonment. The response to her needs during childhood had been unpredictable or rejecting, and her son's demands could have been experienced as persecutory, thus becoming the container for her projected hate. The needs of the child evoked her experience of "impotence," to which she reacted by activating schizoparanoid angst. By identifying herself with the persecutor, she became the perpetrator, and by projectively identifying the child with her persecutor, she became the victim. In both cases, the persecutory behavior—identified in herself or projected onto the child—could have led to violent fantasies or acts, restaging abandonment relationships in which subjective experience was overwhelmed by the emptiness of the relationship.

PSYCHIATRIC FORENSIC ASPECTS

General Considerations

In Italian criminal law, the specific crime of filicide is not considered. The killing of one's own child by the mother or father is regarded as equivalent to the crime of voluntary homicide and is punished according to Article 575 and following of the Penal Code, which identifies the family relationship as an aggravating circumstance. Filicide is considered different from murder of the child caused by a conflict between the parents and adult children and from the killing of a newborn, which configures the crime of infanticide (Fornari 2008).

Filicide is recognized as an aggravating circumstance due to the family relationship with the victim, and from a dynamic point of view, it is often the peak of violent, intrafamilial behaviors perpetrated by parents toward their children. Although no "special treatment" is officially accorded to filicide, *de facto*, especially when mothers are the perpetrators of the crime, insanity or a partial insanity is often recognized as a factor and contributes to the application of reduced sentences or acquittal and admission to a residence for the execution of security measures (REMS) (Bramante 2005; Nivoli 2002, 2006).

Infanticide is recognized by the Italian Penal Code as a specific offense and is punished according to Article 578 of the Penal Code, which identifies it as "the induced death of the new-born immediately after birth or of the fetus during birth, by its own mother, when the fact is determined by conditions of material and moral abandonment connected to childbirth" (Altalex Editorial Staff 2019b). The term *neonaticide* is not prevalent in Italy; *infanticide* is the term for perpetrated death of a child by the mother within the infant's first 24 hours of life. From a legal point of view, infanticide as indicated in the Italian Penal Code has three specific characteristics:

1. Infanticide is considered a less serious crime than voluntary homicide, and the difficult moral and material circumstances in which it occurs are recognized. The applicable penalties are therefore decidedly reduced compared with those for voluntary murder.
2. The perpetrator is identified exclusively as the mother: only mothers can commit infanticide. If others help the mother commit the crime, they are seen as responsible for voluntary homicide, not infanticide.
3. The crime of infanticide occurs at a precise and restricted time—immediately after childbirth, when the victim is a newborn, or during childbirth, when the victim is still a fetus. Greta, for example, was not charged with infanticide but with homicide due to her son's age.

With regard to the ascertainment of criminal responsibility and to the more purely procedural aspects (e.g., ascertainment of commission of the crime, ascertainment of the material causal relationship between the conduct and the occurred event), see Italian criminal law and forensic psychopathology texts (Bandini and Rocca 2010; Mantovani 2007; Nivoli et al. 2019).

Concerning filicide and infanticide, in almost all cases we use the psychiatric evaluation to understand whether the mother was attributable at the time of the index event. Articles 85, 88, and 89 of the Penal Code outline the area of *imputability*: "No one can be punished for a fact foreseen by the law as a crime, if he was not responsible at the time he committed it. Whoever is in full possession of their faculties is imputable" (Altalex Editorial Staff 2019a, Article 85). Also, "[i]t is not imputable who, at the time when they committed the act was, due to insanity, in such a state of mind as not to be in full possession of their faculties" (Altalex Editorial Staff 2019a, Article 88), rendering individuals who were mentally ill at the time of the offense not fully accountable for the crime and therefore not sentenced to imprisonment but to therapeutic-rehabilitative interventions carried out within specific structures, such as the REMS: "Whoever committed the crime, if they were in such a state of mind that could greatly diminish their faculties, without excluding them, is responsible for the crime, but the penalty is reduced" (Altalex Editorial Staff 2019a, Article 89).

The nonimputability renders the perpetrator of the crime not punishable. Consequently, the mother is moved from a sanctioning system that applies a penalty as a consequence of the recognition of responsibility to another juridical dimension that must assess the presence of social dangerousness (i.e., the probability that the mother will commit other crimes in the future) (Padovani 1990). This is called a "double track system" (Bandini and Rocca 2010) that applies a penalty if liability is recognized and provides assessment of social danger and application of a safety measure if nonimputability is recognized. In Greta's case, she was found not culpable and was assessed for level of social danger.

Final Considerations

Greta's case fully reflects the complexity of evaluating a case of maternal filicide. It is useful to remember that the Italian penal system does not consider filicide a specific crime but considers it voluntary murder, aggravated by the degree of kinship. In cases such as this, mental pathology clearly prompted the dynamics of the crime; this was representative of the 19 cases we studied. We believe this case is paradigmatic of the complexity of these clinical situations; the judicial response should regard these factors in excluding a penalty/punishment for the filicidal offender and offer a therapeutic rehabilitative path instead. Indeed, this is the general practice in our penal system. When the ability to understand or know is absent or greatly diminished at the time of the crime, the person is considered not responsible for the crime. This is true even without psychosis present, for example, in the case of a serious personality disorder. The presentation is often brief transient psychotic symptoms, not showing a frank psychiatric disorder.

On the other hand, in contexts in which the motive of filicide is not due to a psychiatric condition (or altruistic reasons) but rather to fatal maltreatment, unwanted child, or spousal revenge (Resnick 2016), the judicial system and outcome of findings will yield a different result. Accordingly, the forensic evaluation needs to be accurate, unbiased by the details of the crime, and performed by an expert professional trained to identify psychopathology as well as the presentation and profile of the accused when the motive did not involve mental illness.

Mothers or mothers to be who are frightened or doubtful about motherhood are often told that "it will come naturally." However, precisely because it *is* a natural event, motherhood can bring to the surface aspects not visible from the outside that are split, removed, or denied because they are not compatible with the external image one wants to present to feel approved by others. Filicide is an event that leaves one appalled and is usually quickly dismissed by public opinion as the extreme act of a sick or psychopathic mind, to be punished to the full extent. Filicide can also be viewed as a representation of a society's failure to protect the safety and right to life of an innocent person and to support the fragility of a mother who collapses, instead of "being happy" and conforming to what is "natural," and is overwhelmed by the emotional short circuit of the mind triggered by the perinatal process.

Greta now is a 40-year-old woman who has undergone treatment for about 4 years at the REMS. At the time of our evaluation at the REMS in May 2019, she appeared as a slight, smiling woman, open to dialogue. She relayed the facts of the day of the filicide with emotional detachment, failing to explain what drove her to stabbing her son. "I was sick, and then I don't know what happened," she claimed. She was on medication at the time of the interview, including venlafaxine, lithium, and promazine, and she believed that at the end of her time at REMS she would be able to rebuild her life. Only her father, who currently had a new wife, and her sister would sporadically visit her. We are grateful for her willingness to share her story.

MAIN CLINICAL/LEGAL POINTS AND CULTURAL PERSPECTIVES

- Greta's case is descriptive of the method of management, from a judicial point of view, of a case of filicide in Italy. Police found Greta *in flagrante delicto*, in a confusional state, showing disorganized language and behavior and delusional ideation after taking the life of her 8-year-old son.

- The judge examined the case and found several elements indicative of a presumable nonimputability for the reason of insanity, such as the presence of psychopathology at the time of the commission of the act, Greta's psychiatric history, and the particular cruelty of the offense. Therefore, he requested a psychiatric evaluation by a forensic psychiatrist as technical consultant.

- This evaluation was supported by a partial technical consultant selected by Greta's lawyer. The two technical consultants examined Greta's clinical records and the documents found in the judicial file in order to detect recent life events that could have played a role in triggering the filicide. They also performed multiple clinical interviews with Greta. The persistence of psychopathology was hence confirmed.

- In Italy, in almost all cases of filicide and infanticide a psychiatric evaluation is required to assess the imputability and social danger of the person. When the ability to understand or know at the time of the crime is absent or greatly diminished, the person is considered not responsible for the crime. This is true even without psychosis, for example in the case of postpartum depression and a serious personality disorder.

- The judge accepted the technicians' report and found Greta not imputable on the basis of a diagnosis of psychotic episode in bipolar schizoaffective disorder. Greta was also found to pose a social danger and sent to a forensic psychiatric facility to carry out the safety measure ruled by the judge.

- Our research group confirmed the presence of a pervasive psychiatric pathology years after the crime with comprehensive psychiatric interviews, which supported the hypothesis of persecutory behavior in a context of projected schizoid fears due to severe disruptions in personality structure and attachment patterns, as assessed by the Adult Attachment Interview and other psychometric evaluations.

References

Altalex Editorial Staff: Of the crimes against the person. Criminal Code, Book II, Title XII. Altalex.com, 2019a. Available at: https://www.altalex.com/documents/news/2014/10/28/dei-delitti-contro-la-persona. Accessed December 13, 2019.

Altalex Editorial Staff: Of the offender and of the person offended by the crime. Criminal Code, Book I, Title IV. Altalex.com, 2019b. Available at: https://www. altalex.com/documents/news/2015/01/15/del-reo-e-della-persona-offesa-dal-reato. Accessed December 12, 2019.

American Psychiatric Association: Diagnostic and Statistical Manual of Mental Disorders, 5th Edition. Arlington, VA, American Psychiatric Association, 2013

Bandini T, Rocca G: Fondamenti di Psicopatologia Forense. Milan, Italy, Giuffrè, 2010

Bramante A: Fare e Disfare…Dall'Amore alla Distruttività. Il Figlicidio Materno. Milan, Italy, Aracne, 2005

Brok EL, Lok P, Oosterbaan DB, et al: Infant-related intrusive thoughts of harm in the postpartum period: a critical review. J Clin Psychiatry 78(8):e913–e923, 2017

Bromberg PH: Standing in the Spaces: Essays on Clinical Process Trauma and Dissociation. Abingdon-on-Thames, England, Routledge, 2001

Butcher JN, Dahlstrom WG, Graham JR, et al: Minnesota Multiphasic Personality Inventory–2 (MMPI-2): Manual for Administration and Scoring. Minneapolis, MN, University of Minnesota Press, 1989

Chandra P, Venkatasubramanian G, Thomas T: Infanticidal ideas and infanticidal behavior in Indian women with severe postpartum psychiatric disorders. J Nerv Ment Dis 190(7):457–461, 2002

Cloninger C, Svrakic D, Przybeck T: A psychobiological model of temperament and character. Arch Gen Psychiatry 50(12):975–990, 1993

Craig M: Perinatal risk factors for neonaticide and infant homicide: can we identify those at risk? J R Soc Med 97(2):57–61, 2004

Fairbrother N, Woody S: New mothers' thoughts of harm related to the newborn. Arch Womens Ment Health 11:221–229, 2008

Fornari U: Trattato di Psichiatria Forense. Torino, Italy, UTET, 2008

Fraiberg SE, Adelson V, Shapiro I: I fantasmi nella stanza dei bambini, in Il Sostegno allo Sviluppo. Milan, Italy, Cortina Raffaello, 1999

Friedman S, Horwitz S, Resnick P: Child murder by mothers: a critical analysis of the current state of knowledge and a research agenda. Am J Psychiatry 162(9):1578–1587, 2005

Giacchetti N, Roma P, Pancheri C, et al: Personality traits in a sample of Italian filicide mothers. Riv Psichiatr 54(2):67–74, 2019

Gutiérrez-Zotes J, Farnós A, Vilella E, Labad J: Higher psychoticism as a predictor of thoughts of harming one's infant in postpartum women: a prospective study. Compr Psychiatry 54(7):1124–1129, 2013

John O, Donahue E, Kentle R: The Big-Five Inventory, Version 4a and 54. Berkeley, CA, Berkeley Institute of Personality and Social Research, University of California, 1991

Kretschmer E: Der Sensitive Beziehungswahn. Berlin, Germany, Springer, 1918

Lysell H, Runeson B, Lichtenstein P, Langstrom N: Risk factors for filicide and homicide: 36-year national matched cohort study. J Clin Psychiatry 75(2):127–132, 2014

Main M, Goldwyn R: Predicting rejection of her infant from mother's representation of her own experience: implications for the abused-abusing intergenerational cycle. Child Abuse Negl 8(2):203–217, 1984

Mantovani F: Diritto Penale. Padova, Italy, Cedam, 2007

Nijenhuis ERS, Van der Hart O, Kruger K: The psychometric characteristics of the Traumatic Experiences Questionnaire (TEC): first findings among psychiatric outpatients. Clin Psychol Psychother 9(3):200–210, 2002

Nivoli GC: Medea Tra Noi. Le Madri Che Uccidono il Proprio Figlio. Rome, Italy, Carocci, 2002

Nivoli GC: Il Perito e il Consulente di Parte in Psichiatria Forense. Torino, Italy, CSE, 2006

Nivoli GC, Lorettu L, Milia P: Psichiatria Forense. Milan, Italy, Piccin, 2019

Padovani T: La pericolosità sociale sotto il profilo giuridico, in Trattato di Criminologia, Medicina Criminologica e Psichiatria Forense, Vol XIII. Edited by Ferracuti F. Milan, Italy, Giuffrè, 1990

Pennebaker JW, Susman JR: Disclosure of traumas and psychosomatic processes. Soc Sci Med 26:327–332, 1988

Resnick P: Child murder by parents: a psychiatric review of filicide. Am J Psychiatry 126(3):325–334, 1969

Resnick PJ: Filicide in the United States. Indian J Psychiatry 58:S203–S209, 2016

Scalabrini A, Mucci C, Northoff G: Is our self related to personality? A neuropsychodynamic model. Front Hum Neurosci 4(12):346, 2018

Wisner L, Gracious B, Piontek C, et al: Postpartum disorders: phenomenology, treatment approaches, and relationship to infanticide, in Infanticide: Psychosocial and Legal Perspective on Mothers Who Kill. Edited by Spinelli MG. Washington, DC, American Psychiatric Publishing, 2003, pp 35–60

Wolkind S, Taylor E, Waite A, et al: Recurrence of unexpected infant death. Acta Paediatr 82(10):873–876, 1993

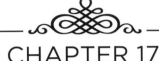

CHAPTER 17

Clinical Case 2: Falling Between the Cracks of Medical Care

A CASE OF INFANTICIDE IN SOUTH AFRICA

Ugasvaree Subramaney, M.B.B.Ch., FCPsych(SA), M.Med. (Psychiatry), B.Sc. (Psychology) (Hons), Ph.D.

Daniel Hoffman, B.A., B.A. (Psychology) (Hons), M.Sc. (Psychology), D.Phil.

In 2017, a family relations unit was established at Sterkfontein Hospital, which is affiliated with the University of the Witwatersrand Department of Psychiatry in Johannesburg, South Africa. This unit was formed in response to an unmet need identified by staff working in the forensic unit. Women who are mentally ill and referred for treatment at Sterkfontein Hospital following a serious criminal charge have challenges reintegrating with their families, especially with their young children. In particular, mentally ill filicidal mothers bear the brunt of stigma and shame. A senior psychologist dedicated to the forensic female ward is responsible for the therapeutic care at this fairly new service, and a forensic psychiatrist, nursing staff, and a social worker support the service at the hospital. Patients and their families are followed up with individual interviews, family therapy, and, if necessary, mother–child bonding therapeutic sessions. Medication for serious mental conditions are routinely managed by the forensic psychiatrist and trainee registrar/medical officer. Preparation for leaves of absence and referrals to community psychiatric services are also provided. In cases in which social difficulties are evident, the ward's social worker liaises with social services in the community as well as with the local jurisdiction. Applications are made to the court when it is thought that the woman is ready for discharge from the hospital.

Ugasvaree Subramaney is a forensic psychiatrist who has worked in the female forensic ward area for the past 12 years and with this family relations unit in particular for the past 2 years. Daniel Hoffman is the principal psychologist responsible for the psychological services and supervision of the psychologist who developed the service initially. The following clinical case represents a mother (MM) who committed infanticide in South Africa. She had an established diagnosis of bipolar disorder and was referred to us following the murder of her baby boy.

The Case of MM

BACKGROUND

MM was 29 years old at the time of the index offense. She had been born by normal delivery in May 1983, with no complications at birth, and had reached expected developmental milestones. MM did not have any behavioral problems; however, she had failed grade 1 due to premature enrollment. She was a very good student and had passed grade 12 with strong marks. Following high school, she attended college, where she attained certification in financial management. MM had worked at a marketing company for 1 month and then experienced mental health concerns; she had not returned to work since then. MM had no history of substance use, epilepsy, or head injury and no family history of mental illness, although she reported her mother to be depressed at times. At the time of the offense and hospital admission, she was living with her mother and siblings in Tembisa, a township in Johannesburg, South Africa. Her parents had an acrimonious divorce when she was 19 years old. Apart from witnessing constant arguments between her parents, she had no history of other childhood traumas or abuse.

MENTAL ILLNESS LEADING UP TO THE OFFENSE

In 2006, MM presented with the following symptoms: screaming, breaking things in the house, singing loudly, and running around naked. South African police officers took her to Tembisa Hospital, where she was admitted and diagnosed with bipolar disorder. She was prescribed lithium, orphenadrine, and risperidone. MM was compliant with treatment and took her medication every night. She also attended the outpatient clinic on a monthly basis and did well on this treatment regimen. In 2008, MM stopped her treatment on the advice of her local clinic doctor, who believed she could function without medication. In 2011, she became pregnant and was very excited and looked forward to being a mother.

During her pregnancy, MM was involved in a very unstable relationship with the father of her child. He was unsupportive and had many girlfriends and children with different women. Despite this, her excitement about becoming a new mother remained. MM was treated for a sexually transmitted disease while she was pregnant. Although much relationship turmoil remained, she stayed with the father of her baby until she was 7 months pregnant. At that time, she moved back to stay with her mother.

According to her mother, MM became very emotional (crying constantly) 2 days after the birth of her son in June 2012. Tembisa Hospital prescribed MM medication to help her with her overwhelming emotions, but the prescription was not enough to last the month. When she went back to the hospital to request more medication, she was referred to a clinic, who referred her back to Tembisa Hospital. At the hospital, the doctor insisted that the doctor at the clinic who first prescribed the medication should renew it. This process of going back and forth, with no one providing the medication MM needed, continued into August 2012, when her baby was 6 weeks old. By that point, MM had relapsed completely. She did not want to eat or sleep, was irritable and unable to cope with the baby crying, became disinterested in participating in activities or conversations, and lacked personal hygiene. She also began to isolate herself, spending most of the time alone in her bedroom, and became paranoid about her siblings, believing they were saying they hated her and did not want her to stay with their mother. MM was also hallucinating, talking and laughing to herself, but denied doing so when her mother asked whom she was talking to.

MM's mother reported that her daughter became very depressed and struggled to cope with the baby. Her mother worked full time and could not assist MM with the baby during the day. She made arrangements with her ex-husband, MM's father, to assist with the baby. He told her that he had a babysitter and that MM and the baby could stay at his home. Her mother took MM and the baby to the father's home on August 2, 2012. Her father's eldest sister (MM's aunt) often visited, and reported that MM had appeared normal when she arrived at her father's house on the evening before the offense occurred. MM later conveyed to her aunt that she was hearing voices. On the following day, MM and her father again went to the clinic to seek treatment.

THE INFANTICIDE OFFENSE

The day prior to the offense, MM remembered feeling she needed to be alone. She was not sleeping most nights and constantly felt tired and sad. Her baby cried often, no matter how much she tried to soothe and comfort him. MM's mother then decided it would be best if MM and the baby stayed on a full-time basis with her father. According to MM, she was taken by force, and her parents shared harsh words on that day. MM said that she felt hurt when her mother told her father that MM was his child and he must take care of her. Her father replied that he would take care of them. Later on, the baby began crying, and her father started praying for the baby. According to MM, her father was drunk and hostile toward her and ordered her to go to sleep. During the night, she went to her father for help with the baby. He became aggressive toward her and demanded that she go back to bed because he needed to complete the ancestral prayers.

The following morning, MM heard her half-brother ask her father about the baby lying on the sofa (her baby). Her father replied coldly, "It is a child." After hearing this, MM wept. She felt rejected, unimportant, and that her son was also being denied her father's love. Her father then helped her bathe her son, but they argued about the baby. Then he took her and the baby to his eldest sister and asked his sister to take care of the baby, without asking MM's permission. Her aunt said that she would find a woman in the township who could look after the boy. MM started to panic at the idea that a stranger would look after her child. She also felt scared to be living with her aunt, because MM did not see her as a caring person. She asked her father to take her to the nearest clinic because she did not feel well, but the clinic again informed her that they were unable to help without a referral letter from Tembisa Hospital. Her father took her back to the aunt's home.

Upon returning from work, the aunt discussed the house rules with MM. MM felt nervous and scared to live there, and when her aunt left to go out again, she was left alone with her baby and felt frightened. During that time, MM's paternal uncle came to see the baby. She asked if he would send a text to her mother asking her to come fetch her and her baby and to buy food for the baby. Her uncle promised he would send the message, but he never did. She recalled feeling very scared and did not know what to do with her baby. She went to the kitchen, where she obtained a knife, and then went to the room where the baby was sleeping and stabbed him in the chest. She said that the baby was crying and that she walked out to the street with the knife in her hand, looking for her aunt. She then sat down in the street and started crying. MM told a person passing by what she had done and asked the person to call the police. An unknown man overpowered her and took the knife. Her baby was rushed to a private physician for surgery, where he was declared dead.

IMMEDIATE: POST INFANTICIDE

MM was arrested by police and taken to the prison cells. The investigating officer reported that MM appeared normal but tired and answered questions relevantly. She told the officer that she had bipolar mood disorder. She did not want to talk about the offense. When her mother came to see her, MM could not recall stabbing her baby. During her mother's next visit, MM apologized for killing her baby and said that she wanted to die and deserved to remain in prison for what she did. Her mother reported that the wardens at prison said all the other inmates were afraid of MM, because they thought she was a witch. MM behaved strangely while in prison. She had scratches on her stomach from crawling across the floor like a snake, and she smeared herself and the cell with feces, although MM could not recall doing this.

LEGAL OUTCOMES

MM appeared in court for the first time in August 2012. Her mother told the court that MM had mental illness. The court remanded the case for an inquiry into her mental state, and her mother provided documents confirming the mental health issues. MM was referred to Sterkfontein Hospital under the terms of several sections of the Criminal Procedures Act (CPA), including sections 77, 78, and 79:

Section 77:

If it appears to the court at any stage of criminal proceedings that the accused is by reason of mental illness or mental defect not capable of understanding the proceedings so as to make a proper defense, the court shall direct that the matter be enquired into and be reported on in accordance with the provisions of section 79. (South African Government 1977, pp. 51)

Section 78:

(1) A person who commits an act or makes an omission which constitutes an offence and who at the time of such commission or omission suffers from a mental illness or mental defect which makes him or her

incapable (a) of appreciating the wrongfulness of his or her act or omission; or (b) of acting in accordance with an appreciation of the wrongfulness of his or her act or omission, shall not be criminally responsible for such act or omission.

(1A) Every person is presumed not to suffer from a mental illness or mental defect…until the contrary is proved on a balance of probabilities.

(1B) Whenever the criminal responsibility of an accused…the burden of proof…shall be on the party who raises the issue.

(2) If it is alleged at criminal proceedings that the accused is…not criminally responsible…the court shall…direct that the matter be enquired into and be reported without hearing further evidence.

(3) If the finding contained in the relevant report is the unanimous finding of the persons who under section 79 enquired into the relevant mental condition of the accused, and the finding is not disputed by the prosecutor or the accused, the court may determine the matter on such report without hearing further evidence.

(4) If the said finding is not unanimous or, if unanimous, is disputed by the prosecutor or the accused…under section 79 enquired into the mental condition of the accused.

(5) Where the said finding is disputed, the party disputing the finding may subpoena and cross-examine any person who under section 79 enquired into the mental condition of the accused.

(6) If the court finds that the accused committed the act in question and that he or she at the time of such commission was by reason of mental illness or intellectual disability not criminally responsible…pending the decision of a judge in chambers in terms of section 47 of the Mental Health Care Act, 2002…. (pp. 53–55)

And section 79(2):

(2)(a) The court may for the purposes of the relevant enquiry commit the accused to a psychiatric hospital…make any other order it deems fit regarding the custody of the accused; or (iv) any other order. (p. 56)

Under the Criminal Procedures Act, MM was ordered to undergo a 30-day forensic psychiatric observation to determine whether she had a mental illness that would affect her fitness to stand trial and criminal responsibility. MM clearly displayed clinical features of dysphoric manic features during the forensic observation period, presenting clear and obvious mental illness. Based on the forensic evaluation, she was found not fit to stand trial and assessed as being unable to appreciate the wrongfulness of her actions. The court then referred her as a state patient under the terms of the Mental Health Care Act, section 42, which states:

Where a court issues an order in terms of the criminal procedures act for a state patient to be admitted for care treatment and rehabilitation services, the registrar of the clerk of the court must send a copy of that order to the Relevant curator ad litem and Officer in charge of the detention centre where the state patient is or will be detained. (South African Government 2002, p. 25)

Legal Issues

In South Africa, forensic psychiatric units offer forensic observation for defendants referred from the courts and provide indefinite detention of mentally ill offenders (Marais and Subramaney 2015). Referral for forensic psychiatric evaluation occurs under Section 79 of the Criminal Procedure Act, as described earlier. This section of the Act deals with *inter alia*, the decision of the court to refer a person for a single or panel observation. For all serious or violent offenses (e.g., murder, rape, or any other offense in which serious violence is involved), the court appoints a panel made up of at least two psychiatrists, one acting on behalf of the state and one on behalf of the defense. The court may also decide to appoint a third psychiatrist who is not in the full-time employ of the state or a psychologist on the panel. The purpose of a forensic psychiatric observation is to determine whether the accused has a mental illness or defect, is competent to stand trial, and is criminally responsible (South African Government 1977).

Based on the findings and recommendations from the forensic observation report, the court decided the outcome of the case. When an accused is found unfit to stand trial or not criminally responsible due to mental illness or defect, the court may decide to admit the accused to a psychiatric hospital, forensic psychiatric facility, or an outpatient facility for further treatment and rehabilitation. State patients are those alleged mentally ill offenders whose charges generally involve serious violence. They are detained at a forensic psychiatric institution, as per section 42 of the Mental Health Care Act described earlier (South African Government 2002).

In this case, MM had experienced a postpartum episode of psychotic depression in the context of bipolar I disorder and was clearly not well at the time of the offense. She was also unable to conduct a proper defense in court and was found unfit to stand trial. She was thus referred as a state patient. In South Africa, if the panel observation determines that the accused is not fit or not criminally responsible for the offense, they are returned to the forensic hospital to be indefinitely detained and treated pending a decision by the judge in chambers. This detention usually involves treatment and rehabilitation, including leaves of absence granted to the patient, such as time away from the hospital to spend with the person's family or equivalent at their home.

Psychiatric Issues

MM had a diagnosed serious mental illness of bipolar I disorder and had been on treatment with a mood stabilizer and second-generation antipsychotic until it was discontinued. She then relapsed with an episode of psychotic depression in the immediate postpartum phase, which very likely evolved into a mixed phase during her incarceration. Despite attempts to obtain her medication from the hospital and clinic, she had not received the care she needed. MM had fallen between the cracks of adequate treatment, which was a significant failure in the system and led to grave consequences for MM and her son.

According to Resnick's (1969, 2016) classification of motivations for filicide, this case falls within the category of acutely psychotic filicide. Peripartum mood disorders are notoriously common, with antenatal depression being the most prevalent of psychiatric disorders in pregnancy and postpartum (Duko et al. 2019). Mothers with bipolar disorder are particularly vulnerable to relapses in the peripartum. Sit et al. (2006) found that nearly three-quarters of women with postpartum psychosis (PPP) had a previous diagnosis of bipolar disorder or schizoaffective disorder.

The relapse MM that experienced within 2 days postpartum is typical; onset of PPP usually occurs in the first 1–4 weeks after delivery (Sit et al. 2006). The added tragedy is that MM previously had been treated in 2006 with the appropriate medication. Her need for ongoing antipsychotic treatment (risperidone), even after the first episode, raised questions about complete mood stability when MM was on treatment. It was clear that she had identified the need to seek help from the clinic prior to the offense but had been shunted back and forth between the clinic and the hospital, receiving treatment from neither. This grave tragedy of miscommunication led to the failure of health services to provide medication and support services when emerging (and historical) mental health illness was clearly evident in one most at risk for PPP: a mother with a history of bipolar disorder.

Psychosocial support and medication are of utmost importance in preventing relapse of mood disorders in the postpartum period. MM had attended monthly sessions at the outpatient clinic in 2006 and received appropriate medication but had stopped a few years prior to delivering her son. In addition, she had no support from the father of her child, experienced disrupted relations between her parents, and had been transitioning between living with each parent and her aunt, which each brought on stressors that played a role in promoting her symptoms. She rapidly deteriorated, resulting in the tragic infanticide death. MM's symptoms were clearly evident in the prison where she was initially held, with behavioral disturbances in the context of severe psychosis that was mood congruent.

In a nationwide study of female offenders in South Africa in which the records of 573 women were reviewed, researchers found that child victims made up 42% of the sample population; of those, 66% of the deaths had been perpetrated by the mother (Nagdee et al. 2019). Of these, 33% of victims were younger than 1 year of age, and 17% were younger than 1 month of age. This population had high rates of psychopathology, especially psychosis. In South Africa, perpetrators of child murder are officially charged with murder, not neonaticide nor infanticide; there is no legal recognition of nor a distinction made between neonaticide and infanticide.

The Expert Witness in This Context

In the case of MM, expert witnesses were not called to court to testify about her symptoms related to the stabbing death of her son. It was clear to the courts that MM was not fit to stand trial, and from the collateral information supplied by her mother, it was clear that MM was acting in accordance with symptoms related to her psychiatric disorder. An expert team of psychiatrists, psychologists, social workers, occupational therapists, and nursing staff were involved in the forensic observation process. The report was written by a panel of two psychiatrists who confirmed the diagnosis. In cases in which the defense enters an appeal, the diagnosis is not so clear, or malingering is suspected, expert witnesses would be called to testify in court.

Sociocultural Considerations

In South Africa, as in other cultures, mental illness is greatly stigmatized. In our experience, it is not uncommon for this stigma to impede treatment, such as in MM's case. Health professionals are often remiss in their treatment of individuals with mental health struggles. Most notably, this stigma does not exist with other illnesses; for example, a person with a perforated ulcer or significantly raised blood pressure who presents at a clinic would not be turned away and referred elsewhere. However, mentally ill individuals often are shunted away on the pretext of administrative issues (e.g., inability to prescribe medication). When MM sought help from the hospital and the medical clinic to provide the medication that had relieved her symptoms before, she was turned away several times, leading to a catastrophic result.

South Africa is a diverse society, with more than 50 million people and 11 officially recognized languages. Black Africans make up the majority of the population (79.5%), and there are different ethnic groups. Madigoe et al. (2017) noted that various scholars have described the traditional world view and cultural belief systems among the Zulu communities of KwaZulu-Natal (e.g., Cheetam and Griffiths 1980; Edwards 1985; Ngubane 1977), which is similar to that of most Sub-Saharan African ethnic groups. Its main structural elements are: 1) two interconnected cosmological realms within the natural world (the elements, plants, animals, humans) and the supernatural world (evil spirits, ancestors, God), and 2) traditional healers, diviners, and sorcerers who mediate between these realms (Madigoe et al. 2017).

The resultant ancestral displeasure is believed to render the person and his/her societal system vulnerable to disaster, misfortune, or witchcraft, the latter being ostensibly administered by community members motivated mainly by jealousy and often construed to be mediated by evil spirits. Within this world view, external attributions are generally favored over internal attributions with regard to the causality of adverse events (Madigoe et al. 2017). The belief is that when the natural and supernatural realms are in equilibrium, the community, families, and individual members experience good health and prosperity. Disequilibrium between the two realms results in illness, misfortune, and disaster. Such disequilibrium principally results from loss of protection by the ancestors, itself caused by individuals failing to perform rituals to honor their ancestors and violating societal taboos (Madigoe et al. 2017).

MM belonged to the Sesotho ethnic group, had been well educated, and was from a family in which her parents had undergone an acrimonious divorce. The cultural belief system was illustrated at various points in this tragic case: Before the offense, when MM was in the throes of a relapse and her baby would not stop crying, her father had begun praying to the ancestors and became aggressive when MM disturbed him; after the offense, inmates in the prison had been afraid of MM, believing her to be a witch due to her bizarre behavior.

Conclusion

Although this clinical case of infanticide in South Africa is a grievous error of the mental health system, it is a story of success from a legal perspective that honors the psychiatric findings. MM did not have to stand trial, the charges were dropped, and she was appropriately referred for care, treatment, and rehabilitation. MM is currently mentally well. She has visited the grave of her deceased infant and has made peace with her parents. With intensive individual therapy, including exposure therapy for PTSD, she has been discharged as a forensic state patient and is currently awaiting placement at a residential facility.

MAIN CLINICAL/LEGAL POINTS AND CULTURAL PERSPECTIVES

- The reproductive and mental health of young women with bipolar disorder are essential to monitor. Fertility issues and pregnancy possibilities are often neglected in the South African context.

- The postpartum period is an extremely vulnerable period in patients with documented bipolar disorder and is known as one of the greatest risk factors for postpartum psychosis.

- Severe depression with psychotic features (i.e., psychotic depression) is common in the postpartum period in patients with bipolar disorder.

- Treatment protocols for bipolar disorder I are paramount following an index episode of mania.

- Early detection and referral are essential when postpartum mental health symptoms occur.

- Failure of the health services to provide adequate care to a mentally ill young mother and a lack of social support played a pivotal role in this case of infanticide.

- Interpretation of psychiatric pathology from a sociocultural perspective is crucial. The strong cultural belief systems of illness behavior included her father praying to the ancestors when MM was at the height of her mental illness and the prison inmates believing her to be a witch due to her bizarre behavior.

- Stigma of mental illness played a large part in this clinical case. Negligence on the part of the health professionals to recognize serious illness in the postpartum period is often manifested by deference to other health establishments, often not seen in other illness settings.

References

Cheetam RWS, Griffiths JA: Changing patterns in psychiatry in Africa with special reference to southern Africa. South Afr Med J 58:166–168, 1980

Duko B, Ayano G, Bedaso A: Depression among pregnant women and associated factors in Hawassa city, Ethiopia: an institution-based cross-sectional study. Reprod Health 16(25):1–6, 2019

Edwards SD (ed): Some Indigenous South African Views in Illness and Healing. Richards Bay, South Africa, University of Zululand, 1985

Madigoe T, Burns J, Zhang M, Subramaney U: Towards a culturally appropriate trauma assessment in a South African Zuly community. Psychol Trauma 9(3):274–281, 2017

Marais B, Subramaney U: Forensic state patients at Sterkfontein Hospital: a 3-year follow-up study. South Afr J Psychiatr 21(3):7, 2015

Nagdee M, Artz L, Correl-Bulnes C, et al: The psycho-social and clinical profile of women referred for psycho-legal evaluation to forensic mental health units in South Africa. South Afr J Psychiatr 25:1230, 2019

Ngubane H: Body and Mind in Zulu Medicine. London, Academic Press, 1977

Resnick PJ: Child murder by parents: a psychiatric review of filicide. Am J Psychiatry 126(10):1414–1420, 1969

Resnick PJ: Filicide in the United States. Indian J Psychiatry 58:S203–S209, 2016

Sit D, Rothschild AJ, Wisner KL: A review of postpartum psychosis. J Womens Health (Larchmt) 15(4):352–368, 2006

South African Government: Criminal Procedures Act No. 51 of 1977. Pretoria, South Africa, Government Printer, 1977

South African Government: Mental Health Care Act No. 17 of 2002. Pretoria, South Africa, Government Printer, 2002

Glossary

actus reus   Latin for the "criminal act." Almost all crimes require both a criminal act and a criminal intent to perform that act. For example, the crime of murder requires a homicide (*actus reus*) and the mental state to do harm, such as intent to kill (*mens reus*)

acutely psychotic filicide   An acute episode of mania, psychosis, or delirium; may include command auditory hallucinations. Per Resnick (1969, 2016), this designation is given when no comprehensible motive for the killing of the child has been determined. For example, a mother might kill her child in response to a command hallucination or while in a confused delirium. Although some women who commit altruistic filicide are psychotic, they have an understandable altruistic reason, whereas acutely psychotic filicides have no comprehensible motive. *See also* command hallucination; altruistic filicide.

adverse childhood experiences (ACEs)   Potentially traumatic events that occur in childhood. Derived from the landmark study by the Centers for Disease Control and Prevention (2019) and Kaiser Permanente, with participants recruited in 1995 and 1997 for longitudinal study. Ten ACEs were identified in three categories of abuse, neglect, and household dysfunction. Toxic stress from ACEs can change brain development and affect how the body responds to stress (www.cdc.gov/vitalsigns/aces/index.html).

Adverse Childhood Experiences Scale   A validated questionnaire that looks at seven categories of adverse childhood experiences, addressing the graded relationship between early trauma and later mental health outcomes.

Adult Attachment Interview   Semistructured interview that assesses state of mind with respect to attachment. Interview is structured to elicit the attachment system through questions related to early childhood experiences, relationship with parents, and memories of moments when the attachment system tends to become more active (i.e., separations, diseases, accidents). The interview also aims to elicit memories of traumatic experiences and grief, both in childhood and in adulthood. *See also* attachment.

affective pregnancy denial   A disconnection from the pregnancy in which the mother has intellectual acknowledgment of the fact of the pregnancy but lacks the expected heightened emotional sensitivity of a normal pregnancy. Often appears like a difficult adjustment.

altruistic filicide   Taking the life of a child "out of love" to protect the child from real or imagined suffering. Usually occurs in the context of severe suicidal depression or delusional beliefs, to prevent the child from experiencing imagined (usually) intolerable suffering. May be accompanied by suicide/ attempted suicide of the offending parent. Per Resnick (1969, 2016), there are two subtypes. The first occurs when a mother with young children plans to commit suicide and decides to take her children to heaven with her. Due to her depression, she often perceives her children as also having miserable lives, especially because they will be motherless after her suicide. The second is motivated by a desire to protect the children from severe suffering, which is perceived by the mother as "worse than death." *See also* filicide.

amicus brief   Document prepared by a person or persons with strong interest in or views on the subject matter of an action who is not a party to the action.

anxiety disorders   Clinically significant levels of anxiety consistent with criteria defined by DSM, including worry, fear, difficulty relaxing, or fears of losing control.

anxious-ambivalent attachment   A type of insecure attachment style in which children show high levels of emotion dysregulation, are less able to use their caregivers as a secure base from which to explore, and vacillate between clinging to caregivers and resisting comfort during times of reunion. Typically develops when caregivers are chronically unreliable or distracted. *See also* attachment.

attachment   A deep and enduring relational bond formed by a biological motivation to seek proximity to caregivers, especially when one has a need for comfort or safety. *See* anxious-ambivalent attachment; disorganized attachment; insecure attachment; organized attachment.

avoidant attachment   Type of insecure attachment style in which children show very limited distress and high exploratory behaviors and do not seek proximity to caregivers during times of reunion. Typically develops when caregivers are chronically detached or emotionally unavailable. *See also* attachment.

la belle indifférence   Seeming indifference or lack of emotional concern for the seriousness of one's symptoms. In cases of pregnancy denial, absence of appropriate concern for the seriousness for a particular situation or circumstances.

Big Five Inventory   A 44-item self-administered questionnaire that measures the factors (dimensions) of personality. Items are rated on a five-point scale ranging from 1 (disagree strongly) to 5 (agree strongly). Factors are seen as dual-personality characteristics (i.e., extraversion vs. introversion, agreeableness vs. antagonism, conscientiousness vs. lack of direction, neuroticism vs. emotional stability, openness vs. closeness to experience).

bipolar disorder   Mood disorder that includes clinically significant changes between extreme highs and lows of mood.

bipolar schizoaffective disorder   Mental disorder characterized by symptoms of both schizophrenia and a mood disorder, which includes mania or depression. "A diagnosis of schizoaffective disorder requires that a major depressive or manic episode occur concurrently with the active-phase symptoms and that the mood symptoms be present for a majority of the total duration of the active periods" (American Psychiatric Association 2013, p. 104). In the bipolar subtype, episodes of mania can occur; during these episodes, the person may fluctuate between overt excitement and intense irritability.

brief dissociative episode   An acute transient reaction to stress that can last only hours and includes constriction of consciousness, perceptual disorder, microamnesias, and transient stupor. Fits best under DSM-5 other specified dissociative disorders for which the criteria do not meet depersonalization or derealization disorder (American Psychiatric Association 2013).

brief psychotic disorder   "[D]isturbance that involves the sudden onset of at least one of the following positive psychotic symptoms: delusions, hallucinations, disorganized speech…or grossly abnormal psychomotor behavior, including catatonia" (American Psychiatric Association 2013, p. 94). DSM-5 defines *sudden onset* as a "change from a nonpsychotic state to a clearly psychotic state within 2 weeks" (p. 94). Episode typically lasts at least 1 day and no longer than 1 month; individual returns to previous nonpsychotic status thereafter.

burden of proof   Obligation to provide compelling evidence supporting one's argument. A defendant must prove a defense of insanity by clear and convincing evidence. *See also* insanity; insanity defense. *See* M'Naghten rule; Model Penal Code; not criminally responsible on account of mental disorder; not guilty by reason of insanity.

child maltreatment filicide   Fatal "battered child syndrome" in which homicidal intent is lacking. Most common cause of both maternal and paternal filicide in the United States (Resnick 1969, 2016). *See also* filicide; maternal filicide.

Childhood Trauma Questionnaire   A 28-item self-report questionnaire exploring traumatic experiences of childhood. For each item, the interviewee selects an answer from among possible alternatives ("never true" to "often true") corresponding to a numerical score between 1 and 5. Total scores of each subscale give a quantitative index of the intensity of the traumatic experience in each area under examination. Traumas explored are emotional neglect, physical neglect, emotional abuse, sexual abuse, and physical abuse (Pennebaker and Susman 1988).

command hallucination   False sensory perception in which a person is directed to carry out an act.

common law   The common law began with a set of laws imposed by William the Conqueror beginning in 1066. These had their basis in Anglo Saxon law and precedents from earlier Greek and Roman laws. Those laws, modified over the centuries, are a tremendous influence on the current laws of each state. Uniformity developed over the years as a consequence of the written decisions of the King's Court, a central court in London.

compulsions   Repetitive behaviors related to an obsession. *See also* obsessions. *See also* obsessive-compulsive disorder.

concealed pregnancy   Mother has conscious awareness of the pregnancy but hides it from others.

***Daubert* challenge**   Legal challenge requiring experts to describe what scientific, technical, or other specialized knowledge they can provide to help the court understand the issue. Experts must show that their opinion is based on sufficient facts or data, that it is the product of reliable principles and methods, and that those principles and methods have been applied to the facts of the case. *See also* expert witness.

death penalty   Restricted to homicide offenders since *Coker v. Georgia* (433 U.S. 584 [1977]), attempts have been made in Texas (Bill HB 8 [Leg. Session 80R]), Louisiana (La.Rev.Stat.Ann. sec. 14:42 [D][2]), Oklahoma (10 Okl.St.Ann.ss 7115[1]), South Carolina (S.C.Code Ann. Ss 16-3-655 [C][1]), Montana (Mont.Code Ann. Sec. 45-5-503), and Georgia (Ga.Code Ann. Sec. 16-6-1) to expand it to crimes other than homicide. The death penalty has been criticized as ineffective, racist, often arbitrary in its application and unjust. In the United Kingdom, the death penalty for mothers who commit infanticide was abolished in 1922.

death qualified jury   A jury of individuals not opposed to the death penalty. Individuals who do not believe in or would not be comfortable applying the death penalty in a particular case are excluded from trials in which the defendant is eligible for the death penalty. *See also* non-death qualified jury.

delusions   Fixed, false beliefs that are resistant to change despite conflicting evidence.

delusions of control   False belief that another person, group of people, or external force controls one's thoughts, feelings, impulses, or behaviors.

delusions of reference   False belief that innocuous events or mere coincidences have a strong personal connection or relevance.

depersonalization   Dissociative experience of feeling detached from one's thoughts, feelings, sensations, or actions or feeling unreal or absent. Individual feels like an observer and not a participant in his or her own actions. Psychological separation from the self.

depersonalization/derealization disorder Dissociative disorder involving numbing of emotions and bodily sensations along with a feeling of unreality, detachment from self, and distortions in time and perceptions.

derealization Dissociative experience of feeling unreal or detached from one's surroundings. Objects or individuals are experienced as unreal, dreamlike, foggy, lifeless, or visually distorted. Perception or experience of the external world is altered so that it seems unreal.

***Diagnostic and Statistical Manual of Mental Disorders* (DSM)** Authoritative text that provides diagnostic categories and criteria for generally accepted mental disorders. The current version at the time of this writing is DSM-5 (American Psychiatric Association 2013).

disease of the mind Mental disorder as defined by Canadian law.

disorganized attachment Attachment style in which children fail to show any organized pattern of behavior toward caregivers. Relational and behavioral responses tend to vary and may include contradictory, disoriented, and fearful responses to caregivers. Typically develops when caregivers are chronically hostile, confusing, or withdrawing. *See also* attachment.

dissociation An alteration in conscious awareness that creates a temporary detachment from reality as evidenced by perceptual disturbances, sensory distortions, and time lapses.

dissociative disorder Per DSM-5 (American Psychiatric Association 2013), a "disruption of and/or discontinuity in the normal integration for consciousness, memory, identity, emotion, perception, body representation, motor control, and behavior" (p. 291). Divided by the core dissociative component into identity disorder, amnesia, derealization/depersonalization, and, where symptoms do not meet these criteria but still cause dysfunction, into other and unspecified.

Dissociative Experiences Scale Validated questionnaire examining the frequency of dissociative experiences in the lives of respondents.

disturbance of mind One element of the *actus reus* of the Canadian infanticide law. All that is required for an infanticide defense is to establish that the disturbance is connected to childbirth and/or lactation consequent to the birth of the child victim (see Chapter 4).

dyadic intervention Treatment method focusing on two individuals, often the parent and child, as a "dyad," or unit. Also commonly referred to as a two-generation treatment approach.

ecological framework Enables understanding of human development and social life as arising from the interaction of individuals, relationships, communities, and societies. At the *individual* level, biological attributes and personal history contribute to development and the likelihood of becoming a victim or a perpetrator of violence. At the *relationships* level, the presence of parents, siblings, a spouse, a sexual partner, extended family, and friends, as well as the quality of these relationships, can protect from or promote experience of violence. At the wider *community* level, neighborhoods and workplaces provide supportive contexts or contribute to marginalization and risk; adverse factors include unemployment, high population density, need for frequent relocation, and easy access to illicit drugs. At the *societal* level, influence comes, for example, from macroeconomics, social policies, the degree of gender equality, cultural norms, legislation, and politics (Bronfenbrenner 1979; see Chapter 14).

ego-dystonic   Ways of thinking that are not consistent or acceptable with an individual's typical self-identity.

ego-syntonic   Ways of thinking that are consistent or acceptable with an individual's typical self-identity.

emotion dysregulation   Inability to control or regulate one's emotions, often resulting in high reactivity and distress.

ethnographic content analysis   Method of qualitative data analysis in which the research goal is centered around the discovery and verification of information. Data collection and analysis are reflective and circular, with research rigor focused on validity and generating an understanding of the narrative data (Altheide and Schneider 2013; see Chapter 12). *See also* frames; themes.

expert witness   Person permitted to testify, either at a deposition or a trial, whose education, training, or experience is relevant to the case at hand or desired field of inquiry. *See also Daubert* challenge.

familicide   Act of killing one's whole family (more commonly perpetrated by a father).

fatal maltreatment   Unintentional killing of a child in the context of either anger triggered by behaviors (e.g., colicky crying) or cumulative neglect. Can be associated with personality disorder, substance abuse, or intellectual impairment but not usually with serious mental illness.

federal insanity standard   Affirmative defense to prosecution under any federal statute that the defendant, at the time of the commission of the acts constituting the offense, was unable to appreciate the nature and quality or the wrongfulness of the acts as a result of a severe mental disease or defect. Mental disease or defect does not otherwise constitute a defense. *See also* insanity.

filicide   Killing of a child at any age by a parent, stepparent, or established parental figure. Can be used as an umbrella term for all children whose lives are taken by a parent or guardian. Filicide also refers to the killing by a parental figure of a child who is older than 1 day and younger than 18 years of age.

frames   Broad, overarching category in which to organize meaningful units of data in ethnographic content analysis (Altheide and Schneider 2013; see Chapter 12). *See also* ethnographic content analysis, themes.

gender bias   Prejudice against or preferential treatment of an individual based on gender (usually a woman or a man, but now extending to nonbinary gender).

Gender Inequality Index   Purpose is to measure gender inequality. Constructed by the United Nations Development Programme (2019; see Chapter 14) from three dimensions of women's development: reproductive health (the maternal mortality ratio, adolescent fertility rate), empowerment (educational attainment at secondary level and above, parliamentary representation), and economic activity (gender-specific labor force participation). Value ranges from 0 to 1, with 0 indicating perfect equality of women and men and 1 indicating total inequality of women's status and development in comparison with those of men.

guilty but mentally ill   Verdict indicating that defendant has not met one or all of that state's not guilty by reason of insanity elements. Defendant may be found "guilty but mentally ill" (GBMI) if, after trial, the trier of fact finds all of the following:

1. Defendant is guilty of the offense beyond a reasonable doubt.
2. Defense has proven by a preponderance of the evidence that defendant was mentally ill at the time of the commission of that offense.
3. Defense has not established by a preponderance of the evidence that defendant lacked substantial capacity either to appreciate the nature and quality or the wrongfulness of the offending conduct or to conform conduct to the requirements of the law.

Codified in the Insanity Defense Reform Act of 1984, which was passed by the U.S. Congress in response to the trial of John Hinckley Jr. for the attempted assassination of President Ronald Reagan. The previous federal standard employed the phrase "lacks substantial capacity to appreciate," which the Act replaced with "unable to appreciate." This language is specifically drawn from the Michigan GBMI statute enacted in 1975. Michigan uses the American Law Institute Model Penal Code test for insanity as is reflected in the third prong of this standard. Approximately one-quarter of U.S. states now have a similar verdict alternative. *See also* Hinckley, John Jr.; insanity; M'Naghten rule; Model Penal Code; not guilty by reason of insanity.

Hinckley, John Jr.   John Hinckley Jr. was found not guilty by reason of insanity in 1982 for the attempted assassination of President Ronald Reagan the previous year. The jury's completely justifiable decision was so unpopular that the Model Penal Code standard fell out of favor, and most states reverted to the M'Naghten standard. *See also* guilty but mentally ill; insanity; M'Naghten rule; Model Penal Code, not guilty by reason of insanity.

homicide   Intentional killing without lawful justification. This definition fits both murder in the first degree in all U.S. states and murder in the second degree in some states but not others. In several states, murder in the second degree differs from murder in the first degree only in that the death penalty applies to first- but not second-degree murder. In all states, a conviction of murder mandates many years in prison at a minimum.

hudud   Under Islamic law, divine punishments, or those mandated by God, for the four crimes of theft, armed robbery, illicit sexual intercourse, and slander. Punishments are the most severe corporal and capital punishments and include stoning to death and amputation of a hand.

Human Development Index   Measure of human development in each country. Made up of three indicators: average life expectancy, average educational attainment (measured by mean years of schooling), and proportion of population with access to resources needed for a decent living, a measured by gross national income per capita. Data are taken from public international sources that are the best statistics available for those indicators at the time (United Nations Development Programme 2015; see Chapter 14).

iatrogenic participation   Process of projective identification in which a woman's denial of her pregnancy is projected onto others, particularly the physician, so that the pregnancy is never discovered, which serves to confirm the woman's denial of the pregnancy.

infanticide   Killing of a child within 1 year of birth, often at the hands of a parent and involving extreme emotional disturbance. Mothers who commit infanticide are most often experiencing a psychotic episode. Defined in New Zealand legislation as a mother killing a child younger than 10 years of age.

Infanticide Act   Refers generally to the second of two Infanticide Acts. In 1922, England enacted a law barring the death penalty from being imposed for mothers who kill their infants. In 1938, that law was expanded to reduce the charges in such cases from murder to manslaughter and to emphasize treatment over punishment. Probation was permissible. A survey of 34 countries found that 27 had some form of Infanticide Act, with a maximum average penalty of 6 years in prison. In the United States, depending on the state in which is occurs, infanticide is seen as a capital offense, which could mean the death penalty or a sentence of anywhere between 25 years to life imprisonment.

Infanticide Law (Australia)   Killing of a child younger than 12 months of age (<24 months in Victoria) by the biological mother, whose balance of mind at the time of the offense was disturbed from the effect of giving birth to that child or from the effects of lactation.

infanticide law (Canada)   According to the *Criminal Code of Canada* (1985), a "female person" is guilty of infanticide when "she causes the death of her newly born child" if, at the time of the act, "she is not fully recovered from the effects of giving birth to the child and by reason thereof or of the effect of lactation consequent on the birth of the child her mind is then disturbed." An indictable offense in Canada, infanticide carries a maximum sentence of 5 years. The Supreme Court of Canada heard a challenge to the infanticide provision in 2016 during the trial of Meredith Borowiec and affirmed the interpretation of the provision for infanticide in the *Criminal Code* (see Chapter 4).

insanity   Legal term based on the concept that certain people are so severely mentally ill that they cannot be held accountable for their crimes. Term has no analogue in psychiatry. Laws of insanity have not been modified on account of any scientific discovery in more than a century; they tend to require proof of lengthy and continuous severe mental illness or psychosis and hold that severe mental illness or psychosis alone does not establish insanity. *See also* burden of proof; federal insanity standard; guilty but mentally ill; insanity defense; insanity standard; M'Naghten rule; Model Penal Code; not criminally responsible on account of mental disorder; not guilty by reason of insanity.

insanity defense   Affirmative but most difficult of defenses, also called not guilty by reason of insanity (NGRI), in which defendant acknowledges committing a crime but denies legal responsibility due to mental disease or defect. Most U.S. jurisdictions require defendants to not know the wrongfulness of their conduct due to a mental disease or defect in order to be found NGRI.

A minority of states also allow an insanity defense if the defendant was unable to refrain from the act due to a mental disease or defect. Exact wording varies from state to state. In Canada, the insanity defense is called not criminally responsible. *See also* insanity; not criminally responsible on account of mental disorder; not guilty by reason of insanity; wrongful act.

insanity standard   Specific statute of each state with regard to defense of insanity in a criminal trial. *See also* federal insanity standard; insanity; insanity defense; Model Penal Code.

insecure attachment   Overarching term to describe disrupted attachment patterns that may arise from consistently insensitive, harsh, unpredictable, or neglectful interactions with caregivers. *See also* attachment.

intergenerational trauma   Transmission of trauma from one generation to the next (e.g., from parent to child). Can occur through a combination of direct and indirect pathways.

internal working model   Cognitive schemas and affective memory traces of caregiving relationships, including expectations of comfort, security, and safety. Early parent–child relationships create the template for the model, which is then carried forward into subsequent relationships.

International Classification of Diseases (ICD)   World Health Organization's classification system for medical and mental disorders used for medical billing and classification. Current version is ICD-11 (World Health Organization 2019).

to know/knew   Critical legal element that must be proven in a criminal case. In cases in which mental illness is claimed, what the defendant "knew" may be proven through expert witnesses. In general, when a mental illness is not claimed as a defense, the defendant's state of knowledge is typically proven by either that person's statements or by inference. When proof is by inference, it is presumed that the defendant knew the natural and probable consequences of his or her conduct (i.e., if a defendant shoots a gun at a victim, it can be inferred the defendant knew it would severely injure, and perhaps kill, the victim). Jurors are often not given this definition in court instructions. When jury instructions are given, the jurors are instructed that a person "knows" or acts knowingly when they are consciously aware that this conduct carries results practically certain to occur. If the issue is whether they knew certain facts, the jury is instructed that the defendant "knows" those facts exist. If a person is psychotic, their perception of reality is distorted, and the normal inference of "knowing" or intent may not be accurate. The psychotic person may not even be aware a gun is being fired.

major depressive disorder   Clinically significant symptoms of depression as defined in DSM that lead to impairment in the individual's functioning. Also known as major depression.

malice aforethought   Referring to defendant's state of mind or intent, if any, in committing the act. Does not require advance planning and can occur in the moment of the crime. Evidence of the interpretation, and even the requirement of, malice aforethought or premeditation is sparse until recent centuries. Use of these terms developed early in the common law until their more recent replacement with more specific terms. *See mens rea*.

malingering   Intentional production of false or grossly exaggerated physical or psychological symptoms, motivated by external incentives such as avoiding military duty, avoiding work, obtaining financial compensation, evading criminal prosecution, or obtaining drugs.

manslaughter   Generic offense from the common law that applies in either of two situations: 1) self-defense in which the case's particular facts have defects, but not enough to be disregarded, and a murder conviction is imposed; or 2) an act, provoked by the victim, that causes unreasoned and uncontrolled passion resulting in homicide. May meet an individual state's definition of second- or third-degree murder (see Chapter 3). Carries significantly lesser penalties than murder, and probation is often granted.

mariticide   Act of killing one's husband.

maternal filicide   Killing of a child or children by the mother. Umbrella term that encompasses neonaticide, infanticide, and a mother killing her child who is of any age. *See also* filicide.

maternal neonaticide   Killing of a newly born infant less than 24 hours old, committed by the biological mother. *See also* infanticide; newly born.

mens rea   Latin for "a guilty mind." Usually refers to the guilty state of mind required for a crime in conjunction with the prohibited act (e.g., intentional, reckless, or negligence homicide). To be found guilty of most crimes (other than strict liability), defendant must have been found to be guilty of committing a criminal act with a specific mental state. For example, to be guilty of murder, defendant must have intended to cause the victim's death and not have been merely reckless in conduct. *See also actus reus*; malice aforethought.

mental disorder   A mental, behavioral, or emotional disturbance resulting in serious functional impairment, which substantially interferes with or limits one or more major life activities (National Institute of Mental Health, n.d.). It is not always the case that a mental illness will exempt an accused from criminal responsibility. The *Criminal Code of Canada* (1985) defines a mental disorder as a disease of the mind. The accused may be found not criminally responsible on account of mental disorder or found unfit to stand trial. Diagnosis of a mental disorder does not exempt the accused from criminal responsibility. *See also* disease of the mind; not criminally responsible on account of mental disorder.

mentalization   Capacity to understand ourselves and others in terms of underlying mental states and intentions in order to make sense of our actions and behavior. Can be implicit or explicit.

Minnesota Multiphasic Personality Inventory–2   A standardized, self-administered test consisting of 567 items for which "true" or "false" dichotomous answers are given. Items are divided into 13 scales: 3 control scales, which provide indications about test validity, and 10 clinical scales, on the basis of which the subject's profile is constructed. T scores are used for evaluation; a score ≥ 65 suggests the presence of psychological problems or pathology.

M'Naghten rule   Very restrictive standard for legal insanity, sometimes referred to as the "right or wrong" test. Name comes from the trial of Daniel M'Naghten in England in 1843. To establish a defense on the ground of insanity, it must be clearly proven that, at the time of committing the act, the defendant was laboring under such a defect of reason as to not know the nature and quality of his or her actions or, if the defendant did know it, that the defendant did not know those actions were wrong. Best-known definition of insanity in states and countries under the common law or with common law histories. Mothers with postpartum mental illness who know it is wrong to kill their children but do so because they are deeply depressed or to protect the children from a lifetime of suffering do not meet this standard, but on rare occasions can have a jury sympathize sufficiently to get such a finding (see Chapter 3 and others). *See also* insanity; to know/knew; wrongful act.

Model Penal Code   Collection and model of criminal laws by the American Law Institute comprised of criminal offenses and sentencing and punishment. Expanded the definition of *insanity* to situations in which severe mental illness caused the defendant to lack "substantial capacity" to appreciate the criminality (in some versions wrongfulness) of the offending conduct or to conform conduct to the "requirements of the law." Allows defense of insanity for a defendant whose mental illness was akin to many with postpartum diagnoses. *See also* insanity; to know/knew; wrongful act.

neonaticide   Killing of a newborn, usually by the biological mother, within the first 24 hours of life.

newly born   In Canadian law, a child is considered *newly born* until its first birthday for the purposes of an infanticide defense. *See also* infanticide law (Canada); maternal neonaticide.

no acquittal unless act or omission not willful (Canada)   Part of the infanticide framework of laws designed to clarify the interpretation of Section 233 by courts and medical experts providing evidence in these cases. According to Section 663,

> Where a female person is charged with infanticide and the evidence establishes that she caused the death of her child but does not establish that, at the time of the act or omission by which she caused the death of the child,
>
> (a) she was not fully recovered from the effects of giving birth to the child or from the effect of lactation consequent on the birth of the child, and
>
> (b) the balance of her mind was, at that time, disturbed by reason of the effect of giving birth to the child or of the effect of lactation consequent on the birth of the child, she may be convicted unless the evidence establishes that the act or omission was not wilful [sic]. (*Criminal Code of Canada* 1985, c. C-46 s. 633)

> *See also* infanticide law (Canada).

non-death qualified jury   Jury consisting of individuals who are willing and able to entertain the entire range of punishment if a conviction occurs, as long as the death penalty is not an option. *See also* death qualified jury.

not criminally responsible on account of mental disorder   According to Section 16 of the *Criminal Code of Canada* (1985, c. C-46): "No person is criminally responsible for an act committed or an omission made while suffering from a mental disorder that rendered the person incapable of appreciating the nature and quality of the act or omission or of knowing that it was wrong." Provision only applies when the individual has a guilty verdict entered. *See also* disease of the mind; guilty but mentally ill; insanity; mental disorder; not guilty by reason of insanity; to know/knew; wrongful act.

not guilty by reason of insanity   Plea by a criminal defense meant to establish that at the time of the commission of the offense, due to a mental disease or defect, the defendant lacked the mental capacity necessary to be convicted of the criminal offense. *See also* guilty but mentally ill; insanity; not criminally responsible on account of mental disorder; to know/knew; wrongful act.

nulliparous   A woman who has never been pregnant or who has never carried a pregnancy beyond 20 weeks.

obsessions   Persistent thoughts, impulses, or urges that are recognized by the person as inappropriate, such as repeated thoughts about contamination (e.g., becoming contaminated by shaking hands); repeated doubts (e.g., "Did I lock the door?"; "Did I turn off the stove?"); a need to have things in a particular order; and horrific impulses (e.g., to hurt one's child or to shout obscenities in church). *See also* compulsions; obsessive-compulsive disorder.

obsessive-compulsive disorder (OCD)   Clinically significant disorder in which the individual has an abnormal number of unwanted and intrusive thoughts, images, or urges (obsessions) and/or behaviors (compulsions). *See also* compulsions; obsessions.

organized attachment   Overarching term used to describe attachment styles in which the child demonstrates consistent and predictable attachment behaviors. *See also* attachment.

PA 100-0574   First criminal law passed in the United States referencing postpartum mental illness. Enacted into Illinois law in 2018 and intended to allow for a sentence reduction for women whose postpartum mental illness was overlooked.

partner revenge filicide   Taking the life of a child in order to cause extreme psychological pain to the partner/other parent, thereby exacting revenge for abusive behaviors, such as infidelity or particularly acrimonious child custody proceedings. Although a significant personality disorder may exist, serious mental illness is seldom evident.

paternal filicide   Killing of a child or children by the father. *See also* filicide.

patriarchal society   Social structure in which men hold authority over women, including political leadership, social privilege, and personal relationships. *See also* gender bias.

perinatal   Time period including pregnancy and up to 1 year postpartum.

persecutory/paranoid delusions   False belief that one is being followed and/or that harm is imminent, resulting in heightened paranoia.

postpartum depression   Clinically significant depression with onset in the postpartum period.

postpartum psychosis   Episode of psychosis with onset following pregnancy. Current proposed criteria include psychotic symptoms, mood instability, and cognitive disorganization.

pregnancy denial   A dissociative process in which both the fact and emotional acknowledgment of the pregnancy are so outside of the mother's conscious awareness that normally expected pregnancy symptoms are absent, or symptoms are misattributed to another cause. *See* affective pregnancy denial; concealed pregnancy; iatrogenic participation; *la belle indifférence*; psychotic denial.

premeditation   *See malice aforethought.*

projective identification   An unconscious defense mechanism originally theorized by Melanie Klein (1946), in which the individual externalizes (i.e., projects) aspects of the Self perceived either as good or bad onto someone else. At the same time, the person who receives these projections acknowledges them as legitimate and incorporates (i.e., internalizes) them, ending up thinking and acting accordingly.

psychotic denial   Defensive psychological process in which the mother perceives the fact of the pregnancy in a delusional way.

reckless homicide   Reduced charge from murder; typically applies to reckless driving that results in death.

reflective functioning   Operationalized form of mentalization. Describes a parent's understanding of the child in terms of the child's underlying thoughts, feelings, intentions, desires, and attitudes. Parents with high reflective functioning can effectively make sense of and anticipate their child's needs. *See also* mentalization.

secure attachment   Healthy formation of attachment wherein a child can use the caregiver as both a safe haven in times of danger or distress and a secure base from which to explore. *See also* attachment.

spouse revenge filicide   Killing of a child or children for the purpose of making the spouse suffer. Often occurs after discovery of spousal infidelity or after one parent loses a bitter child custody battle. Least frequent type of filicide, occurring in only 4% of cases. *See also* filicide; partner revenge.

Syariah law (Malaysia)   Limited to matters of personal status (family, inheritance, and crimes against Islam). Family laws apply to marriage, divorce, custody and guardianship, maintenance of children, matrimonial properties, and spousal support. Laws of succession apply to probate and associated matters. Syariah criminal law is limited to offenses in relation to polygamous marriage, kin marriage, "indecent" dressing and sexual behavior, violation of the pillars of Islam (e.g., not fasting during Ramadan, not attending Friday prayers, desertion by either spouse), and apostasy (i.e., renunciation of Islam or expression of views at odds with Islam). In Malaysia, Syariah law does not impose *hudud* punishment. The Federal Constitution of Malaysia provides that Islam is the religion of the Federation, but other religions are permitted. Syariah law applies exclusively to Muslims, whereas civil courts administer civil law to Hindus, Christians, Buddhists, and other religious minorities. *See also* hudud.

Temperament and Character Inventory–Revised   A 240-item inventory of seven dimensions of personality traits: four temperaments (novelty seeking, harm avoidance, reward dependence, persistence) and three characters (self-directedness, cooperativeness, self-transcendence). Respondents indicate the extent to which they usually act or feel, using a five-point scale ranging from "very false for me" (1) to "very true for me" (5) (Cloninger et al. 1993).

thanatophoric dysplasia   Severe skeletal disorder that results in stillbirth or death of the infant from respiratory failure shortly after birth.

themes   Recurring idea presented within data in ethnographic content analysis. Several themes can compose a single frame (see Chapter 12). *See also* ethnographic content analysis; frames.

trauma   Overwhelming or shocking experience involving either actual or perceived threat of death, injury, or bodily harm that may negatively impact an individual's functioning, beliefs, and ability to cope. *Relational trauma* is more specifically an experience of trauma that occurs within the context of an interpersonal relationship.

trauma-informed approach   Treatment approach intended to foster a culture in which traumatized individuals feel safe and empowered to work toward healing. Recognizes and understands the pervasiveness of trauma and changes the conversation from "What's *wrong* with you?" to "What *happened* to you?" *See also* trauma.

traumagenic neurodevelopmental model of psychosis   Model that integrates current knowledge of biological and psychological processes to describe the relationship between childhood trauma and psychosis. *See also* trauma.

Traumatic Experience Checklist   A 29-item self-report questionnaire investigating different types of traumatic experiences. Measures severity of the experience, investigating four variables: presence of the event, age at which the event occurred, duration of the trauma, and impact on the subject. Also investigates contexts in which the experience occurred. For each type of traumatic experience (sexual abuse, sexual harassment, physical abuse, emotional abuse, emotional neglect), a composite score from 0 to 12 is calculated (Nijenhuis et al. 2002).

unwanted child filicide   Often occurs simply because the child is in the way of the parent's goals. Frequently denied or concealed; mothers may have hidden previous pregnancies and killed and hidden the infants' bodies. Seldom related to mental illness prior to the killing, but the offending parent may experience depression and symptoms of trauma related to the killing. Most common motive for neonaticide. *See also* filicide, neonaticide.

uxoricide   Act of killing one's wife.

voir dire   Process of screening potential jurors that is held at the beginning of trial to determine whether individuals possess a bias for or against either of the parties.

wrongful act   Something done, usually voluntarily, by a person that is prompted by intention and proximately caused by a motion of the will and goes against the laws of the state or government. The act for which a person is criminally charged and prosecuted. *See also* to know/knew; malice aforethought.

References

Altheide DL, Schneider CJ: Qualitative Media Analysis, 2nd Edition. Los Angeles, CA, Sage, 2013

American Psychiatric Association: Diagnostic and Statistical Manual of Mental Disorders, 5th Edition. Arlington, VA, American Psychiatric Association, 2013

Bronfenbrenner U: The Ecology of Human Development: Experiments by Nature and Design. Cambridge, MA, Harvard University Press, 1979

Centers For Disease Control and Prevention: Adverse childhood experiences. Vital Signs, November 2019. Available at: https://www.cdc.gov/vitalsigns/aces/index.html. Accessed August 31, 2020.

Cloninger C, Svrakic D, Przybeck T: A psychobiological model of temperament and character. Arch Gen Psychiatry 50(12):975–990, 1993

Criminal Code of Canada, R.S.C. 1985, c C-46

Klein M: Notes on some schizoid mechanisms. Int J Psychoanal 27:99–110, 1946

National Institute of Mental Health: Mental Health Information: Mental Illness (webiste), n.d. Available at: https://www.nimh.nih.gov/health/statistics/mental-illness.shtml. Accessed August 31, 2020.

Nijenhuis ERS, Van der Hart O, Kruger K: The psychometric characteristics of the Traumatic Experiences Questionnaire (TEC): first findings among psychiatric outpatients. Clin Psychol Psychother 9(3):200–210, 2002

Pennebaker JW, Susman JR: Disclosure of traumas and psychosomatic processes. Soc Sci Med 26:327–332, 1988

Resnick PJ: Child murder by parents: a psychiatric review of filicide. Am J Psychiatry 126(3):325–334, 1969

Resnick PJ: Filicide in the United States. Indian J Psychiatry 58:S203–S209, 2016

United Nations Development Programme: Human Development Report 2015: Work for Human Development. New York, United Nations Development Programme, 2015

United Nations Development Programme: Human Development Reports: Gender Inequality Index. New York, United Nations Development Programme, 2019

World Health Organization: International Classification of Diseases, 11th Revision. Geneva, World Health Organization, 2019

Index

Page numbers printed in **boldface** type refer to tables and figures.